My Banar
Stuart

G000141755

© Stuart Moss
stuartmoss@gmail.com

ISBN 978-1-5272-9773-9

Derefeld Books, Leeds, UK
First published 2021

Cover design by Leah Cole

All rights reserved. No part of this publication may be reproduced, stored in a retrieval system or transmitted without prior consent of the author.

i

To my dear family and friends, I love you all.

To everyone that I have met along the way, if you have been in my life, you have been a part of my journey, whether I mention you in this text or not.

To everyone that has ever struggled to accept the way that they look in the face of socially constructed ideals of beauty.

To every superhero fighting the good fight in the NHS.

To Linda, the most perfect woman and wife, what would I do without you?

Foreword

If I said that nobody likes being fat, I would of course be wrong. I'm certain that some people like being fat; sumo wrestlers for example must surely pride themselves on being built like mountains. In some parts of the world size equates to status, the bigger you are, the more elevated in society you are, such as in Ethiopia where the Bodi tribe hold an annual 'fat man contest', for which men prepare by drinking copious amounts of cows' blood and milk to enlarge their bellies. In the Pacific island nation of Fiji, it is a compliment to tell somebody that they have gained weight, and an insult to tell somebody that they are looking thin. This is quite the opposite of the societal norms in most Western nations, where weight loss is considered under most circumstances to be an admired achievement. In Europe, the socially constructed ideals about what constitutes a beautiful body have traditionally been one that is either slim or muscular and athletic, and the Romans and ancient Greeks immortalised toned muscular bodies in their public art.

In Fiji, food forms a central part of the nation's traditional culture and eating large amounts is considered healthy living. This all changed in 1999 when MTV arrived on the island; the relatively skinny role models in music videos and on teen melodramas made young people (particularly girls) question their traditional cultural values and themselves. This was followed by a rise in body dysmorphia and eating disorders such as anorexia.

The media is responsible for promoting people with slim or athletic bodies over those that aren't. Sex sells, and the media relies on viewers and audiences of its output being attracted to it, so that they stay fixated and return for more. In the 1990s, television and printed media were the main culprits in distorting the mindset of viewers, in the 2020s the internet has conquered all other forms of media and particularly social media now seems to be responsible for telling people what they should look like, further encouraging body dysmorphia amongst those who interact with it. Most people don't look like celebrities, which is a word that is now largely meaningless when anybody can get 15 minutes of fame with their followers, likes and sycophantic 'fans'.

How we are supposed to look has of course changed over the years; the aforementioned ancient Greeks set in stone the images of male gods as being highly muscular and rugged, while women had the odd exposed boob on their slender figures. Jump forward to the 18th century when romantic poet and writer Lord Byron bemoaned Italian food for making him gain weight, a century before the first photographic technology was available to accurately capture what people looked like. In the 1960s and swinging London, being slim or skinny was desirable for both women and men who followed role models such as stick thin model Twiggy and skinny superstars such as The Beatles. That was largely the status quo for the next 20 years until big screen Hollywood movies encouraged men to bulk up and be muscular and women to have small waistlines and big boobs (just about every superhero). In the 2000s, the emphasis for women changed to the backsides and lips, which were encouraged to be fatter. As crazy as it may seem, if you are fat in the right places then that is absolutely fine, with the oxymoronic term 'slim-thick' being used to describe this look. The long overdue integration of black popular culture into mainstream popular culture, particularly in music, brought to the fore a new set of role models, as ordinarily Eurocentric images of artists were replaced with more Afrocentric ones. The Africanisation of body image in popular culture can be highlighted for men with the rapper 50 Cent and his muscular tattooed body and for women with Beyoncé with her long legs and large rear end (rebranded as a 'bootie' by marketers) as well as her full lips, small waist and ample bosom. Such an impossible look to achieve naturally for many, has led to a rise in surgical procedures for those fans wanting to emulate their role models, such as butt lifts and injections of Botox into lips. Girls started going to the gym to do squats in the hope that it would give them a larger backside, a physical feature that would have been considered hideous 40 years before. Fads and fashion driven by popular culture, which once made the 'trout-pout' a social media 'look', have led to a large backside on girls being considered something to point towards the camera when having a photograph taken, which is truly a symptom of a media-influenced mind.

For men it is a very different story; if you're fat in popular culture, then you can only be one of three characters: a villain (Tony Soprano), an object of comedy or stupidity (Peter Griffin), or a powerful uncaring boss person (The Fat Controller). If you are a fat man in real life, then you've failed at life, and it's your fault. How many genuinely cool, male fat role models can you think of from popular culture? The media is guilty of enforcing fat negativity in the psyche of the masses who absorb it.

My mate Skip (whom you'll read more about later in this book), isn't at all fat by typical British standards; sure he has a little bit of a beer gut, and there might be an extra chin lurking beneath his face, but in the UK he wouldn't be considered as being fat at all. Put Skip in another country however, such as India, and beer- and curry-loving Skip might as well be nicknamed 'Ten-Ton Terry Tikha', that's because by typical Indian standards Skip might be considered to be fat. He likes his cricket, he plays regularly and he enjoys following the England cricket team when they play in India. He's been to India many times, he loves the country and he loves the admiring attention that he gets there for his fuller figure.

Writing this from the perspective of a fat person is bizarre, because the last thing that I as a genuinely fat person ever want is special attention for being fat, I'd rather that you please just ignore me and carry on with what you're doing. Not Skip though, he loves the almost celebrity status that being considered fat gets him in some parts of particularly rural India. Skip being a Yorkshireman likes a bargain, which is one of the reasons that he likes going to India, "you just can't spend your money there" he often tells me. Sometimes when Skip goes to India he goes to a small town in the northeast of the country away from the big cities where by British standards the prices are truly very cheap. Here in the town, next to a modest sized marketplace is a bustling street of shops and traders, one of which is a tailors. Skip will visit the tailors and be fitted for a made-to-measure suit. He's had them all from there, including pinstripe, wedding attire, a tuxedo and even a cream coloured colonial era type suit that looks like 'The Man from Del Monte' (remember him, he said yes).

When Skip visits the tailors, it is a special occasion indeed, the tailor makes a fuss of him and uses the opportunity of having a large white man in his shop to drum up some publicity. When Skip gets measured up, it isn't in a dressing room or in a private fitting cubicle, Skip is put in the front window of the shop to be measured. The tailor's dummies are moved out of the way, samples of materials and textiles are shifted, and the space is cleared for a showing of the heavy-set white man to passers-by, who become an audience to the spectacle of the show being performed in front of them. Skip is a novelty, the town doesn't get a lot of portly, white British visitors and as such he attracts attention. Each and every one of Skip's body measurements is taken theatrically by the tailor, with Skip performing not so subtle Bollywood style dance moves in-between each application of the measuring tape. After each measurement is taken, the tailor writes the numbers down on a large blackboard with a piece of white chalk for all to see (there is no data protection here), and as he does this, one of his understudies who is standing in the shop doorway announces to the gathered crowd what each of the sizes is. Whistles are blown by members of the crowd outside of the shop, who also clap and cheer their appreciation of the stout white man performing before them. The tailor takes his time; whilst he is an extremely busy man, he does not want to rush the event, which gains his business valuable attention and publicity. After the show has ended, Skip leaves the tailors with his arms and hands aloft as if he has just hit a six for England. The crowd gathers around him, his hand is shaken numerous times, he is patted on the back, selfies are taken with him by members of the crowd, and his local celebrity status is cemented simply for being full-bodied. As I sit here writing this, I'm smiling at the thought of this fairly ordinary middle-aged British man becoming a cult figure for having a bit of a paunch and a double chin. In Indian society, a bit of extra body padding is a sign of wealth, which in turn is a sign of success. Skip is admired for being a successful fat man.

In Britain if you are fat, the chances are that you are not admired in the slightest, in fact if you are fat or overweight, it is likely that many people will consider you to be a failure in life. Somebody who is either stupid and doesn't know the difference between healthy and unhealthy foods, lazy and can't be bothered to exercise or cook for themselves, or greedy and always wants more than their fair share. Stupidity, laziness and greediness are in the mindset of many Britons synonymous with being fat.

I have been overweight for most of my life, I'm one of those people who has a large frame and can carry a bit extra without it being obvious how much extra I'm carrying. If I asked you to guess my weight, you would likely guess 2 stones (28 pounds/12.7 kilos) less than what I actually weigh. Even when I wasn't fat, I was overweight, or at least I felt overweight. All of my life has been spent with a weight gremlin sitting on my shoulder whispering nasty thoughts about myself into my ear. *I have failed at life because I'm fat, I'll never find a beautiful wife because I'm fat, I'll never be successful because I'm fat, I'll never be a professional footballer because I'm fat.* Yet none of these negative things about my future came to fruition, apart from not being a professional footballer. I have had a fantastic life, I've travelled the world, I am successful in my career and with my creativity, I married a beautiful wife and I did once get a touch of the football at Oakwell, the home of Barnsley FC after it hit me flat in the face at home versus Crewe Alexandra 2002. Well it gave everyone around me a laugh as a fat man getting hit in the face by a football is funnier than a thin man getting hit in the face by a football. "Hahaha nice one, fatty, surprised it dint go in thi gob."

In adulthood I gained weight on a daily basis, at least that's how it felt. I stopped getting on the weighing scales, not because it was depressing, but because the needle went right to the end and there was nowhere else for it to go. I was quite literally off the chart. I lost a bit of weight here and there, but always managed to find it again, and usually with a bit more to go with it.

Of course, there are some upsides to being fat. When I started boozing in my late teen years, which incidentally made me fatter, people would assume that the big bloke was a hard bloke, so I didn't get much hassle. I'm soft as shite actually, and I say shite and not shit intentionally, as that's how we say it in Yorkshire. The downsides are basically everything else; painful joints, can't find clothes that fit, nobody wanting to sit next to me on the bus or train (that's not so bad though), the social stigmas attached to being a fatty and of course other associated health problems caused by being overweight. These, dear reader, are some of the reasons why I began this journey, this banana journey to try and fix my physical health and mental wellbeing permanently. I needed to find peace with myself so that I would live not just a longer, but a happier life.

This book will take you through several months of my life, on either end of having weight loss surgery, a procedure that I had in October 2019 under the NHS at St. James's Hospital in Leeds. I will reflect upon the factors, contributors and aspects of my whole life that made me fat, I will discuss the preparation physically and mentally for the procedure that I underwent, and also the impacts that the surgery has had on me afterwards, the good, the bad and the very, very, ugly. This will be intertwined with stories, anecdotes and incidents that have occurred throughout my life, from growing up in Barnsley, backpacking around the world, living and working in Australia and settling in Leeds, where I met and married the most beautiful and perfect wife, my PW.

This book isn't particularly intended for those undergoing a weight loss journey of their own, (although I'm sure it would be most helpful), it is my intention that mostly anyone will get some sort of enjoyment from reading it. Truthfully if it makes you think twice about mentally judging somebody else for having a larger frame than you, then hopefully this book will have served its purpose.

Let the banana journey begin!

1 – Early life

1972 was quite an eventful year: the events of 'Bloody Sunday' took place in Derry, Northern Ireland where British soldiers shot 26 unarmed civilians during a protest march resulting in 15 deaths in January; the Soviet Union took a step forward in the 'space race' by landing a spacecraft 'Luna 20' on the moon in February; in the midst of the Vietnam War, 'The Easter Offensive' began after North Vietnamese forces entered the Demilitarised Zone (DMZ) of South Vietnam in March, on the same day that the British Government suspended the parliament of Northern Ireland; women were officially allowed to enter the Boston Marathon in April; the Dominion of Ceylon became the Republic of Sri Lanka in May; United States (US) President Richard Nixon was tape recorded talking about using the Central Intelligence Agency (CIA) to obstruct the FBI's investigation into the Watergate break-ins in June; 22 bombs that were planted by the Provisional Irish Republican Army (IRA) exploded in Belfast, Northern Ireland, killing nine people and injuring 130 more in July; Ugandan President Idi Amin announced that he would expel 50,000 British Asians from Uganda in August; 11 Israeli athletes were murdered at the 1972 Summer Olympics in Munich by members of the Arab terrorist group Black September who invaded the Olympic Village in September; riots in the Maze Prison in Northern Ireland led to most of the prison burning down in October; the last executions by guillotine took place in Paris, France in November, and; the last manned mission to the moon took place aboard Apollo 17 in December.

The events of 1972 made it a pretty typical year in terms of the years that I've lived through so far. People murdered other people because they had different political or religious viewpoints, the competition for global dominance between Eastern and Western superpowers was ongoing as was the struggle for equal rights by women and minority groups who faced discrimination and persecution. Countries broke up with their friends and went separate ways, and politics at the highest level was dirty and corrupt. Yes, 1972 was just another year on planet Earth, sandwiched between 1971, which was the year that the UK adopted the decimal currency of Sterling pounds and pence (what came before was just weird), and 1973, the year that the UK joined the European Community (EC), which went on to become the European Union (EU). One thing did set 1972 apart from the other years, which was that in the midst of this 366-day (1972 was a leap year) socio-political shit-storm, I was born in Barnsley District General Hospital (BDGH) in the month of July, just on the Cancerian side of the crab/lion divide of the astrological charts. I entered a world where Donny Osmond was number one in the UK singles chart with his song 'Puppy Love' and the UK had a Tory government led by Ted Heath. I obviously don't remember being born or when I first heard mop-topped Donny, and I certainly wasn't born political, but I was almost certainly born hungry as I entered the world and screamed my first breath, I usually am hungry, so I was probably born that way.

I was the first-born to my parents, Wendy and David, neither of whom are from Barnsley. My mum is a southerner, from Pangbourne in the Royal County of Berkshire and my dad from Hebden Bridge in West Yorkshire. I'm not quite sure how between them they ended up in Barnsley. I don't even think a straight line on a map from Pangbourne to Hebden Bridge would go through Barnsley, but end up there they did, and it was in Barnsley, in the 'Socialist Republic of South Yorkshire' that I spent the first 22 years of my life.

I was a sickly baby and toddler, quite intolerant of a lot of food these days people talk about allergies and food intolerances, in the early 1970s, people weren't clued up on things such as the need for some people to be gluten free, or dairy free, or having a nut allergy. In the early 1970s, people puked, shit themselves and dropped dead without explanation. If you'd asked the average Briton in the 1970s what a coeliac was, they'd probably have said somebody from 'Seelier', and if you'd asked them to spell coeliac…well let's just not go there, because most Britons wouldn't be able to spell coeliac even today. Not that I am a coeliac mind, I'm just making this point to raise the fact that education around food in the 1970s wasn't what it is today. I do remember my mum telling me what a 'sicky' toddler I was, who could only tolerate mashed banana or mashed chips. I do remember once being sick at the dinner table, probably aged around 4 years old straight onto the dinner plate of 'Uncle Earl', who was a close friend of my parents and was stopping at our house with 'Auntie Sandra'. In those days, food wasn't wasted, and this happened to be one of my mum's incredible Sunday roast dinners. I got shouted at for being sick, and my dad ended up swapping dinners with Uncle Earl. The sick was just on one side of the dinner plate, so my dad just washed that bit off under the sink tap and then ate from the other side of the plate. With hindsight I probably had some kind of intolerance to food, which over time I outgrew as my digestive system and general health developed and improved. As a toddler I was a skinny little thing with a mop of blonde hair, but as I became tolerant of more types of food, the weight went on, I grew and for some reason my blonde hair turned brown.

My sister Carla was born in June 1975 on the very same day that the United Kingdom first held a yes or no referendum over whether or not to remain a member of the EC. On this occasion the electorate voted to stay in the EC by a decisive margin of 17,378,581 to 8,470,073. I was 3 years old, and the first time I was aware that I had a sister was having my Nan make me breakfast, because "Mummy had gone to have her bump taken out of her tummy." I remember being fascinated by my mum's big tummy when she was pregnant, I knew a baby was in there, and the bump was something that was about love that everyone adored it and wanted to touch, stroke or gently pat it.

I developed an awareness that I was 'fat' when I was between 3 and 4 years old. It fell upon my dad to have to take me to the doctors for a standard toddler check-up appointment, as my mum had to stay home to look after my baby Sister. I can't remember what the name of our normal doctor was, but I do remember the name of the doctor that we saw on this particular appointment, Dr Galvin, a name etched into my brain. I think the appointment was just a general health-check, but during this appointment the doctor told my dad that I was overweight, that I was 'fat' for my age. This is my earliest memory of being fat, except that I had no idea what fat was. How many 3-year-olds have an understanding of body image, and how many 3-year-olds have responsibility for their diet? I remember my dad being annoyed at me on the long walk home from the doctors for being fat, but he blamed my mum for it. When we got home, my parents rowed about me being fat, which made me upset, I didn't know what I'd done wrong, I didn't know what this fat word meant, but I knew strongly that it was negative, that it was something bad. The outcome of this argument was that my mum vowed that my dad would never take me to the doctors again and that I would never ever see Doctor Galvin again. I've never ever forgotten that day, which was my fat awakening, even though I didn't really understand what fat was.

I went to a junior school in Darfield, called Darfield Upperwood Junior and Infant School. It was quite a new school and the majority of children who went there were from the estate upon which I lived. I was the tallest and heaviest child in my class, I knew this because we had to measure ourselves every so often and the teacher would make comments about the measurements. My weight always came up as a topic of conversation for the class to discuss, before the teacher would have a moralistic talk about 'good foods' and 'bad foods'. The eyes of the class were always on me because I must be eating the most bad foods, which made me feel like a bad person, and it made some of the other children not want to be friends with me because only bad people ate bad foods and got fat. I didn't have that teacher forever, and it was mostly a really nice school, but it wasn't always easy.

Darfield was in the thick of Barnsley's coal mining industry. Darfield had its own colliery as did the nearby villages of Little Houghton, Stairfoot, Elsecar, Grimethorpe and Wath. There were numerous other collieries around Barnsley and beyond, and the majority of dads in Darfield seemed to work underground in dangerous conditions, sending coal to the surface above to burn in power stations and keep Britain generating electricity. Coal was also a solid fuel that was burnt in the home. Almost everyone who worked in the coal mines had a coal fire in their house, as miners were entitled to a free coal delivery each month as a benefit of the job. I was one of the few children in Darfield whose Dad didn't work in the coal mines. My dad, after an early career on the railways where he had been a fireman on steam trains and a driver of diesel trains, was working in a town called Rawmarsh near Rotherham in a furniture shop. We didn't have a car in those days, and from our home in Darfield, my dad would have to walk 1.5 miles (2.4 km) to Wombwell, where he would catch a bus from Wombwell to Rawmarsh. In this day and age, very few people would make that physical effort to get to work; if they don't drive, they would use public transport or get a taxi. It's hard to imagine in 21st century Britain anyone walking a significant distance in order to get to work, but my dad did this walk twice per day (there and back) as well as working in a job role where he was actively walking around a large furniture store in order to both keep it running and make sales with customers. In the 1970s, people led more active lifestyles, not through choice, but through necessity. People didn't need to go to the gym to run on treadmills (which there probably weren't very many of in 1970s Britain anyway) as they weren't sitting on their backsides for the majority of their waking lives.

Money was tight, and we only had the one income for our family in the early days. My mum didn't work, she had children to raise, a house to run and in 1970s Barnsley, there just weren't that many jobs for women. My mum not working was not at all unusual, most mums in Darfield didn't work during that era either. Mum did the weekly shop in the nearby town of Wombwell. She would have me walking by her side and Carla in the pram for the 3-mile (4.8km) round-trip to Hillards supermarket, which was centrally located on Wombwell High Street close to butchers, bakers and greengrocers. Wombwell was bustling in those days, but today the High Street is a shadow of its former self, just as it is in many towns around the UK. More people work, fewer people go to shops, more people buy online and fewer people are on the High Street as their satnavs take them around it on a bypass. Mum shopped around, she was money-conscious because she had to be and always looked for the best deals. Rain, sunshine, sleet or snow, Mum would make the trek, week in and week out, returning not just with two grumpy tired kids, but laden down with heavy bags of shopping. Just like my dad, my mum had a physically active life not through choice, but through necessity, people did in that era.

Because money was tight, food was regimented into four meals per day, and there was never any snacking in-between. Breakfast was either a bowl of cereal or two slices of toast and jam with a cup of tea or coffee. Lunch was always sandwiches, crisps and orange squash, followed by a sweet treat such as a chocolate biscuit or piece of cake. My sister and I would eat lunch sitting on a blanket on the floor in front of the TV while *The Flumps, Trumpton* or Bagpuss' was on. Our main cooked meal of the day, dinner (which was served at 16:45 like clockwork) consisted of meat and two veg type meals, one of the veg being potato, which we ate almost every day. My parents bought potatoes by the sack load, literally huge paper sacks of potatoes that stood around 4 feet (120 cm) tall. My favourite potato-based food was of course chips. My mum and dad had the greatest chip pan in the world ever, which made absolutely incredible chips. They still have that chip pan too, and it still makes incredible chips, as well as my dad's signature onion and potato fritters coated in calorific crispy batter. Apart from meat and two veg type meals, we ate a lot of pies, stews, hotpots, liver with onion and fish. My mum was a brilliant cook (she still is) and she could cook just about anything. Most meals were British type meals, we rarely had rice or pasta (few people did in Barnsley in the 1970s and early 1980s), and pizzas were something that you occasionally saw on TV, but I think I was probably a teenager before I'd actually tried one. We hardly ever ate ready-meals, they were expensive and just not that good compared to what my mum could make.

The final meal of the day was supper, which was a regulation two biscuits with either a glass of milk or a cup of hot chocolate. When we got a little older, we were allowed to substitute our two biscuits for a slice of toast and jam. Supper was the only meal of the day that we would get ourselves (from me being around 8 years old anyway), but we would always ask permission first. Mum and Dad would be watching *Emmerdale* or one of the other soaps, so would largely be happy to leave us to it. However, when Carla and I would be alone in the kitchen getting our supper, we could guarantee that Dad would come into the kitchen under the pretence that he was looking for something, when what he really was doing was checking up on what we were eating. We would be chastised if he suspected us of eating more than two biscuits or even if I had too much jam on my toast. This wasn't just about 'being greedy', as a family we genuinely didn't have a lot of money to spare and food was an expense. My mum would then be brought into it and would often stick up for us, stating that my dad would be dipping into the biscuit box multiple times per day (which he did) therefore setting us a bad example. This caused conflict between them, which was upsetting for us; we associated food with conflict. Therefore we became sneaky, and if we wanted a third biscuit, we would wait until Dad had been in on his reconnaissance mission, and we would then hide it in our clothing. Carla even went to the extreme measure of going outside to the front of the house and posting a biscuit through the front letterbox, which would go into the hallway. She would then collect the biscuit on her way up to bed, our parents being none the wiser. We progressed from sneaking an extra biscuit to sneaking packets of crisps up to our bedrooms, which was much more difficult as crisp packets made a crackling sound when disturbed. If you put a crisp packet in your pocket it would make a noise as you walked, so the answer was to go and get our supper, wearing a dressing-gown, then when leaving the kitchen to go to bed, carry the dressing gown in a bundle, a bundle of swag! A dressing gown wasn't just good for hiding crisps, it would be good for hiding biscuits, chocolate bars, pieces of cake wrapped up in kitchen roll and yoghurts, the dressing gown was the tool of choice for the dedicated supper smuggler. Like alcoholics with hidden bottles around their houses enabling them to drink in secret, Carla and I became secret eaters at supper time. Any crisp packets or biscuit wrappers would be screwed up inside a toilet roll or paper before being put in the bin so as not to give us away.

My family was small, just myself, my sister, Mum and Dad at home. In Hebden Bridge was my Nanny Moss (my dad's mum). My Grandad Moss died when I was a toddler before my sister was born. I don't have strong memories of him as I was so young when he died. Nanny Moss was a funny woman, quite eccentric and very practical in all sense of domesticity, particularly needlework and cooking. She worked in one of the many sewing factories in Hebden Bridge, sewing 'Spencers' trousers before retiring and then working voluntarily for Oxfam. She was a very social and fit person who would go out dancing on an evening with her friends. In Pangbourne were my Nanny and Grandad Kent (my mum's parents). Nanny Kent never worked in my lifetime that I can remember, she was a smoker when I was very young (she eventually gave up) and her daily routine involved domestic chores, a gossip with the women from next door and lots of television soaps and dramas, including *The Sullivans* an Australian World War II drama, which was my Nan's favourite afternoon programme. Grandad Kent was a tall, broad and very strong athletic man, a bit like *Tarzan* actor Johnny Weissmuller. Grandad Kent worked as a gardener for a doctor in Pangbourne, Dr Martin, who had a large house and lots of garden to maintain. Grandad Kent was an expert gardener, and also very practical in terms of DIY and mechanics.

I used to love visiting my grandparents for holidays; we didn't have a great deal of money, so a fortnight in Hebden Bridge or Pangbourne was a standard family holiday for us. We would travel by train with heavy suitcases, not suitcases with wheels on the underside, they hadn't been invented at this point. From Hebden Bridge railway station it was a long and winding walk uphill to my Nan's house above the main part of the town. We were always red-faced and slightly 'out of puff' when we arrived. We'd be greeted with either cups of tea or home-made lemonade with home-made parkin, flapjack and Eccles cakes. I loved my Nan's cooking, but it would sometimes have a bitter taste when she would tell me that I'd "spoiled myself" by being fat. By the time I was 8 or 9 years old, I understood fully what these words meant, and the negative connotations of fatness. It used to upset me, but I would keep this hidden inside. I never talked about how I felt, you just didn't in those days, and I'd come to accept that it must be me in the wrong, because I was the fat one, nobody else in my family was fat. Even though I loved my Nan to bits, there were times that I would dread seeing her, knowing that the first comment she would make to me would be about my weight. I must emphasise though, that the many happy memories I have of visiting my Nan in Hebden Bridge by far outweigh those sad ones. My Nan loved me unconditionally, and her digs at me about my weight however misplaced were because she cared and she wanted me to grow up to be healthy. She also wanted me to work in a bank when I grew up and that was definitely never going to happen! Her house was a terrace on four levels, on the lower ground floor was the kitchen and cellar, on the upper ground floor were two sitting rooms, on the first floor were two bedrooms and a bathroom and on the second floor was the attic complete with a proper slate bed snooker table. Carla and I had a great time playing hide and seek in the house, which with all its stairs gave us a proper workout. Often when my Nan and parents were watching TV in the living room, we'd either be playing old records and snooker in the attic or in the kitchen tucking into endless tins of my Nan's home-made sweet-baked treats, in secret of course, we had become quite adept at being secret eaters.

We would go for many family walks around Hebden Bridge, up hill and down dale, quite often we'd go picking blackberries, bilberries and edible dock leaves. My Nan would turn blackberries and bilberries into pies, crumbles and jams. The dock leaves would be de-stalked, chopped, boiled with onion, have oatmeal added and made into absolutely delicious 'dock pudding'. This truly is a Hebden Bridge delicacy; these days people add all kinds of ingredients to dock pudding to make it 'contemporary', there are even dock pudding competitions, but back then dock leaves were a regular part of the foraging calendar that nearly almost all Hebden Bridge locals followed as a matter of course. Not only was this wild-growing food cost-free, getting it involved a good deal of exercise. People in Hebden Bridge weren't just thrifty financially, they were physically fit and lean, as people walked long distances up and down hills to get to and from work and had physical jobs in factories. The people of Hebden Bridge actually needed food that was calorific as they led such physically active lives, my Nan's dock pudding would be fried in bacon fat and served with bacon, eggs and fried mushrooms. Still to this day my dad makes an annual pilgrimage from Barnsley to Hebden Bridge to pick dock leaves, and he makes dock pudding the traditional way, just like my Nan did; he always saves me a tub too, and yes I still fry it in bacon fat.

When we were at Hebden, we'd sometimes walk to a place called Kittling Bridge, where we would make a campfire, and fry sausages in a frying pan to make sausage sandwiches. I was always the chef with the blackened frying pan and fat-spattered burnt arms, but I absolutely loved doing this. My sister would be somewhere nearby halfway up a tree, she was so much more active than I was in those days. Despite me being fat, my Nan would always make us eat everything on our plates, leaving food was simply not an option. I remember once leaving half a grilled tomato because it had gone cold and I wasn't that keen on it, and honestly the fuss that was made about it was just ridiculous. Days later my Nan was still talking about that uneaten half a cold tomato (which incidentally I ended up eating anyway just to shut everyone up). Nan was telling me that there were starving children in Africa, so I told her that she should have just posted it to them. I got a rare clip around the ear for that bit of cheek.

Visiting my Nan and Grandad Kent's house in Pangbourne took all day on the train with several changes along the way. Their house was also a good walk from the railway station, albeit on the flat rather than being uphill. Pangbourne was always hot in summer, it was akin to going abroad for me, plus everyone talked funny there too. Nan Kent was also a great cook, and there would always be jars of homemade jams, marmalades, and pickles to try. My Nan and Grandad had a walk-in pantry, with shelves and shelves of all kinds of food. I used to love just standing in their looking at what was on the shelves, it was like being in a shop and I'd be in awe.

My grandparents had a large garden and Grandad Kent grew many different vegetables, which would invariably end up on the dinner table. I remember mountains of runner beans on the kitchen worktop, hundreds of green tomatoes left to turn red on window ledges and huge bunches of onions tied together in braids, just like you'd see in France (well I'd seen it on TV in France). My weight was never an issue in Pangbourne, it was seldom mentioned by my grandparents. Food was a big part of every day, and the first cup of tea was served by my grandad to us in bed at 07:00 before he went to work. Breakfast was at 08:30 served by Nan, and this would be toast and jam followed by cereal, and hot coffee from a percolator with both milk and coffee whitener in it, which at the time was a real luxury.

In the mornings, Carla and I would walk down to the shops with my Nan's shopping list and a purse full of coins. We would also call into Oxfam, where I'd scour the books looking for a science fiction bargain to buy from my spending money. Back at my grandparents' house, lunch would be served at 12:30, and my Nan used to cook it on a Rayburn stove, I was fascinated by the Rayburn, which had a full coal fire integrated into it, I'd love messing around with the fire (with or without consent). Lunch was the main meal of the day and would be a hearty affair with meat, vegetables and potatoes usually featured. Lunch was always followed by a 'pudding', which might have been fruit in jelly, tinned fruit and custard, ice cream, fruit pie or a crumble with custard. My grandad used to drive home for lunch, and as soon as we saw his brown Rover P6 (which was akin to a tank) pull up, we knew that it was time to go and wash our hands. My grandad had a physical job and he would arrive home for lunch hungry. I would be in awe of the mountain of food on his plate, which was always much bigger than everybody else's plate (I was also slightly jealous of his plate too), my grandad Kent was truly my hero, a big strong man with a heart of gold, a very gentle manner and a lion's appetite, I wanted to be just like him.

Even though my weight was rarely mentioned, my grandad would encourage me to be active by doing jobs in his garden for him while he was at work or going for walks down to the River Thames, where there was 'the rec', which was a play park with climbing frames, swings and roundabouts. Carla and I spent many happy hours on the rec as kids. At tea-time we would have sandwiches and crisps in front of the TV followed by cake and fizzy pop. For supper, a cup of tea or hot chocolate with biscuits was the norm. Truthfully though, while grandparents and parents were sitting in the living room watching TV, Carla and I would be pantry raiding. Instead of having a regimented and measured supper, we would sneak into the dining room and shut ourselves in the pantry where we would feast upon whatever we could open and devour that wouldn't be noticed. There were foods there that we just didn't have at home and everything was just so tasty, our night-time secret eating continued unabated.

Home life in Darfield was good, and my parents did what they could to ensure that we had everything we needed. We had a nice house, which was warm and comfortable. We had the odd holiday outside of visiting grandparents, we even went to Portugal when I was 8 years old, I'm not quite sure how we afforded that, but I do remember that we flew there with the now defunct Laker Airlines. My parents were very allocentric when they were younger, they were not afraid to travel to the continent and get on a train. Before I was born, they once went all the way to Faro in the south of Portugal by train. I have adopted that trait from them now and have become something of a serial traveller in later life, something that I will discuss throughout this book.

At some point in the late 1970s the furniture shop that my dad worked at in Rawmarsh closed down. Faced with redundancy my dad was proactive and found himself a job in a carpet shop on Wombwell High Street called Broadheads. He would walk to work and back every day and spend most of his day at Broadheads on his feet too. My dad worked with a friendly bloke called Cyril who lived in a village called Cudworth. My dad, my sister and I used to go swimming at Cudworth swimming baths every Saturday morning. Mum was a non-swimmer and would spectate. Because my dad got on well with Cyril we would sometimes be invited over to their house for lunch after we'd been swimming. Cyril was married to Dorothy, a very kind lady who always smiled and spoiled us with fancy sandwiches and cream cakes. Carla and I used to call them 'Uncle Cyril' and 'Auntie Dorothy', as the uncle and aunty prefix was the polite way to address adults in those days. Cyril had a yellow speedboat called Flipper, and every summer we would be invited to join them on a boat ride along the River Ouse and into the centre of York on the boat. It was such an adventure to us, and we were very lucky to have this opportunity, but even those days of happiness were tinged with sadness and upset for me. I remember Uncle Cyril once saying to me "you know what you are, you're a good little lad, but you're a fat little bugger, you are you know, you're really fat." There it was again, the fat word, the f-word. I don't think for one minute that Cyril meant to hurt my feelings, but I just wanted to cry when I heard those words. He was such a nice man and always did nice things for us, but even he called me fat, and after that I stopped wanting to go around to their house after swimming. I'd say I had a headache or felt sick. Sometimes it worked and we'd go straight home, sometimes it didn't and I'd just sit there quietly trying to blend into the background, so as not to be seen so that my size wouldn't be commented upon.

My mum passed her driving test in 1980 and my parents bought a second-hand blue Mini Clubman. This opened up a whole new world to us; not only did it mean that we could drive to our grandparents instead of spending hours on trains, it meant that we could go on family holidays to such exotic destinations as Lampeter in Wales and West Auckland in County Durham. At Lampeter, we stayed in university halls of residence flats that were unused in summer and therefore cheap, and at West Auckland we stayed in a red-bricked holiday cottage in the middle of nowhere on a farm called Brackenberry Leazes, I loved it there. By the time I'd started high school (I went to Darfield Foulstone) the whole family would go together on an annual holiday, all of us under the one roof in a red-bricked cottage just outside of West Auckland. There would be Mum, Dad, Carla, Nan Moss, Nan Kent and Grandad Kent. I would spend 51 weeks of the year looking forward to this week, it was just so brilliant having my whole family together, and even better, every now and again my cousins Andrew and Maxine along with my Aunty Judy and Uncle Keith would drive up from Barnsley for the day to visit us there.

The cottage had an open coal fire and my daily job was to use a small axe to split kindling, which along with scrunched-up newspaper was used to light the fire. Then coal would need to be brought in, in a scuttle from an outside coal shed. I took responsibility for the fire, supervised by my dad and grandad. I have always been fascinated by fire, anthropologists believe that the minds and imaginations of early human ancestors were shaped by fire. Think about the last time you just sat and stared into mesmeric dancing flames. An open fire was the 3D 4K HD TV of its day, except unlike television you have to work to keep a coal fire going, and that involves movement. We've now become less active in the home with TVs to stare at and gas fires and central heating taking over how we keep our houses warm.

At West Auckland there was a barbecue, and we would cook outside on the open flames. Again, that was my responsibility, I loved barbecuing sausages and burgers, while my sister looked jealously on, too young at that point to be allowed so close to the flames. I had grown up into a tall young teenager, and a lot of my weight had come off as I grew older. When I look back on photographs of myself from this era I look positively skinny, but I must have suffered from some form of body dysmorphia, because in my head I always thought that I was fat, I was never happy with my appearance, and was always sad in my own skin. I felt like I had tree trunk legs and a great big belly, but in reality I really didn't.

20 years after we had stopped going to the holiday cottage in West Auckland, my parents bought a week at a time-share lodge at Slaley Hall in Northumberland. Every year since then we have gone there on an annual family holiday. Nowadays my parents, sister, nephew, wife and I spend a week together there every February, and I count down the weeks and days to visiting, just like I did as a child when we went to West Auckland. Do you want to know what's really bizarre about this though? The drive from our house in Leeds (I left Barnsley in 1994) to Slaley Hall takes us on the A68 road, and as we drive north along the A68, there to our left sitting alone in the middle of a farmer's fields is the West Auckland holiday cottage. I always smile and get a warm, happy feeling inside when I see it in the distance. So many very happy memories from an era when I wasn't fat, even though I thought that I was.

Around 1980, my dad lost his job at Broadheads, which closed down. He was then forced to do what nearly all Barnsley dads did and he became a coal miner. It was a job that he hated with a passion, but it paid well and kept food on the table and a roof over our heads. Come rain or shine he would cycle from our house and back to Houghton Main Colliery, a distance of about 4 miles (6.4 km) in each direction. The calories burnt getting to and from work and then working 12 hours in a physically demanding job, must have really kept him in good physical shape.

In 1984, the National Union of Mineworkers (NUM) led by Arthur Scargill called their members out on strike for a whole year in protest at proposed pit closures by the then Tory government, which was led by Margaret Thatcher, or Bastard Thatcher as she was (and still is) known in Barnsley. I could write an entire book about my experiences through the miners' strike, and maybe one day I will, but I don't want to detract from my banana journey story too much right now. Suffice to say, that the year that the miners went on strike, was the worst year of my life. It was heart-breaking seeing the strain that my parents were under, as the financial pressures grew. It was a frightening and intimidating time to live in Darfield. I used to walk past a bus shelter on Barnsley Road that was daubed with the words 'Robson is a scabby bastard'. I've no idea who Robson was, but he's probably still referred to as a scab to this very day. My dad didn't work for an entire year, he never scabbed but he rarely went picketing either, it was cold, miserable and he thought it was a waste of time. Instead he put his energies into DIY and gardening. That year he built Carla a new wooden bed that had storage inside it, and he grew more vegetables in the garden than ever before, he needed to, or we would have gone hungry. When donated food parcels were handed out to miners' families from Darfield Working Men's Club, we were at the back of the queue because my dad hadn't picketed enough. I think over the entire year we might have had one food parcel. That year my parents obliterated all of the savings that they had, and they were helped financially by grandparents and my dad's brother Gordon. Without their help we would likely have likely lost our house. As it was, we never once went hungry and there was always a meal on the table at tea-time. The house was cold in winter, but at least we had a house.

Throughout my childhood and teenage years I grew up with a soundtrack of music, politics and dieting. Mum liked The Beatles, Queen and Michael Jackson, Dad liked Abba and I developed a taste for hip-hop from when I first heard Grandmaster Flash aged 10 years old. I used to listen intently to the lyrics of the music, which were often about societal issues such as crime, violence and injustice. I learned more from hip-hop than I ever did from school! I could see the social injustices rapped about 1980s New York reflected in some ways in 1980s deprived Barnsley. I was a fairly average school pupil, I achieved nearly all Grade Cs in my GCSEs. I wasn't thick, but I certainly wasn't a striver either, career prospects in Barnsley weren't exactly great and I had no clue what I wanted to do with my life. When the careers adviser came to my school to interview us, I told him that I wanted to be a radio DJ, so he advised me to look for jobs in light rigging in theatres. I never really did work that one out, nor did I follow his advice.

My weight in my mid-teen years yo-yo'd up and down, I wasn't excessively fat but I was certainly overweight compared to all of my friends, who were mostly skinny, and while they all wore medium-sized t-shirts, mine were large. For some reason, my mum always seemed to be on a diet, and I would often follow her lead counting calories and eating salads. Like me, Mum never seemed to be happy with her weight, even though she wasn't ever fat. The bathroom weighing scales would be out almost every day. I hated those bloody scales, it was never good news. Try as I did to diet, I just wasn't very good at it. I wasn't an active teenager and calories consumed usually surpassed calories burnt. Teenage weight gain caused me to grow breasts, these days people call them 'moobs' (man boobs), and back then they became a reason to pick on me for one or two arseholes at my school. The moobs made me miserable, and in the end my mum took me to the doctor from where I was referred to a specialist at Sheffield's Northern General Hospital. Aged 12 I actually had 'plastic' or cosmetic surgery, via an operation called a gynecomastia, which was basically a male breast reduction. Amazingly I somehow managed to keep this a secret from everybody at school for years including my closest friends.

By the time I was 14, my mum had got a job in Rotherham at Cooper's Toy Shop, followed by a secretarial job for the 'Stop it don't drop it' anti-litter campaign. She then got a job for Barnsley College, where she spent most of the rest of her working life, until some crooked bastards that ran the college caused it to go into financial meltdown in the late 1990s, which led to numerous redundancies, including my mum's. When my mum first got a job, she was concerned that Carla and I would become 'latchkey kids' (kids who were left to look after themselves). This never happened, but what did happen was that my responsibility in the kitchen became heightened and I would often make dinner for the family. I particularly liked making pots of stew. By my mid-teens I was a very competent cook who wasn't afraid to experiment with flavours including herbs and spices. My family would often compliment me on the meals that I made, although my dad would moan if it was spicy and of course if I was cooking it, I'd make sure that I had a good portion of it.

I was never sporty, I rarely exercised, and I don't come from a particularly sporty family. My Grandad Kent was an athlete in his younger days, winning medals on track and field, but neither of my parents were into sport, and that was largely the same for me, apart from a bit of a mid-teenage obsession with golf. One of my best mates at school, John Boocock (Booky) turned out to have a real talent for golf and that rubbed off on me. Booky and I would spend every summer evening hitting golf balls on playing fields. The clubs and balls belonged to Booky, but he would let me borrow them in return for some company while he played. Eventually I saved up enough money to buy a second-hand Sondico seven iron, something which Booky ribbed me for, because apparently Sondico wasn't a brand to shout about, but I didn't care, I was happy to have my own golf stick! Golf turned out to be great exercise, we would walk for miles and this stabilised my weight, in fact it helped me lose weight. I appreciated the value of exercise from this point onwards and would run home from school every day, my logic being that if I did this I wouldn't need to diet. I must have looked a state in my ill-fitting school uniform, puffing and panting with a red face as I ran up Barnsley Road, but it did do me some good. In third year, I was press-ganged by my classmates into running the 1,500 metres at the school sports day, basically because nobody else wanted to. So I took on the challenge and you know what? I came third, which was a huge achievement for me, I actually won a sports medal. It's the only sports medal that I've ever won in my entire life, and I very much doubt that I'll ever win another. But there you go, that was my brief brush with sporting athleticism, a bronze in the 1,500 metres at the 1986 Darfield Foulstone Sports Day event. I think I stopped running home from school not long after that though, instead favouring messing about with my mates as we tramped up Barnsley Road and across the Inkerman Fields.

Sixth form college was a waste of 3 years for me educationally, but I had a great time socially making fantastic friends and listening to bands and artists including Public

Enemy, Beastie Boys, Ice-T, NWA, Run DMC and LL Cool J. I was heavily into music, especially hip-hop, which apart from food and girls was the essence of life. Yes, I'd also discovered the joy of sex while at Barnsley College, and somehow A-level physics didn't seem to be that fun anymore. This was in the late 1980s, the rave scene (the second summer of love) was in full swing, and I was more interested in music, partying and meeting girls than anything else, anything else apart from eating that is. I loved my food and was always hungry, I was gaining weight, but at the same time I was keeping it in check with regular daily gym workouts. Sixth form college had a free gym, and I really got into pumping iron, as a pumped body was good for attracting the ladies, and thanks to my gynecomastia operation, I could move my pecs up and down as if by magic after a gym work-out, which was always a good talking point at parties. I had a solid group of mates from school, Skip, Skel, Fez, Gaz and Col, most of whom went to sixth form and most of whom I hung about with. Still to this day we meet up, not regularly admittedly (most often on WhatsApp or Zoom), but when we do see each other, it's like we've never been apart. I also had other mates at Barnsley College who were massive hip-hop heads like me and we've since reconnected on social media.

My first proper paid job was at Ardsley House hotel, where I worked in a number of roles relating to the bar area. I started as a glass collector but progressed to barman and then bar supervisor, before taking on the role of cellarman. These roles gave me ready access to food and drink, and I definitely abused this. Whilst my role as a cellarman was physically demanding, I'd be drinking fizzy pop and snacking on crisps and nuts while I worked, and drinking beer at the end of my shift, so the weight just went on. People at work would tell me that I was "getting as wide as you are tall," or that I was "putting on timber." I'd developed a thick skin by this point (no pun intended) and had got used to my weight being a topic of conversation. I just batted away weight-related comments with another pint and another bag of crisps. I liked working, but my education at Barnsley College suffered as I concentrated on earning money instead of on my studies, much to my mum's dismay.

From Ardsley House hotel, my next step was to a record shop, before going back to Ardsley House and then taking a slightly larger step, in fact a step that was truly globe-spanning, right across the planet to Australia…and that, dear reader, is where I will leave this first chapter, as my Australia stories as well as further stories about my childhood, early years, eating habits, weight and life will be intertwined and reflected upon throughout the rest of this book.

2 – Things get bad before they get better

"If you don't do something to drastically improve your health, you're looking at having a major event in the next 10 years." The tall, slim and very matter-of-fact doctor looked me straight in the eye as he gave me his prognosis. His use of the word 'event' wasn't referring to any fun kind of event such as a festival, concert or pub crawl, quite the opposite, it was in relation to me heading fat-belly-first towards a heart attack or a stroke. It wasn't what I wanted to hear, but it was the wake-up call that I needed. The year was 2014, I was 42 years old and just tipping the weighing scales at 26 stone (364 pounds/165.1 kilos). I'd been overweight for most of my adult life, but my weight had now got to a point that it was causing both me and my wife some major concerns. It wasn't difficult to see that I was overweight, but few people would have guessed how much I actually weighed. I have always weighed more than what people might have guessed, I have a large and solid frame, just like my Grandad Kent. Unlike my Grandad Kent though, my frame is coated in excess timber cladding, and lots of it. I had made the appointment to see my doctor as I wanted and needed some help to lose weight and keep it off. I'd tried dieting over the years, and whatever came off as a result of me cutting down, seemed to go back on twice as fast and with interest. Yo-yo dieting had been a part of my life for nearly 30 years, and it just wasn't working for me as my net weight had increased and I continued to get larger and larger. The doctor had just taken my blood pressure and it was high. I can't remember exactly how high, it wasn't in the 'dangerous' range, but it was higher than it should be, and I wasn't surprised by this, I knew that my health was suffering.

My joints permanently ached, basic movement and walking hurt, I had difficulty climbing a flight of stairs, which would leave me out of breath, going downstairs hurt my knee joints, my ankles were permanently sore and swollen, I sweated when I ate, I had a burning sensation in my left upper thigh, my feet were often numb and always cold, I would wake up most mornings screaming in agony with severe leg cramps, I was always tired, my mood was low, I was lethargic and depressed and scariest of all I was stopping breathing while I slept. I had come to the doctors today with a shopping list of ailments that I suspected were all down to my weight, and that I wanted to get help with.

The doctor told me that he was glad that I'd had this 'epiphany' and finally come into the surgery, noting that I hadn't seen a doctor in over 4 years previously; how that was about to change! The doctor told me that where I was health-wise was something that was becomingly increasingly common in his experience, but I could do something about it, particularly with help. He told me that heart attacks caused by heart disease were the biggest killer in the UK and indeed globally. Heart disease is where the arteries carrying blood to the heart narrow and harden through fatty deposits in the blood, which causes blood flow to the heart to diminish and in some cases stop, and when the blood flow stops, that is when a heart attack happens. Similar to a heart attack, a stroke can also be caused by an interrupted arterial blood supply, but this is to the brain rather than the heart, as blood carries oxygen and when the brain is starved of oxygen a stroke can happen, causing part of the brain to die. The doctor told me that strokes were the third biggest killer in the UK, and as with heart disease both high blood pressure and high cholesterol were attributing factors. As a result of my visit, the doctor sent letters off to The Weight Management Service and The Sleep Service, two departments of Leeds NHS, and he also booked me in for an overall health check with a practice nurse at the surgery, which would include blood tests.

I needed to sort myself out and I needed help in doing this, thank God for our National Health Service (NHS). The implications of me facing a heart attack or stroke in the next 10 years were extremely worrying to me. I didn't want to die young, I actually love my life, apart from my health, my life is fantastic. I have a happy marriage to an amazing wife, a loving family, a very nice home, a great job, and a fantastic leisure life, which includes a lot of socialising, gigs and holidays. I have everything to live for, yet I seemed to be killing myself slowly through overindulgence and a lack of exercise. I accept that death is a part of life, everybody dies, but I was also aware that the average age that people in the UK die is around 82. The way I was heading at this point, I would be lucky to see 52 and that was something that I simply couldn't contemplate. I hate death, I hate anything coming to an end, a life, a film franchise, a television series, a really good book, a pint of beer or a packet of crisps, it's all heartbreaking to me! I know that everyone dies and that everything does come to an end eventually. Whilst I accept that, it doesn't make it any easier for me to mentally deal with.

I remember when John Lennon was shot dead, I was 8 years old, and had been brought up on a diet of music by The Beatles, and besides this I had just bought my first vinyl album, from my spending money that I had been saving for weeks, which was the album *Double Fantasy* by John Lennon and Yoko Ono. I was devastated by Lennon's murder, how could anybody want to hurt such a nice man who made lovely music and only wanted peace for other people? I remember one night lying in bed as a youngster, unable to sleep thinking about life and death and shouting for my mum, when she came up to my room to ask me what was wrong. I asked her, "am I going to die one day?" and she told me that "everybody dies, but you won't die for a very, very long time," before tucking me tightly under the covers and kissing me goodnight. I always slept with the door slightly ajar with the landing light on outside of my room, which gave my bedroom a sliver of light for reassurance and protection, just in case any ghosts, monsters or the Grim Reaper might be lurking around.

I didn't handle death well as a child, like I mentioned in the previous chapter, I was too young to remember my Grandad Moss passing. I remember going to my Nanny and Grandad's house one day and suddenly he wasn't there. I remember approaching the house with my mum, Dad and Nanny Moss with me, I ran ahead of them banging on my grandparents' front door saying "Grandad will open it, Grandad will open it," but of course he didn't. He had died of a heart attack 3 weeks previously, and my Nan had been stopping with us in Darfield since, something that as a 3-year-old I had never even questioned. My Nan was of course very upset at what I had done, I remember her crying and I was confused. Nobody had told me that Grandad had died, not that as a 3-year-I had an understanding of what death was anyway. My parents had to sit me down and explain to me that my Grandad had gone away on a long journey and that he wouldn't be coming back. I remember thinking that maybe this was on a ship, as ships went on long journeys. I pictured in my mind a tall ship with white sails on a rough sea with dark stormy skies and in the early years of my life, that was how I imagined death, a long difficult journey on a tall ship.

I next got first-hand experience of death when I was around 6 years old. I went to give my beloved goldfish 'Bubbles' some fish food and there he was lying still on the water's surface. I was a bit slow to understand that Bubbles had died, maybe it was denial, maybe it was wishful thinking. I spent a period just looking at him floating there, before I blew on him in the hope that my magic breath would fix him; it didn't and Bubbles just bobbed on the surface. I was devastated and cried my eyes out. I had 'won' Bubbles on a hook-a-duck game at a fun fair in Mytholmroyd around 3 years previously, and with hindsight, Bubbles had a pretty good innings, as most goldfish won at fun fairs barely survived the journey home in the plastic bag of water that they were in. I thought about Bubbles and all the fun times that we'd had, which was basically me feeding him and tapping on the glass bowl as I said his name (I had decided Bubbles was a boy fish in the early days). I cried myself to sleep at night for days afterwards, I missed him terribly. We held a funeral in the back garden for Bubbles; he was buried in a match box under the shade of large leaves from my dad's rhubarb plant, and I said a few words before being overcome with tears. I made a cross out of two lollipop sticks and wrote 'RIP Bubbles' across the horizontal stick. I also wrote on a piece of paper torn from an envelope 'best fish ever', and put this beneath the lollipop stick cross, holding it in place with a pebble. The lighting and placement of a birthday cake candle by Bubble's grave marked the end of the ceremony as we retreated indoors to a funeral tea of cups of tea and jam sandwiches.

Not wanting to see their boy upset, a few days later my parents bought me a new goldfish, which I called 'Bubbles 2', I never really bonded with Bubbles 2 like I had done with Bubbles though, he (another boy fish obviously) just wasn't the same. Bubbles 2 didn't last very long either, so another funeral followed and another burial in the rhubarb patch. 'Bubbles 3' was a similar story and followed by Bubbles 4, 5 and 6. After which I stopped getting goldfish as pets. I'm not even sure that we had a proper funeral for Bubbles 6, who may have been unceremoniously 'buried at sea' with a toilet flush. Having fish as pets had helped me to understand what death was, though I still found it upsetting when they went. So from goldfish, we progressed to rabbits, (which I shared with Carla). We had 'Dixie', then 'Pixie', then 'Pebbles'. I was annoyed at Carla for naming our third rabbit Pebbles, it being the third rabbit should obviously have been called 'Trixie'. Dixie was a brilliant rabbit, a grey and white Hollander; he had a very loving personality, he seldom bit or scratched us, he loved being stroked and fussed, and he genuinely felt like a companion. We would play with him before and after school and walk all over Darfield picking dandelion leaves for him. When Dixie died, I was heartbroken, he was buried at the top of the garden in a rough patch of grass that we didn't really walk on. After this, I took a step back from the pets, as losing them was just too painful. Carla took over rabbit ownership responsibilities in our young teens. I wanted to avoid getting upset at the death of future pets by not getting too close to them. It was a bit of a strange tactic, but I hated death so much that evasion was how I chose to handle it.

You cannot literally evade death though, and the sad fact is that as I have got older, more people I have known have died, including my three remaining grandparents, each of whom I have the happiest of memories of, and each of who's passing hurt enormously. I am lucky however, in the fact that three out of four of my grandparents passed when I was an adult, so at least they had been in my life throughout my entire childhood.

Anyway, back to my 42-year-old fat self. I went straight to work from the doctor's where I consciously avoided the tasty things that were going to end my life early and tried to take my mind off a premature death by getting on with the daily toil. At the end of the working day, my perfect wife Linda (who is a nurse), came to collect me and drive me home. Linda knew that I had been to the doctor's about my weight and she wanted to know what the outcome of my visit was. As we drove up Otley Road I gave her the news that my blood pressure was high and that I'd been referred to both The Weight Management Service and The Sleep Service, as well as having an appointment with the nurse made for a health check and blood test. I decided to withhold the information about the possibility of me facing a heart attack or stroke in the next 10 years, which was something that I needed to come to terms with more myself before I could talk about it, and I also knew that this would hugely worry her. In the previous 8 years, my wife had lost both of her parents as well as one of her brothers. I had been with her throughout all of this and did not want to put on her the worry of possibly losing her husband in the next 10 years. I don't like withholding information from my wife, it feels dishonest and she deserves better, but I conscientiously made this decision to protect her and to avoid having to talk about the one thing that I hate talking about, which is death.

We got married in 2011, having been together since 2006. I waited for the right woman to come along before taking the plunge, and she really is the perfect woman for me. Linda has made a perfect wife, hence I call her the PW. She is the same height as me (6 foot/1.8 metres) although much taller in heels, she is slim, has a beautiful face and flowing blonde hair. Her physical features are what I noticed first, but then when I got to know her, I knew that she was the one. Not only is she the perfect wife, she is a brilliant mum to two lovely girls (Hannah and Becky, both now *our* grown-up daughters), a fantastic home-maker, extremely funny – we laugh together A LOT – she is a professional woman (another reason for the PW tag) with a great job and the most caring of personalities. Above all of this, she puts up with me (which isn't always easy) and loves me unconditionally, so I am an extremely lucky man to have her in my life. I think by not telling her of my potential 10-year prognosis that I was also wanting to protect her too.

Things don't usually happen overnight with the NHS, but my health check and blood tests took place on the following week, which was good. Having gone into the room to see the nurse on duty I was asked to stand on the weighing scales. I knew that this wouldn't end well as the scales only went up to 22 stones (308 pounds/139.7 kilos), but I stood on them anyway and the needle immediately flew clockwise all the way around the dial hitting the maximum weight like a car hitting a crash barrier, thunk. "Oh," the nurse exclaimed, looking slightly surprised (I don't know why). I told her what my actual weight was, which she took my word for and duly recorded on the computer, and next came my blood pressure. I have no idea what it was, but it was high, the nurse noted it down before telling me "we need to do something about that," "we" being me. I then had a blood test. I hate needles, which is something that goes back to childhood trauma (you'll find out about that later), so I always look away rather than at the needle going in. I try not to jolt or do a sharp intake of breath, but I usually end up doing one or both of the above.

The nurse gave me advice on diet and exercise (which I'd been given many times before), before sending me on my way. I would need to make a follow-up appointment with a doctor, once my blood test results came back. Feeling like I needed to do something positive upon leaving the surgery, I walked home, which was a distance of around 1.5 miles (2.4 km). I was a slow walker, the kind of slow walker that faster walkers might want to punch in the back of the head, especially when they get stuck behind me on a narrow pavement. The walk took me a while, I never used to walk this slowly, but at this very heavy point in my life I lumbered with a limp from very painful ankle joints and sore aching feet, with each footstep feeling like I was walking on frozen peas or Lego bricks. By the time I had got home I was breathless, my feet felt like they had been smashed in with hammers and my ankles were on fire. I sat in my chair (like I did each day for far too long) in order to recover. Eventually I painfully pushed myself upwards and towards a drawer that we have in the living room, which contains medical supplies. I took two ibuprofen and two paracetamol, washed down with a cup of tea. I had been popping these tablets several times daily for a number of years at this point, just to manage the pain in my feet and ankles, which in recent years had become debilitating and disabling. The heavier I got, the more it hurt to move, the more it hurt to move, the less I moved and the heavier I got. It was a truly vicious circle.

A week later my mobile rang while I was teaching, the screen flashed up 'Doctors', but I couldn't answer it. I left it vibrating on the table in front of me while I carried on talking about entertainment marketing in front of a small but fairly keen class of first-years. The phone vibrating was a slight distraction for all concerned, it slightly threw me off my thread, but I joked to the class "it's OK, it's just my GP ringing to tell me when I'm going to die." I got a few looks of mild amusement at this line, and then carried on. My phone ceased vibrating, then a few moments later vibrated twice to tell me that I had a voicemail. This did seem a little unusual as I didn't often get voicemails from my doctor's surgery, but I carried on with the class regardless, putting thoughts of my phone-call to one side. This day, like most days, the PW came to collect me from work and drive me home. On the drive up Otley Road I suddenly remembered my missed phone-call, so I listened to the voicemail that had been left. The voicemail was from a female doctor and whilst there wasn't overt concern in her voice, there was something about the words she used and the tone of the message that gave me some cause for concern. She wanted me to call back and make an appointment to talk through the results of my health check and blood test. The PW was right next to me whilst I listened to the message, so I couldn't avoid telling her about it. She was obviously a little concerned too; although she tried not to show it, I know her well enough to know though. It was too late for me to call back that day, but I called back on the following day and made an appointment to go in and see the doctor.

A few days later I was sitting in the office of the doctor. I don't seem to have a set GP at my surgery, it seems to rotate, which I don't actually mind. I was slightly nervous about what I was going to hear, but whatever the message was going to be, I needed to hear it. The doctor began by discussing the numbers on my blood test. I was listening but it felt as though there was loud static playing between us, nothing was sinking in even though I was robotically nodding my head. Then the doctor started talking about the medication I could take to reduce my blood sugar and I suddenly snapped to attention and asked, "so am I diabetic?" to which she looked extremely sympathetically at me and nodded her head, maybe she thought I was a bit slow. Maybe I was being a bit slow, maybe I was in denial. This was another Bubbles moment. I was coming to terms with hearing that I might be a bit closer to the heart attack or stroke that the other doctor alluded to than I had expected. I was in shock and needed to get my head together, I'd just been told that I had Type II diabetes, or lifestyle diabetes as I had seen it referred to in the press and on social media. These things didn't happen to me, this happened to fat people in gossip magazines, the kind of fat people who slobbed on their sofa in a onesie all day, drank 10 litres of full sugar cola per day and lived on a diet of fast food and bulk-bought supermarket chocolate. These were the fat people that got diabetes, the ones who were gossip magazine worthy, the ones who made the sad sacks who read such publications feel better about themselves and their own depressing lives. These were the people who get diabetes, not me, I'm not gossip magazine worthy, I was just a boring ordinary fat bloke, who didn't even own a onesie, but I was now in the diabetic gang, amongst sweet and syrupy blood brothers and sisters. I was officially diabetic and prescribed Metformin, which I had to take daily for the rest of my life, unless I stopped being diabetic. The doctor gave me good advice about exercises that I could do to help me overcome my diabetes as well as weight loss and diet advice.

It took me some coming to terms with the fact that I was diabetic, but it did give me a kick in my fat backside into taking my health seriously. I had to break the news to the PW, who was also shocked, but as always with my poor health news was pretty wonderful about it and vowed to help me. I was feeling motivated, so I decided that exercise was the obvious place to begin. I started walking to and from work, and I started arm exercises using an old pair of dumbbells that I had in my office to try and get my muscles working and excess blood sugar used. The problem with walking though was that it hurt my ankles, and whilst I walked, I walked slowly with a limp, and I was taking a vast amount of paracetamol and ibuprofen to ease the pain and the swelling. After a while, the health benefits of walking became outweighed by the constant pain that walking so much left me in and I started to walk less and less until I stopped walking altogether. I got bored with the dumbbells too; they were sort of fun at first, but the lack of physical difference that they seemed to make to me made their novelty wear off. Eventually I was back where I was before, fat, inactive, diabetic and taking Metformin, which incidentally also gave me the most putrid stinking sludge shits, each of which took about 50 wipes just to cut through the grease. My poor arse was red raw.

The Leeds Weight Loss Service were the next people to get in touch with me, and I began a 12-week programme of counselling and exercise. This consisted of me attending a group counselling session at Holt Park Medical Centre, where a member of the weight loss team would show us a plate and then divide it up into sections for vegetables, whole grains and healthy proteins, basically all of the types of food that we should be eating. There were six of us attending the session, and we sat on classroom style chairs in a circle with the group host, a young man in his 20s, probably not long out of university and evidently keen and motivated to want to make a difference to people's lives. The problem with these people, however, was that at least half of them were completely disinterested in the process and sat there sullenly with blank expressions or rudely looking at their phone screens. Three of the group were evidently there either as something to do, or as a box-ticking exercise of some sort. The other half, which included myself, were genuinely interested in the advice being given, and tried to offer input, conversation and questions. It felt like being back at school and I was one of the geeks in the class. I would leave each class motivated and wanting to make changes to my life, but over the days this diminished, the classes were on Tuesdays and by Saturday I would find myself overeating and over-drinking again. The weeks became peaks and troughs of good and bad eating behaviour, except the bad behaviour seemed to be intensified at the weekend.

Alongside the classes were individual 1-to-1 appointments with a dietician (also on a Tuesday), and then an exercise class, which took place at Holt Park Leisure Centre on a Thursday. I don't mind admitting that I felt completely humiliated doing bends, stretches and star jumps in a room full of women pensioners plus me. The class was some sort of local authority/NHS initiative to get people moving for their health. I was the only bloke there and it was obvious to all that I was there because I was fat. I just smiled through gritted teeth and got on with it. The staff were all great and liked a chat as well as a bit of banter and by the time I went to the third class I largely felt at ease, although I still stuck out like a sore thumb, but that's nothing new to me. The total length of the program of group sessions, 1-to-1s and exercise classes was 12 weeks and by the end of this period, I was 2 pounds (907 grams) heavier than I was when the program began.

I felt at a loss for a few months as I waited for the next NHS step along my weight loss journey to trigger, I was in a long queue of people who all had similar problems to myself. During this period, my weight went up and down, but generally in an upward trajectory. My health deteriorated in all senses, my pain increased, my stress levels increased and my exercise lessened. During this period, however, I was contacted by the Leeds Sleep Service, a department of the NHS at St. James's Hospital in Leeds, and then invited in for a consultation about my suspected sleep apnoea. I met with a kind fellow, but I did feel that he thought that he was speaking to an idiot, so at some point in the conversation I explained who I was in a professional capacity, which didn't make a difference, I still felt that he thought I was a dunce. During our conversation he revealed the thousands of people in Leeds with sleep apnoea and how the team was extremely stretched.

This was in the midst of David Cameron's Tory government where George Osborne was Chancellor making everyone in the public sector do more for less under the banner of austerity. Public sector workers felt the squeeze, for the NHS it was another nail in the coffin and for their overburdened and underpaid staff, another knife in the back, so shame on the Tories as they made sure that their billionaire friends and benefactors enjoyed generous tax breaks. The upshot of our meeting was that I was equipped with a set of bodily attachments for my face and chest, which connected to a small computer. That night I had to attempt to go to sleep whilst wired up. This was much easier said than done, but eventually sleep I did. I had no idea what the attachments were monitoring, but the next day I had to return the kit to St. James's Hospital, where the results would be analysed.

Around 10 days later I was back at St. James's Hospital for my follow-up appointment. The news was not good, I had severe obstructive sleep apnoea. It hit me like a punch in my fat gut, even though I already suspected that I had this condition. Not only was I fat, not only was I in constant joint pain, not only was I stressed, not only was I diabetic, I now had severe obstructive sleep apnoea to add to my long list of ailments and conditions all caused by my weight. Obstructive sleep apnoea is when your breathing stops and starts while you sleep. Breathing is stopped by the soft tissue in the mouth and throat blocking the airway. This is common amongst people who are overweight where the soft tissue contains excess fat. In essence, my fat mouth and throat were choking me while I slept, and I needed assistance to prevent this from happening. The test revealed that for every one hour that I was asleep, I was having 38 apnoea episodes, this meant that for every hour that I was asleep that I was only actually having 20 minutes of quality sleep, so for 7 hours of sleep I was actually only asleep for around 2 hours and 20 minutes. In the months leading up to this appointment I had been falling asleep at my desk at work and having a lot of headaches, and this was the reason. When you experience an apnoea episode, you stop breathing, but your body still needs oxygen, so your heart takes over the job of oxygenating your blood by beating faster, and in severe cases this can lead to a heart attack, particularly amongst those who are unfit and may already have a weak heart. I had woken up numerous times each night for years gasping for breath with my heart racing caused by the apnoea. Sometimes this woke me up, sometimes it didn't, sometimes it woke my wife up who was very concerned by what she was witnessing.

To manage the apnoea, I was equipped with a continuous positive airway pressure (CPAP) machine on long-term loan from the Leeds Sleep Service. A CPAP machine blows air into your mouth and nose with the use of a mask that is worn over the face whilst sleeping. The mask is connected via a plastic hose to the CPAP machine which blows air continuously. The model that I was given was quite an old one, it was fairly bulky and quite noisy. It took a lot of getting used to, not just for me as the wearer but also for my wife, who now found herself sleeping with somebody who looked like a cross between an intensive care patient and a Cyberman from *Doctor Who*. The first night that I wore this device, I had a panic attack, tearing it off my face in the early hours of the morning and knocking over my bedside lamp in the process, breaking the lamp at the neck beneath the lampshade. Every morning I would wake with a dry mouth and gulp down water before getting out of bed. Every night for weeks I would dread going to bed and having to wear the mask. Over time, however, I did get used to wearing the mask up to a point that I would not want to fall asleep without it.

The next step on my banana journey was to climb another rung on the ladder of the Leeds Weight Loss Service. I was sent an appointment to speak to a dietician at Leeds General Infirmary (LGI). The dietician that I met, Janine, was a friendly and very down-to-earth Leeds lass, for whom I developed the utmost respect. I could tell from the outset that Janine was on a mission to help people, and her role as a dietician wasn't just a job to her, it was a mission in life. Janine would keep a model of a 1 pound (454 grams) lump of fat in her desk drawer, and when we spoke about fat and weight loss she would often get the lump of faux fat out, so that I could physically see what a pound of fat looked like. It wasn't pretty, the model was rubbery but squishy to the touch. I imagine that over the years hundreds of people had sat in Janine's office either poking or holding the lump of fat in the palm their hand, lifting it up and down to evaluate how heavy a pound in weight felt. When I had lost or gained a pound the lump of fat enforced a feeling of either jubilation or disappointment, in what was a process of kinaesthetic learning and reflection. Janine encouraged me to eat healthily and exercise more, again the classic 'food plate' model came out, demonstrating exactly the portions and proportions that I should have on my plate.

I discussed bariatric surgery with Janine and indicated that this was something that I was interested in pursuing. There were three options available in Leeds: a gastric band, a gastric bypass, and a sleeve gastrectomy. Janine gave me information about all three of these procedures and encouraged me to read and research them all to be sure that I wanted to proceed in that direction. Janine agreed to add me to a list of potential candidates for this surgery in Leeds, and I would be contacted further down the line to discuss this with a specialist.

Whilst seeing Janine I tried calorie counting and had some moderate success with this, although after a while I got bored with this process and started cheating and lying to myself as if in denial that I'd just eaten those crisps or drunk that beer. Then I adopted a cheat strategy, which was a modification of the 5-2 diet, if you don't know what this is, the 5-2 diet is pretty much eating normally for 5 days, and then having an extremely restricted diet of 600 calories per day for 2 days. This process is known as intermittent fasting, and does have some proven results of success, but not all dieticians (including Janine) approve of it. My version of the 5-2 diet was a 7-3 diet. On my 3 days of intermittent fasting, I would follow a diet sheet, which according to the header on it was originally from St. Mary's Hospital in London and was designed to help patients who were awaiting an operation lose a lot of weight very quickly. I'd had this sheet for over 30 years, I've no idea where I originally got it from, but I suspect my mum might have acquired it at some point and then I 'borrowed' it. I had in the past done the '3-day diet' in the 3 days leading up to an event such as a holiday or my birthday. The 3-day diet would have some remarkable results for me, I could lose 10 pounds (4.54 kilos) in 3 days, then over the following week I would gain back most, but not all of this weight. So if I was seeing Janine for a weigh-in every month, and I did this diet 3 times during the month, I could almost guarantee that when I went for my 'weigh-in' I would be at least 3 pounds down on my previous weigh-in, sometimes I would be as much as 6 pounds down. The weight did start to come off and I did begin to show results, but – and this is the but – the 3-day diet just wasn't sustainable for me. After several months, I started to do it less and less until my weight loss plateaued and then eventually went into reverse, showing month by month gains. In the end I confessed to Janine what I had been doing, and she was very understanding, she had heard it all before. Successful weight loss has got to be sustainable in terms of lifestyle. The 3-day diet did show results, but it just wasn't something that I would ever be able to keep up for the rest of my life. As a post-note, I'd like to add that the 3-day diet seems to have been adapted online now with some modifications and re-badged as 'the military diet' for people who want to 'shred'. It isn't something that I would ever recommend to other people on a weight loss journey, it's nothing more than a quick fix, which unless you do it as a part of your lifestyle forever isn't going to be helpful in the long-term.

I was at a loss as to what to do next on my weight-loss journey, so Janine suggested that I consider giving Slimming World a try. There was some logic in this. Slimming World involves a weekly weigh-in, and I was quite target orientated in terms of my monthly weigh-in with Janine, so maybe having something that was more frequent would be good for me, alongside my monthly weigh-in. The other potential benefit of Slimming World is that it is a group therapy experience, so rather than just being one-on-one with a consultant, participants have the benefit of listening to the shared the experiences of others as well as sharing their own experiences. I signed up with a group that was local to me at Cookridge Holy Trinity Church. The group met once a week on a Tuesday morning. I don't mind admitting that I was nervous when I got there. I met the consultant who talked me through the process in about 3 minutes flat, the words went in one ear and out of the other; this was going to be a case of learning by doing. Just like with my aerobics class I was the only male here, with the rest of the class equally divided into older ladies mostly post-retirement age, and younger mums, some of whom brought their annoyingly noisy kids and babies to the group with them.

Listening to the conversations going on around me, I immediately grasped that this group was for some participants as much a part of a social experience and getting out of the house as it was about health and weight-loss. Some of the women in the group had been attending Slimming World for over 20 years, and had paid £5 per week for the privilege; to put this into context, they had paid £260 per year to be in Slimming World, 20 years' membership cost £5,200, which is roughly the same as a gastric band done privately. After 20 years in Slimming World, some of these ladies were still very overweight, which made me wonder if they had ever really been serious about losing weight, or if they just wanted to be a part of something that gave them a social distraction, albeit for 90-120 minutes per week. There were also the 'lovely target ladies' who attended the group, and these were the Slimming World deputy sheriffs, who all other members aspired to be like. A lovely target lady, or in proper speak a

Slimming World Target Member is somebody who has reached their weight loss goal and has remained within 3 pounds (1.36 kilos) of their target weight (up or down) thereafter. Target members do not have to attend the group sessions weekly, but must attend at least every 2 months, and for being role models to the other members, they do not have to pay a weekly membership fee as long as they remain within their target range.

On my first day at Slimming World I was asked what my target weight was, and I replied 17 stone (238 pounds/108 kilos), which meant that I would have to lose 8 stone (112 pounds/51 kilos). I'd never lost more than 2 stone (14 pounds/6.4 kilos) in my life before, so to immediately set myself this huge target wasn't just a bit ambitious, it was pretty stupid, and almost guaranteed that I'd be paying £5 per week for the rest of my life. Don't get me wrong, Slimming World like any other healthy eating and lifestyle program (I won't use the word diet), DOES work, if you stick to it and follow it, and if every single person who joined Slimming World did stick to it and followed it, then Slimming World would have to think of a new business model, because if everyone reached their target, nobody would pay anything for membership. But humans are in the most part weak, and like myself they begin Slimming World with good intentions, but soon find themselves straying from the path. There are of course those who stay on the path and stay completely motivated, going on to achieve excellent results. Two of my own ex-students have featured in the *Slimming World* magazine, in fact one of them even made the front cover for her amazing weight loss and body transformation. I'm extremely proud of both of them, because I know first-hand just how hard a challenge this is, and ultimately, Slimming World proved to be another journey into a dead-end for me, although I did have a good deal of success before this particular part of my banana journey ground to a halt.

Slimming World classes are quite fascinating from a psychological standpoint. They begin with the weigh-in, which cannot begin one second before the advertised class time begins. Here, seasoned members chomp at the bit to get a good place at the head of the queue so that they can be weighed quickly and then proceed to have a cup of tea and a snack often consisting of either a banana, sandwich or nutrition bar. Many class participants had not eaten and barely drunk before the class so as not to tip the scales in the wrong direction, and members often arrived at the class both hungry and thirsty, so a speedy weigh-in meant that they could then enjoy something to eat and drink without the risk of it contributing to weight-gain. The weigh-in process was a long, boring and sometimes painful one, the aroma of cheesy feet and body odour would begin to permeate the air after around 5 minutes into the weigh-in and there was no getting away from it, as everyone proceeded to remove their footwear and take off layers of clothing before climbing onto the scales. The Slimming World class was held only a 10-minute walk from my house, so I would walk there in all weathers wearing flip-flops on my feet and shorts or very lightweight trousers with a T-shirt on and a jacket. Like all of those being weighed I would kick off my footwear, empty my pockets and remove my jacket before getting on the scales. If I was wearing a heavy wristwatch, I'd take that off too – every little helps (as the supermarket slogan goes). Once near the front of the queue you hand over your Slimming World ID card, Slimming World booklet and your weekly £5 (unless you have paid an advance subscription, which can save money) to either the group host or one of their trustees (often a target member). Then you patiently wait your turn to climb onto the scales. I used to dread that last few seconds of waiting time, which felt more like minutes. Some weeks the scales gave out good news (a loss), some weeks the scales gave out bad news (a gain) and some weeks the scales were indifferent, which meant that I had maintained (stayed the same weight). In all honesty, most weeks I would have a reasonable idea if I was going to be up or down, and maintaining nearly always came as either a good surprise (when I thought I might have gained weight) or a bad surprise (when I hoped that I might have lost weight). Weigh-in could take up to an hour, particularly at peak-times such as after Christmas, when the class was very busy with new members. On quiet weeks such as around bank holidays weigh-in could be done and dusted in 15 minutes. Some people disappeared straight after weigh-in (a tactic for those not wanting to be named and shamed as weight-gainers), and others stopped for the group discussion, particularly those who had made a good loss and wanted bragging rights.

Following weigh-in came the group discussion/therapy part of the class, and depending on the shape of the venue and the number of members, we would usually sit in some sort of circle with the group host in the centre. If you've ever seen TV's satirical sketch show *Little Britain* where Matt Lucas plays the character of Marjorie Dawes who hosts 'Fat Fighters' then you might have a good idea of what follows, albeit without the vicious cruelty. The host would stand in the circle and then go through the attendee names on her list, which would appear in the order in which people got weighed…imagine the scene:

Host: "Now where's Pamela?"

Pamela: <raises hand>

Host: "Pamela has lost 2 pounds this week."

Host: <claps>

The room: <claps>

Pamela <smiles and looks around the room>

Host: "Right so next on my list is Judith, where are you, Judith?"

Judith: <raises hand>

Host: <tilts head to one side and nods sympathetically> "Judith, you've maintained this week, so what's been happening for you this week?"

The room: <silent, all eyes on Judith>

Judith: <gulps> "Well I don't know really, I've followed the plan, but it just doesn't seem to be happening for me." <sad face>

Host: "Would you like a food diary?" <frantically waves a piece of paper in the air>

Judith: <begrudgingly> "I'll take one, yes."

Host: <hands piece of paper to Judith>

Nobody wants a food diary, ever. First of all it makes you confront your wrongdoings or abstention from the Slimming World plan, secondly it's a pain in the backside remembering to complete it, so you just end up fudging it last minute and thirdly it is a confession to the host of what you've really been putting in your mouth – if you complete it truthfully, which I never did and I suspect lots of others didn't either.

Host: "Now where's Stuart?"

Stuart: <the only male in the room looks around at everyone else in the room who are female and laughs before raising his hand>

Stuart: "I'm here."

The room: <laughs>

Host: <tilts head to one side and nods sympathetically> "Stuart, you've made a gain this week."

Stuart: <nods head and frowns> "Yes, I was expecting it this time unfortunately."

Host: "And why is that then, Stuart?"

Stuart: "Because I haven't tried this week as much as what I should have done and I went out drinking Friday and Saturday night as well as Sunday afternoon, I also went out for an Indian buffet."

The room: <wide eyes, open mouths and expressions of horror>

Host: <wide eyes and look of surprise before nodding head> "Well I can see how that wouldn't have helped you, so what's your plan for this week to get you back on track?"

Stuart: "Not to go out drinking and to try a bit harder, I think I just had an off-week last week."

The room: <nods and murmurs>

Host: "Would you like a food diary?" <frantically waves a piece of paper in the air>

Stuart: "Erm no thanks, I know where I went wrong." <nods head>

The majority of the time that I went to Slimming World I just couldn't see the point in telling lies if I had made a gain, if I'd not bothered one week I just confessed. In all honesty, I did try most of the time that I was a part of the group and the weight did come off slowly, but it was a bumpy ride and there were periods where the weight didn't come off at all and sometimes went back on. What irked me about Slimming World was the absolute rubbish that some people would use as excuses as to why they hadn't lost weight, and if I could make a Slimming World bingo card, it would contain the following excuses for not losing weight.

I haven't drunk enough water throughout the week	I did some exercise so have gained muscle, which weighs more than fat	Family member(s) came to visit	Family occasion such as a birthday or wedding	I've had a bit of a cold/I've been feeling under the weather
I had a glass of wine one night in the week	I went out for a meal one night in the week	I think it must be my hormones	I've been taking this medication, which makes me gain weight	My husband cooked dinner this week and I think he used cooking oil instead of Fry Light
I think it's genetic with me	I've got a really slow metabolism	I've been really busy this week	I haven't had time to cook this week	The weather has been really bad, so I haven't been able to exercise

There are plenty more excuses too, but these are just the ones that immediately come to mind. I would hear this week in and week out, the people who were saying it knew it was rubbish, the host knew it was rubbish, everyone in the room knew it was rubbish, yet the collective cynicism within the room seemed to be masked by an unspoken acceptance and sympathy when one of the above phrases was used, because most people in the room had used one of those excuses themselves at some point during the time that they had been attending classes. My thoughts were a bit more pessimistic – basically Karen, you've enjoyed the chocolate, chips and wine this week so just bloody admit it – and the excuses annoyed me.

The Slimming World classes had a competitive element to them, with the biggest loser each week winning a prize, which was often a bowl of fruit or something healthy to eat. During my time in the group I won the prize on several occasions, proudly taking home to the PW either a bowl of fruit or a pumpkin or something similar.

The Slimming World plan that I followed was one where certain foods were given points that were called 'syns', I was allowed to have 15 syns per day, so for example a Kit Kat Chunky chocolate bar had 13 syns, so if I had one of those, then I only had two syns remaining, a 25g bag of Hula Hoop crisps was 6 ½ syns, leaving me 8 ½ syns remaining on my daily allowance. Fresh fruit and vegetables were syn free, as were some lean meats and fish, and on the Slimming World plan it was permissible to eat as much of these types of food as you wanted. This was a key advantage of Slimming World for me. I could eat large portions of food, providing they didn't carry syns. I liked this idea, I could eat until I was full and not feel hungry, providing I didn't eat the wrong foods. The other thing that I liked about Slimming World was that syns could be banked, so if I had completely syn free weekdays, it meant that at the weekend I could be a 'synner'. Now I must stress, that this wasn't promoted as being good practice by my group host, but she did acknowledge that it was within the rules, so immediately I was happy that I had found a sort of loophole, that still allowed me to enjoy my food and drink at the weekend, where I would enjoy a full week's worth of syns (105 syns) over Saturday and Sunday.

I like to drink strong real ales, usually around 5% alcohol by volume (ABV) or above. One pint of beer of around this strength was about 11.5 syns, which meant that over the weekend I could enjoy nine pints of beer, which would translate into a Saturday night and Sunday afternoon session. In some respects, it was a bit like a reverse of the 5-2 diet, so instead of having five bad days and two good ones, I would have five good days and two bad ones. But of course, when you drink beer, you get hungry, and after five pints, I wouldn't be craving tuna and cucumber on a rice cracker, I would want onion bhajis or a kebab. This is the reason why my Slimming World journey was a bumpy one, it was nobody else's fault but my own. My mindset was never fully in the right place, and at times my motivation severely waned.

During the time I spent attending Slimming World classes, I was given an appointment to see Dr Barth, who was a senior figure within the Leeds Weight Loss Service and who ultimately would have a major say in whether or not I would be eligible for bariatric surgery. Dr Barth was no-nonsense and straight down the line, he had heard every excuse under the sun for not being able to lose weight. I got this impression as soon as I met him at St. James's Hospital in Leeds and knew that honesty would be the best policy if I was to convince him that I should have NHS funded bariatric surgery. The PW had also come along with me to the appointment, so I knew that there was no point in being untruthful with her sitting there next to me. Dr Barth was very to the point with me; "if you have bariatric surgery you will struggle with food for the rest of your life," and my reply was that "I've struggled with food all of my life so far, so the future will just be a different kind of struggle, whether I have the surgery or not I'll be struggling one way or another." Dr Barth seemed satisfied with my response, in that he seemed to realise that I had given this some thought and wasn't just looking for a quick fix. We discussed the types of surgery on offer, and I explained that I expressed a preference for a sleeve gastrectomy.

I had read plenty, I had watched YouTube videos, and the PW had recorded numerous programs about weight loss surgery over the preceding few months, so I felt pretty-well informed about the direction in which I wanted to go with the surgery. For me the gastric band was a non-starter, I hated the thought of a band around my stomach with a control mechanism under my skin, it made me feel sick thinking about it, I would never accept that. Reviews of this surgery online also revealed a number of people who had had the surgery and who then struggled to eat anything afterwards.

The gastric bypass looked horrific. In this surgery the stomach is divided into a small upper pouch and a much larger lower pouch with the small intestine rearranged to connect to both. This was a huge operation and I judged out of all three surgeries that it was the one with the greatest likelihood of something going wrong (based upon nothing scientific, it was just a feeling). Another reason that I didn't want this surgery was that I had read reviews from several people online who had had the surgery but were still obese as they felt that it didn't restrict them enough. This operation was also for some people a second choice operation, when their first choice operation (usually a gastric band or a sleeve gastrectomy) had for whatever reason failed. In the back of my mind, I considered that this could also possibly be a fallback for me if the sleeve was not successful.

The sleeve gastrectomy seemed to be somewhere between the band and the bypass, in that it would restrict the amount of food that I could eat, but hopefully not to the point where I wouldn't be able to eat anything at all. There was also a greatly reduced amount of rearranging internal pipework with this operation, compared with a bypass. In terms of foreign bodies left within me, this would only be some staples that would be needed to close my stomach. You see a sleeve gastrectomy involves trimming the stomach down to a smaller size so that the amount of food that it can hold is less as the stomach is physically smaller. Imagine the stomach as a small ball (probably not so small in my case), the ball is cut into the shape of a banana, with food entering the top of the banana and exiting the bottom of it. The physical volume that the stomach can hold is thereby reduced meaning that a feeling of 'fullness' will register more quickly when eating. If you don't stop eating when you're full, you'll likely be sick or feel quite ill. This operation meant that there might also be some restrictions on the types of foods that I could eat in future, but this seemed to vary a lot from person to person whom I had read reviews from. Some people couldn't tolerate any meat after the operation and ate largely a vegetarian diet, but this prospect didn't bother me at all as I had previously been a vegetarian in my teenage years and twenties. Some people couldn't tolerate anything stodgy such as bread, pasta or pastry afterwards as it seemed to get stuck on the way into the stomach and left them feeling sick. Some people had no restrictions whatsoever, they just chewed their food really well before swallowing, and could eat anything they liked, just much less of it. I really felt that this last scenario would apply to me, but of course I had no idea where I might end up on the post operation food tolerance spectrum.

Over the duration of my appointment with Dr Barth, I shared my thoughts on all of the above with him, and genuinely felt that he was pleased with the thought that I had put into this. Next came a discussion around exercise, which I blatantly didn't do enough of. Dr Barth made me realise that I would need to up my game in order to make my heart stronger for the operation. I explained about the severe joint pain that I experienced so Dr Barth suggested swimming. "I was too embarrassed," I admitted to the doctor, who again had heard this all before and suggested to me that I try attending one of the disabled swimming sessions at my local leisure centre, Holt Park. "Nobody will be looking at you there" he assured me, and he was right.

The disabled swimming session at Holt Park was held on a Monday evening, I wasn't registered disabled and I felt like a fraud for being there, but upon balance I did have severe mobility issues through joint pain, I was diabetic and I had sleep apnoea. You are disabled under the Equality Act 2010 if you have a physical or mental impairment that has a 'substantial' and 'long-term' negative effect on your ability to do normal daily activities. By this definition I did feel that I qualified as being disabled enough to be able to attend the Monday night session, and nobody at Holt Park questioned me being there. Nobody looked at me as I came out of the changing cubicle, nobody looked at me as I got into the pool. I was just another person there to swim. I actually really enjoy swimming, it was something that I did weekly as a child and I used to be pretty good at it. In adulthood the story was a little different for me, swimming was limited to holidays to hotels that had a swimming pool and where nobody apart from the people that I was with would know me. I would also spend more time doing forward and backward rolls in the water and messing about, than I would spend swimming. This was about to change, I wasn't here to mess about, I was here to exercise in order to make my heart stronger. So I began to swim up and down the lanes of the 25 metre Holt Park Leisure Centre swimming pool. I stuck to the breast-stroke on this day, I didn't want to try anything fancy and I didn't want to draw attention to myself. The exercise was a struggle, it absolutely drained me and over the duration of an hour I only managed a very pathetic 12 lengths, with lots of breaks to catch my breath at the end of each length. I was completely out of shape, but I actually enjoyed myself.

The week after I returned and did 15 lengths in an hour. The week after that I managed 17 lengths in an hour and the week after that I managed 20 lengths in an hour. I felt that both my swimming technique and my stamina was improving, but that I needed to swim more often. So I bit the bullet and took the very brave step of attending general swimming sessions four times per week, sometimes early morning, sometimes in the afternoon and sometimes in the evening. I would swim around my work schedule and when I felt that the pool wouldn't be too busy (which it very often was). After a year of swimming, I was managing over 40 lengths per hour and would set myself an hourly target of 40 lengths minimum, which represented 1km of swimming. To a good fast swimmer this isn't particularly good, but I'm not a good fast swimmer, I'm a steady swimmer, who maintains a pace and sticks to it. I'm more of a whale than a shark in the water, but that didn't bother me and I didn't try to hide it.

All this while I carried on with Slimming World and seeing Janine, and slowly, slowly the weight started to come off consistently. I went down to 22 stones (308 pounds/140kg), which for me was an absolute victory. I was feeling much healthier, and I knew that I was climbing the waiting-list ladder to having the surgery that I needed.

In the New Year of 2017, I was sent a letter for a routine appointment for a blood test to check my blood sugar levels for my Type II diabetes, which I duly attended. A week later I was summoned by the doctor to go in and discuss my results. I didn't know what was going to happen here, the last time that the doctor and I spoke it was very bad news concerning my diabetes, so should I expect more of the same? The answer was an emphatic no. The swimming combined with the weight loss had reduced my blood sugar level to below the diabetic range, and the doctor was delighted for me. I got the impression that she didn't see this happen very often and was almost in disbelief that somebody had heeded her words and improved their diet and increased their exercise in order to improve their health. No more Metformin for me, no more greasy 50 wipe shits, my arse definitely thanked God or whoever for that small mercy.

I was on a high, I was improving my health and I was losing weight, my monthly meetings with Janine kept me focused on my longer term goal, as did the weekly Slimming World meetings, although the expense of £5 per week was something that I began to question. I also began to question at one of my appointments with Janine whether or not I actually needed the surgery, as I had seemingly discovered a new lust for life and health, and maybe, just maybe I could achieve my goals without having an operation. Janine told me that my case had been discussed and I should soon expect an appointment to meet the surgeon, but that it was not too late to put this on hold for the time being. I discussed this with the PW, who was pleased with my progress and confessed to being a little worried about me having what was major surgery. The doubts then began to surface and truthfully, I began to worry about whether I would survive an operation and whether or not I would be miserable after the operation, if I was unable to eat properly. I poured my heart out to Janine and explained my doubts, at the same time playing up how happy I was with my current physical state as I was seemingly already doing what the operation was meant to do for me. I made the decision to come off the appointment list, but to continue seeing Janine on a less frequent 6-weekly basis to see how I got on. With hindsight, this was a big mistake, but like everyone else, you need to make mistakes in life to learn from them.

The next mistake that I made followed a negative experience that I had at Slimming World. I had missed a week through being on holiday and despite my protestations that I had booked this in, it wasn't showing on the system and it was a case of "computer says no," so I had to pay £5 for the week that I had not attended (you are allowed six holidays per year, which means you can miss six sessions per year, providing you have booked them in advance). I wasn't happy about this, I also wasn't happy about the fact that I had made a significant gain whilst on holiday, despite some attempt to moderate my eating and drinking behaviour, but what really made me blow a stack was that the group part of the session was going to be delayed after the weigh-in so that the group could have a 'swish'. I'd never heard of a swish before, but apparently on the week that I was away the group had decided that they were going to have one this week.

A swish is basically a clothes swapping session, where those people who have lost weight bring in the clothes that are now too big for them to swap with other people for their old clothes that are currently too small for them. So basically, the most overweight people get to wear the clothes of those who have lost weight, and those who have lost weight get to wear the clothes that the most overweight people might wear again in future if they did lose weight. I hope you get my drift here. I didn't like the concept of the swish at all, it felt like an 'I'm doing better than you' competition. I couldn't participate in the swish anyway, because I didn't know about it, so I hadn't brought anything and I was the only bloke there, so who the hell would I swish with anyway? I made a cup of tea and went outside while the swish took place, chuntering and grumbling in a pretty foul mood, what a waste of my time. Following the swish came the group therapy, and all eyes were on me as this had to be the only week in Slimming World history where there was only one person in the group who had gained, and that person was me who had seemingly completely let the side down. There were quite a few who had maintained their weight, but I was Gloria gainer this week. I couldn't even be bothered to explain myself as my name was called out, I just said that "I was on holiday and I will be back on track next week, and no I don't want a bloody food diary, thank you."

One of the women who maintained her weight, ended up breaking down in tears over her food cravings and confessed to wanting to eat a digestive. The group assured her that that was fine. Everyone was quite sympathetic until the woman then confessed that she didn't just eat one digestive, she ate the entire packet, but worse still, she put butter on them! There were gasps of horror and disbelief as the poor women sobbed. Suddenly I felt that I'd got off lightly as the only gainer as the woman took the group's attention away from me, at least she hadn't gained on top of this. I left the group that day questioning why I was still a member of Slimming World and there and then decided that I wouldn't be paying £5 per week anymore. I didn't need to go to Slimming World, I could lose weight myself, it wasn't rocket science. I had the Slimming World books, I knew what to do, I could go it alone. With that I quit in early 2017, and that was my next big mistake; there would be many more on this journey.

3 – My banana journey begins

One year later in February 2018, I was at crisis point. My weight had hit an all-time high, I was 26 stone and 7 pounds (371 pounds/168Kg), everyone was worried about me, family, friends, colleagues and myself. I went for my appointment with Janine, which I had allowed to slip to being bi-monthly. I was depressed, stressed and in constant pain. My physical and mental health was not good and I was hurtling faster than ever towards that major event which my doctor had warned me about. The appointment followed the standard process of beginning with me stepping onto the bariatric scales. I had gained again. After the weigh-in I lumbered behind Janine into her office. I was miserable and she knew it. "Can I go back onto the waiting list for the operation please?" was the first thing that I said. Janine agreed to put me forward again for discussion for surgery and also to make my appointments monthly again (it was me that had made them less regular).

I'd had a particularly stressful year at work, which I won't go too much into, but after some major departmental changes and being shafted for a promotion that should have had my name on it, I wasn't in a happy place. On top of this, like every other public sector worker I was expected to do more with less. I'm not complaining, because I love my job, but there can be an image of lecturers as having a cushy job with loads of holidays only teaching for a few hours per week. For a minority this might be true, but let me tell you, I get paid to work 35 hours per week and the reality is that I work at least 50 hours per week and many weeks particularly in the autumn semester I can work 70 hours or more. On top of this, I'm expected to produce publications as well as research and write a PhD. In days of old, lecturers turned up to packed lecture theatres, spoke for 45 minutes and then disappeared having little or no further contact with the students who would often have another member of staff to deliver their tutorials.

These days the role of a lecturer (I'm actually a Senior Lecturer) involves (to name but a few things): lecture and seminar preparation and delivery (1 hour of delivery can take 4-5 hours to prepare); group and one-to-one tutorials; assessing, marking and moderating student work; writing documentation such as module and course handbooks; maintaining international relationships with partner institutions in other countries; speaking at conferences; managing academic programs and developing new ones; mentoring other staff members; research and publication into our specialisms; getting involved in enterprise initiatives for income generation; being a part of panels for mitigation, suspected plagiarism, health and safety and a whole host of other purposes; running field trips and field visits outside of class time; being a complete slave to email; and pastoral care for tutees with problems that lie outside of academia.

The lecturer is always the first port of call for students, particularly with smaller courses where students see fewer staff members. As an extreme example of the type of duties a lecturer can be confronted with, I have over the years on several occasions had to help students suffering from mental health problems. This once happened at 6:30pm on a Friday evening. I was actually still in my office working on a class for delivery on the Monday morning (I wanted to have a work-free weekend), the student was extremely lucky to find me there, God knows what they might have done if I hadn't been there. There are procedures to follow under such circumstances and everything turned out fine for the student involved who even on a Friday night received the help that they needed from the correct people. This sort of emotional labour takes a severe mental toll, I have lost count of the sleepless nights that I've had over the years through work-related stress. Not just through student issues, but also through colleague and management issues. It doesn't help that I'm a stress-sponge, I seem to absorb everyone else's stresses, even though I don't often show it on the outside.

Universities, like political parties, seem to be incredibly adept at promoting poor people into senior positions. Don't get me wrong, there are a majority of good and very competent people in universities, and there are lots of good university managers and leaders too, but they are let down by a minority of ladder-climbing bad apples who shit on those around them and seem to rise too quickly to the surface. I've seen this at universities around the world, but the UK seems particularly good at promoting academics who are little more than salespeople that can talk the talk, but ultimately are rubbish at their jobs and earn nicknames such as 'Plastic Professor', 'Teflon Annie' and 'Billy Bullshit'. Bullshit as an expletive has been used in the English language for over 100 years. Esteemed academic Harry G. Frankfurt once wrote an essay about the usage of the word bullshit, called *On Bullshit* in 1986, which was reprinted as a book in 2005. Frankfurt discussed the concept of bullshit and analysed it from a communications perspective. We are surrounded by bullshit, it is everywhere. Virtually every piece of advertising click bait that we see online is bullshit. 'Everybody is talking about this product'... no they're not, you bloody bullshitter. Frankfurt determined that bullshit is speech intended to persuade without regard for truth, it's like we perpetually live in the fairy-tale story 'The Emperor's New Clothes'. Convince the people, it doesn't matter if it's the truth or not, just make the sale, bullshit, bullshit, bullshit. Politicians, journalists and marketers are absolute masters of this craft and some academics are really not so far behind.

It is one of the tragedies of the higher education (HE) sector, that salespeople often get more respect than genuinely great student-facing educators who are the bedrock of any university. The highly marketized nature of public relations reliant HE is the reason for this. It is also a tragedy that those academics who regularly publish journal articles can be rewarded by being given less teaching. A minority of self-centred academics strive to achieve this goal as quickly as possible; it's completely wrong, if you work in the education sector then you should consider teaching to be central to your role as much or more than what research is. Students are often denied first-hand access to the brightest researchers, who are instead enlisted to help universities in terms of league tables and associated funding streams. How many prospective students to a university even know what a journal article is? I can tell you the answer first-hand, and that is virtually none. I have produced four 80,000 word academic textbooks over the past 15 years, yet my feet are still firmly on the ground, I teach at all undergraduate levels and I wouldn't want it any other way, I'm not a bullshitter. Those academics who strive to be recognised as researchers first and teachers second as quickly as possible are one of the things that is wrong with HE, which should be about giving back and not personal empire building. It is a minority of academics who do this in order to avoid the inconvenience of having to teach, but they leave a bad taste for the rest of us and I'll only ever look at them as a stain on the education system. When universities lose sight of the fact that the bread and butter of their institution is undergraduate students, who are the raison d'être for the university existing, suddenly higher education doesn't seem to be about education anymore. It's about the markets, competition, branding, shiny new signage, space-aged buildings and image. It makes me sad that in some circles, what actually happens in the classroom doesn't seem to matter enough. The frontline teaching staff can be left feeling like poor relations to Plastic Professors, Teflon Annies and Billy Bullshits who keep themselves protected from doing real work in their faux ivory towers. Some of these characters might on occasion lower themselves to teach at post-graduate (PG) levels (heaven forfend they'd have to teach an undergraduate), but even those teaching at PG level are usually teaching classes that are tiny in comparison to their undergraduate teaching colleagues. I'm generalising slightly, but hopefully you get my point that the teaching environment isn't always an even one, and this causes me (and many others) additional stress.

Many years ago, I took my eldest daughter Hannah to a university open day in Sheffield. I won't say which university (there's only two so toss a coin as to which), but the course introduction talk was given by three senior academics (the university had basically rolled out the top brass to impress at a public event). The academics proceeded to talk about themselves, their research and their publications for 30 minutes of the 1 hour session. There were then 15 minutes devoted to the course and modules and 15 minutes for questions. There was no mention of contact hours, there was no mention of class format, there was no mention of types of assessment and there was no mention of whether assessment was group work or individual. This is what prospective students want to know. The academics couldn't answer basic questions about these essential aspects of the course, instead deflecting people to the 'school website', which they then struggled to find and navigate on the PC that was in the room. They were all bullshitters.

I've met some very senior academics over the years who I can honestly say lacked common sense and contemporary industry knowledge around their subject area but were amazing salespeople, who were very adept at saying "look at me I'm great," I call them LAMIGs. They're great persuaders, but ultimately, they are style without substance and further down the line are often exposed. Many years ago, I was asked by a LAMIG professor with good editorial connections if I would like a research paper publishing in a journal that he had involvement with? What a great opportunity, I thought, until he told me that I'd just need to add his name to the paper...I gave him a two-word response, the second of which was 'off'. With hindsight, this is probably why I was shafted for promotion, I wear my heart on my sleeve and I'm honest. You can take the lad out of Barnsley, but you'll never take the working-class Barnsley mindset out of this lad, and I'm not scared to tell people to their face either. If you're wondering what happened to that research paper, I ended up getting it published as a chapter under my own name in a textbook, and many more have followed it. Despite my ranting, I DO love my job: it gives me huge satisfaction seeing young people develop into professionals; I get to travel internationally regularly, and it does pay pretty well, certainly above the national average, but it is a sedentary and at times extremely stressful job. Ultimately it has been a very significant contributor to my banana journey.

I re-joined Slimming World, this time with a different group at Cookridge Old Modernians Sports and Social Club. This was an evening group, and whilst predominantly female in membership, there were a couple of other men there two, one of whom had lost a whopping 8 stone (112 pounds/51 kilos) so far. I was most impressed by his achievement and he was still going with more weight to lose. What he had lost in total represented most of what I wanted to lose at this point, he showed me that it can be done. The format of the Slimming World classes hadn't changed, although the host (a different one) was now using a tablet computer instead of a notepad. The rush to be at the front of the weigh-in queue, the smell of cheesy feet and the same old excuses were all too familiar to me. I persevered though, because I had to. At this point I felt that my life depended on it, because basically it did.

I began the classes highly motivated and stuck to the Slimming World plan religiously, I was only drinking one night per week and would bank a few syns for a synful Saturday, but even then, I didn't go overboard and I completely gave up takeaway food for months. Over time though, my consistently good weight loss decreased and plateaued. I had begun to cheat or just not try as hard, and inexplicably I also stopped going swimming. Over the previous year I had reduced the frequency of my swimming from four times per week to just once and then I just didn't go anymore, so all that hard work was seemingly for nothing. I knew that I needed to do something about this, so I decided to improvise with a hybrid of Slimming World/the 5-2 diet and the 3-day diet. I would do a week of each in rotation and then on my fourth week, which would be the week AFTER seeing Janine for my hospital weigh-in, I would have a 'normal' week with no dieting or restriction, but I would try and be mindful about what was going into my mouth. The weight once again began to come off, albeit slowly; some weeks I lost nothing, but over the course of a month I would be at least a couple of pounds (0.9 kilos) down. I kept going to the Slimming World classes for several months, but after a while I decided that I could do this without attending the classes. My monthly weigh-in meeting with Janine was the goal I was aiming for and I wasn't really following the Slimming World program, apart from 1 week per month. So once again I stopped going to Slimming World, which this time around wasn't the big mistake that it was the first time.

At one of my meetings with Janine I did tell her about my weight loss strategy, but she wasn't too impressed with the intermittent fasting nature of what I was doing, but it was working for me so I stuck to it. Janine gave me good news in that I was back on the surgery list and would hopefully be having the operation in the next 12 months. In the meantime, I would have to meet with Dr Barth again as well as having a couple more hoops to jump through. I would need to see a psychologist for their evaluation, as well as attending a support group for people who were pre or post bariatric surgery.

My psychologist appointments were held at LGI and were one-to-one 30 minute appointments held every two weeks. The psychologist was a slim middle-aged man who worked from a cramped and cluttered office with little natural light in the hospital's Clarendon Wing, which was the same wing in which my monthly appointments with Janine were held, so it was almost a home from home. We discussed my eating habits and the psychologist immediately picked up on the fact that I had hesitated before talking about what I ate. I immediately felt threatened, which was weird, as while we were physically close together, this was a non-confrontational and fairly comfortable environment. Psychologists are good, and this one had got inside my head in about 7 seconds flat. I realised that there was absolutely no point whatsoever in having any kind of defence and that honesty was the best policy. We talked about all aspects of life including of course food and eating, but also childhood, family, relationships, work, stress, exercise, hobbies, holidays, health and even toilet habits!

The key theme that came out of our sessions was mindfulness, which is about keeping aware of your actions with what you are doing. Mindfulness is good to practise for people who have eating disorders of any kind, whether you eat too much or not enough. We went through a program of mindfulness activities and exercises, and I was set 'homework' between sessions, that I must confess appealed to the academic within. I obtained a copy of a 2007 book called *Binge-eating Disorder: Clinical Foundations and Treatment* by several authors (James E. Mitchell, Michael J. Devlin, Martina de Zwaan, Scott J. Crow and Carol B. Peterson), which was a really excellent read and support tool for the work that we did. I'm actually quite surprised that this book hasn't had a more recent edition published. It opened my eyes to the damages of cyclic behaviour that is allowed to go unchecked and becomes a downward spiral with damaging knock-on implications, it was a metaphor for my life story. In fact, this book could have many uses outside of eating disorders, I could even see the underpinning principles of it being applicable for students who got into the habit of missing classes. Being mindful of the causes behind such behaviour can further down the line mitigate the harmful impacts that such behaviour can have. It all made perfect sense, so why couldn't I apply this to myself in everyday life all of the time, in a constant state of mindfulness and self-discipline? If I knew the answer to that and could implement it then I wouldn't need the surgery, I'm certainly not stupid, so maybe I was just weak? Or maybe I had bigger problems that I couldn't tackle by myself, that surgery would help me cope with? In the end that was the conclusion and recommendation made as a result of me attending these classes.

I was told that I have an addictive personality, which means that I can suddenly find myself neck-deep in something and seemingly unable to get out of it. With eating and drinking this can of course be harmful, but I must emphasise that having an addictive personality isn't always a bad thing, it can sometimes be a real positive and a driving force behind me, making me a great person to have on board when it comes to (for example) project work. I live and breathe whatever it is that I'm currently addicted to, and I've gone through my whole life like this since childhood. The sessions that I had with the psychologist made me reflect upon and acknowledge that this has been a major part of creating who I am. As a child I was addicted to Action Man, comic books, *Star Wars*, Lego, reading and television programs. I would get heavily into them and not want to do anything else for long periods until something 'better' came along to be my next addiction.

In adult life, the PW has always jokingly said, "it's another one of Stuart's phases," when I've really got into something (which is often leisure related), and she was completely right, I still go through insane phases of activity that is related to something that I enjoy doing in my own time. Some of the healthy positives of these have been over the years walking, cycling swimming, gardening and even *Pokémon Go* (which as an active game involves walking), each of which, when I really get into them, I hugely enjoy and want to keep doing. Other more creative/educational examples include travel, photography and film-making. I usually go abroad at least monthly for a long weekend, I love absorbing cultures and learning about places. I take tens of thousands of photographs a year, some of which end up on my Instagram (@stumoss). I meticulously film, edit, upload and label hundreds of hours of film per year onto my YouTube channel (www.mosstravel.tv). I spend hundreds if not thousands of hours per year painstakingly editing photos and films, and when it comes to uploading them, they have to be tagged correctly to get the optimum exposure with the right audiences. A single photo on Instagram can take me 30 minutes to edit, upload, label and tag. A YouTube video of a cityscape (basically me walking around a city filming), can take me several days to actually film, and then anywhere between 10 and 40 hours to edit, upload, label and tag. Whilst walking around filming is a healthy activity, sitting in a chair editing definitely isn't and because I'm so project focused and also a perfectionist, I sit there for hours at a time with very little in the way of breaks.

Writing is something which I get heavily into and then shy away from. When I'm in 'writer's mode', there is no stopping me, and sometimes I can't sleep because I just want to get things out of my head and onto paper (substitute paper for Microsoft Word). This book for example is one such endeavour, and once I start writing, I often find it difficult to stop. When I'm in the zone, I am truly in the zone. So apart from working on a computer, which is largely sedentary, you may wonder how else does having an addictive personality have negative impacts on my health? The answer unfortunately is that I have become addicted to eating and drinking behaviours that were not healthy for me. In terms of eating, I would not be satisfied with a normal sized meal, I would always want the king-sized option. I enjoy food just like I enjoy making films, so I would want more of it or to do it more often. I wouldn't be satisfied with a normal burger, I would want the biggest most expensive burger. I wouldn't want to share a pizza, I would want the whole thing to myself, and I wouldn't be satisfied with just having a curry, I would want all of the trimmings and starter accompaniments. Eating for me became more about the experience than it was the sustenance. When I sat down for a meal I would eat until I couldn't eat anymore. Eating was an experience that I enjoyed, so I would want to do it for as long as I could until I didn't enjoy it anymore.

In terms of drinking, I'm not and do not consider myself to ever have been an alcoholic, I've never ever needed to drink to function, I've never got out of bed in the morning and fancied a drink, but I do enjoy the experience of drinking just like I enjoy the experience of eating. So when I do have a drink, it isn't just one or two, it becomes a session, most usually at weekends when the prospect of a next-day hangover doesn't matter as much. This is binge drinking, which the NHS would define as consuming 8 units of alcohol in a single session for men or 6 units of alcohol in a single session for women. I only drink strong beers, I appreciate the complexity of the flavours be they a hoppy IPA or a syrupy Belgian Tripel. I typically seek out real ales that are at least 5% in strength, a pint (568ml) of which contains just under 3 units of alcohol. I would easily drink at least 5 pints on a night out, and quite often more. On a full day session at the weekend, this could be anywhere between 8 and 10 pints. I'm not proud to write that (maybe the big Barnsley lad in my head is), but if I'm not honest about acknowledging where I have gone wrong in my life, how can I make positive changes for my future?

If you're interested to know how to work out how many units of alcohol a drink contains, it is a pretty easy formula. You simply multiply the total volume of a drink (in ml) by its alcohol content, and then divide it by 1,000. So for example 1 pint of beer is 568 ml, if the beer is 5% ABV then 568 is multiplied by 5, which is 2,840, this figure is then divided by 1,000, which is 2.84, so a pint of 5% beer contains 2.84 units of alcohol. Using the same formula, a 250ml glass of wine that is 12% ABV contains 3 units of alcohol, and a single 25ml shot of whisky/gin/vodka that is 40% ABV is 1 unit of alcohol. A pint of 6% beer contains more units of alcohol than a treble whisky, and vastly more calories.

The NHS recommends that men consume 2,500 calories per day and women consume 2,000 calories per day. Herein lies the problem with binge eating and binge drinking; the consumer is taking on board a very large amount of calories in one go, and if the consumer is sedentary, the calories do not get burned off and the result is weight gain. A takeaway 12 inch (30 cm) pizza, drenched in fatty meat and cheese can easily contain 2,000 calories, a 5% ABV pint of beer contains around 240 calories. Can you imagine putting a whole pizza down your neck after drinking 6 pints of strong beer? Well I have done just that on very many occasions, before going to bed.

Alcoholic drinks are made from natural starch and sugar, alcohol contains 7 calories per gram, which is almost as many calories as there are in a gram of fat. When you look at it like this from a scientific perspective, it's very easy to consider making more informed and better decisions about food and alcohol consumption. But we don't look at food and alcohol from a scientific perspective (well most of us don't), we look at them from a fun and social perspective, and suddenly all of those numbers don't matter anymore, they certainly hadn't to me throughout my lifetime. So having an addictive personality and as a consequence of this, being a binge eater and binge drinker, were yet more factors that had sent me on my banana journey.

The support group that I attended for people who were pre- and post-bariatric surgery was held not far from where I lived at Weetwood Hall in Leeds. The group would meet once per month on a Monday evening. Weetwood Hall is a historic Grade II listed building, which has its origins in the 17th century, when it was a part of the Kirkstall Abbey estate. Between 1919 and 1991 it was a halls of residence for women attending the University of Leeds. Nowadays it is a very decent hotel with excellent conference facilities, located on the busy intersection of Leeds Ring Road and the A660 Otley Road. I had been here on many occasions, not just to attend conferences, but also to attend the hotel's on-site pub The Stables (built in an actual old stables building). The Stables is a good venue for a pint of real ale, and I have spent many happy hours there over the years that I have lived in northwest Leeds.

As part of my commitment to weight loss, before I could have the bariatric surgery that I so desperately needed, I had to attend the weight loss surgery support group that was held here. Prior to attending the session, I saw this as something of a box-ticking exercise to get my name on the list of attendees, which was a requirement of having the surgery. Having attended the Slimming World classes, I had decided that group therapy wasn't probably the best option for me personally. I liked to read and learn for myself and I did feel very well informed about the different surgeries that were available. Nevertheless, I had to go to the session, so I went twice. On the first occasion that I got there, I went into the conference reception and completely had what I can only describe as a huge wobble (not a weight related wobble either). I've never had a panic attack before, and I don't know if this was one, but I found myself with a dry mouth, feeling dizzy, hot and gasping for breath. I had to turn around and go outside. I walked back out into the cool night air breathing deeply and sat on a bench for 10 minutes composing myself. By the time that I had decided to go back into the session, the door into the room had been closed, there was no way that I was going to open it and have all eyes on me as a latecomer. I'd been defeated without going into the room, I hadn't heard from or spoken to anybody, I didn't even get my name on the precious attendance register. I felt like a complete failure, so went to The Stables pub and drowned my sorrows with a couple of pints of ale.

My second visit to Weetwood Hall to attend the support group was a more successful one. This time I didn't go alone, I took the PW with me. I felt like a little boy going with his mummy to the scary doctors. It was a bit pathetic that I couldn't do this alone, but I really couldn't, I have no idea why either. Once again, when we arrived my mouth went dry and I felt hot. "It's happening again," I told the PW, who was aware of what had occurred on my previous visit. "You'll be alright," she said reassuringly, as she stood behind me blocking my escape route. So we went into the room. I think I was the only person in attendance who was accompanied by a spouse/partner who wasn't also having bariatric surgery. The room was divided in two, with rows of chairs facing each other and a host at the front. We sat towards the back of one of the rows near the exit, just in case I needed to make a run for it.

The session was hosted by two very friendly women who themselves had undergone weight loss surgery and were actually doing this voluntarily, this was their 'giving back'. It transpired that some years ago there was very little in the way of information and support for pre- and post-operative bariatric patients, and this group had been the brainchild of somebody who had themselves struggled with their own weight loss journey as a consequence. In the room at this session, there must have been 40 people. I was genuinely surprised to see so many attendees, and this made me realise that this type of surgery is increasing in demand as obesity levels continually rise. People hadn't just come to this session from around Leeds, but also from surrounding towns and cities. The makeup of the group was around two thirds of people who had had the surgery and one third like me, who were on the waiting list; the majority of those in attendance were women, in fact there were only four men in the room including myself.

People were asked to share their stories, and that was the purpose of the group, it was group therapy based upon learning by doing and learning by reflecting on the successes and failures of self and others on everyone's weight loss journey. It was very apparent that the vast majority of people in the room who had already had the surgery had undergone the gastric bypass operation. Some people present were still very overweight and the operation had made very little impact on them in the long term. This was a worry for me, but it also enforced to me that the gastric bypass wasn't the operation for me. From listening to people speak, it just seemed to be a consistent issue that the bypass had not modified their behaviour, and that people were still overeating the wrong foods – cake seemed to be a word, which came up consistently. The bypass had worked very successfully for some of the attendees who were clapped when revealing how much weight they had lost and for how long. Fewer people in the room had undergone the gastric band, and in fact some people in the room who had a gastric band fitted, then had a second 'revision' operation, where the band was removed and they had then had a gastric bypass. Barely anyone in the room had had a sleeve gastrectomy, but as it happened out of the other three men who were in the room, two of them did have this operation, and both of them looked fantastic. Looking at them, you would never had known that they had ever been overweight, both were positively slim and certainly seemed to have had the best results of everyone in the room. I knew that I needed to talk to them.

After people had been given the opportunity to address the room, there was then a more social 'mingling' session, where attendees were encouraged to talk to each other and share their stories on a more personal level. "You need to talk to those two," the PW said to me, nodding her head towards the two men who'd had the sleeve gastrectomy. I nodded my head and stood up. "Come on then," I said, as I headed in their direction, with the PW close behind me.

There's a funny thing that some men do, it has become quite irksome to me over the years, but this is something that only men seem to do, at least I've never noticed women doing it (although maybe they do), and this happened at the group. The two men that we were heading towards, were a tall man and a shorter man, and the shorter man did the thing that I find irksome. He looked at me, then he looked at the PW, then he looked at me again, then he looked at the PW again, and I could imagine in his mind he was probably thinking, "what on earth is she doing with him?" I'm going to be honest with you, the PW is a head-turner, she's tall, blonde and has a very beautiful face. I'm tall, fat and most of the time feel like a right ugly bastard. I don't need another man to remind me, that in terms of physical attractiveness, I'm 'punching above my weight', which is a phenomenon that describes mismatched attractiveness between two people. I know the PW is a stunner, and I know that I'm not, but fortunately for me, our very good relationship is based upon more than looks alone (thankfully). This is obviously not the first time that I've noticed this happen, I've noticed it happen on many occasions, and with greater frequency in recent years as I've gained weight. You might think there'd be some camaraderie amongst men, a bit like a band of brothers who are there to support each other, slap each other on the back and say, "well done, mate, your missus is a beauty." I can confirm that there isn't and that men are shits when it comes to judging other men and their better halves.

Everything that I've just identified in the paragraph above occurred in less than a second, because people make judgements very quickly, and maybe I had misjudged, but I suspect that I hadn't. I couldn't let thoughts of negativity creep into my mind, I needed to speak with these men, they were in terms of post operation physique exactly where I wanted to be, and I needed insider info. I introduced myself and the PW and explained where I was in terms of awaiting surgery. The two men were both several years post-surgery and had in fact prior to surgery been as heavy as or heavier than I was. Prior to surgery, they both drank a lot of alcohol and they both had unhealthy diets. Post-surgery, the tall man revealed that he could barely drink alcohol now, and if he wanted a can of Guinness (his favourite tipple), he would open it and consume only a few mouthfuls, having to finish the can the next day. I'm going to be honest with you, that freaked me out a bit, I couldn't contemplate not being able to tolerate even one beer. I didn't mind if I'd have to sip it, but having to drink one beer over 2 days sounded pretty grim to me. The short man prior to surgery had spent every night in his local pub drinking beer, post-surgery he still visited the pub regularly, but nowadays he drank black coffee. He also told me that his favourite tipple was diet cola, but he would have to open a bottle and put it in his fridge to let it go flat before he could drink it. I was aware that post-surgery, fizzy drinks were not advised, but I hadn't realised that they would be so intolerable. Both of the men concurred that they could only eat very small portions, and that if they pushed the limit by eating more than they should, they would be in a lot of pain.

I noticed that the tall man had tattoos; they looked like they were a few years old, but they also looked in good shape. I had wondered if weight loss might mean excess skin, which could make tattoos misshapen in appearance, but his tattoos looked completely fine. I asked about excess skin, and the tall man confirmed that there was a bit here and there, but in the scheme of things, it was a very small price to pay for the benefits that bariatric surgery had brought to him, and the shorter man nodded in agreement. I asked about exercise, and the tall man told me that he didn't do a lot as he had a driving job, which was quite sedentary, but the shorter man told me that he had taken up running and now did this very regularly. It evidently was working for him, because he looked in great physical shape. Both of the men carried with them water bottles, that they were continually swigging from during our conversation. I asked them about this, and one of them told me that they got thirsty very easily, and that carrying a drink around was an essential aspect of life post-surgery. Another thing that they revealed was that they now largely ate a vegetarian diet, as meat often wasn't easy to tolerate. I told them both how much I admired them for what they had achieved post-surgery and thanked them for sharing their experiences. Whilst I didn't like the idea of not being able to manage a single beer or having to carry a water bottle around with me, they both looked in such great physical shape that I was inspired to emulate their achievements. I knew that I had to have this surgery and I knew that changes to my lifestyle were necessary, but I also knew that everybody's weight loss journey was different, from what I had read online and from my meetings with Janine. Just because one person took two days to drink a beer, it didn't necessarily mean that another person would be the same. I didn't want to go back to the days of excess beer drinking, but I would be gutted if I couldn't manage one now and again.

When we got home, I talked at length with the PW about my thoughts after attending the Weetwood session. We both concurred that the two men whom we spoke with looked in the best physical shape of everyone in the room who was post-surgery, and we both concurred that the sleeve gastrectomy was the right way forward for me. "It's not about a quick fix," the PW said to me, "it's a long journey, the operation will help you, but you need to be prepared to make changes to your lifestyle too." She spoke softly and sympathetically, looking me in the eye, and I knew that she was right. I knew that if I wasn't mentally prepared to make lifestyle changes, then all of this would be for nothing and I absolutely didn't want that. This had to be for something, this had to be for a healthier, lighter future and a longer life. The PW was always right, I was so lucky to have her with me on this journey.

I spent most of a year trying not to gain weight, using a combination of intermittent fasting from the 5-2 diet, the three day diet and dipping in and out of Slimming World syn counting. My weight loss slowed during this period, to a point where it had stalled completely but remained fairly constant at just over 25 stone (350 pounds/158.8 kilos). Sometimes it would increase dramatically by as much as 5 pounds (2.3 kilos) over a month, when I didn't try hard enough, and sometimes I would have to up my self-discipline, barring myself from nights out and increasing my intermittent fasting to combat this. Eventually my appointment came through to go and see Dr Barth again. This time however, the rules for having surgery had changed and whatever I weighed when I went to see Dr Barth was to be the maximum weight that I could ever be again. To put it simply, if my weight increased in future from what I weighed when I went to see Dr Barth on this next appointment, I would be taken off the surgery list, and put further back in the queue. This was a prospect that I simply couldn't allow to happen, so from this point onwards I was going to have to be extremely self-disciplined.

The appointment with Dr Barth was very similar to the one that I'd had with him previously, and the PW came along and sat there by my side listening intently and nodding as Dr Barth spoke. Again the doctor told me that I would struggle with food for the rest of my life, and again I told him that I already struggled with food. He quizzed me again about my choice of surgery and my rationale behind it, and once again I told him why I felt the sleeve gastrectomy was the right choice of surgery for me. The weigh-in revealed that I was 25 stone and 5 pounds (355 pounds/161 kilos). I was a little disappointed at this, as it was more than I had expected, although this was my clothed weight, which was always going to be a few pounds heavier than my weight at home, when I would weigh myself naked, first thing in the morning, usually after having a poo! The appointment was over after 30 minutes and now I had to play the waiting game again for my next appointment, which would be with the actual surgeon who would be performing the operation on me, things were now beginning to move and the operation was getting closer.

The appointment with Mr Metha followed a few weeks later, and the PW once again accompanied me to St. James's Hospital as she had done with my previous visits to see Dr Barth. We both felt that it was important that she was there, because not only was she my wife and would invariably be going on this journey with me, she was also a nurse, and had a better understanding of health and medical matters than I did. After checking in, we didn't have to wait very long to see the man who would be saving my life. Mr Metha was an impressive man, tall, slim, good-looking and extremely professional and to the point. He didn't have time for me padding out my answers with waffle, and would prompt me to keep me on track, when asking questions about myself, my lifestyle and why specifically I had chosen the sleeve gastrectomy. He seemed satisfied with what I said to him and made notes as we spoke. He then had to tell me what I didn't want to hear; that as a result of undergoing surgery, I could die, the odds were miniscule, but still I could die, and I had to sign a piece of paper to say that I understood that. This was normal practice, if you're having an operation it puts a lot of strain on your body, sometimes your body can't handle the strain and gives up. It was a stark reality of what I was facing, it was frightening to think that an operation to enhance and extend my life could also end my life, but it was also very unlikely to happen. Nevertheless, I needed to know the risks.

Mr. Metha also made sure I knew about the liver reduction diet (LRD), which all bariatric patients must go on for 2 weeks prior to surgery; this was a very low calorie diet, designed to shrink the liver, which can obstruct the stomach. He told me that I would ordinarily be given a week's notice to prepare myself and my fridge and larder for the LRD.

Following the meeting with Mr Metha, I was then sent on what I can only describe as a 'treasure hunt'. Imagine the entirety of the huge St. James's Hospital as an escape room. I was given a map and a detailed set of instructions and then sent off with the PW for a pre-operation assessment. Navigating our way along corridors, up and down lifts, through green doors to the left and second blue doors on the right, we eventually found where we needed to be. The pre-operative assessment involved me filling in a very long questionnaire; having an electrocardiogram (ECG), which is a test that measures the electrical activity of the heart to show whether or not it is working normally (thankfully mine was); being weighed; having a blood test, and having an interview with a nurse. Everything went very smoothly, and I was moved along the assessment conveyor belt with the utmost efficiency. At the end of the assessment I asked the nurse who interviewed me how long it would likely be between me having the assessment and the operation, and she told me 6 weeks. This was getting very, very real. When you're a kid, 6 weeks feels like forever, but in my very busy life, 6 weeks was no time at all. I was suddenly quite daunted by what was ahead of me, and admittedly more than a little afraid.

Time was counting down, and I had to face telling my parents about the operation that I was due to have. So far only the PW, our girls and a few of my close mates knew. We went over to my parents' house in Barnsley for my birthday weekend in July. My parents now live in a village called Silkstone Common, a lovely little village, very rural although like many places constantly expanding with the continual demand for housing, which then eats up green spaces. We went for one of my mum's incredible Sunday lunches, which are quite literally legendary. In the UK, everyone's mother's Sunday dinners are legendary, everyone thinks that their mother can cook a better Sunday dinner than everybody else's mother. What none of them know is, that my mother's Sunday dinners are actually the very, very, very best. In football terms, my mum would easily beat Brazil at the World Cup of Sunday dinners without the need for extra thyme (did you see what I did there?). My mum could put to shame any Michelin Star chef when it comes to cooking roast beef, Yorkshire puddings, roast potatoes, mashed potatoes and a grand assortment of boiled and roasted vegetables, all smothered in thick beefy gravy. If my mum had a superpower, it would be to defeat the enemy by overfeeding them the most delicious of Sunday roasts until they fell asleep in the armchair for the sheriff to come and capture. Anyone undefeated by her Sunday roasts would almost certainly succumb to her puddings (desserts to anyone not from up north). My mum's puddings don't come out of a box or from a packet, everything is made from raw ingredients, her specialities are trifles, cheesecakes, apple pies, fruit crumbles, chocolate pralines, all manner of cakes and buns, and egg custards. It is impossible to go to my parents' house for Sunday dinner and leave hungry, in fact it is impossible to go to my parents' house for Sunday dinner and not feel as though you are having a food baby afterwards. I haven't even mentioned my father's incredible home-made mushy peas (which he refers to as 'Yorkshire Caviar'), which are also served as an accompaniment to the main meal (it's a Yorkshire thing).

It's always lovely to see my parents, we are physically only 30 miles (48 km) apart, but as the PW and I lead very busy lives, our weekends are often time to get domestic jobs done at home, as well as for leisure. We try and visit my parents around once per month, and they usually come and visit us around once per month also, we see them around every 2-3 weeks. The format of the day is usually welcome/greetings hugs and kisses; giving gifts (flowers/wine/chocolate); a cuppa and a catch-up; loading up the car with firewood (my 78-year-old dad cuts up discarded wood for fun for us as we have a wood burner at home); my mum's amazing Sunday lunch, with my dad's home-made 'Yorkshire Caviar' (mushy pea) accompaniment; me trying not to fall asleep in the big comfy chair as the food digests; another cuppa and more conversation, and then finally gathering our things before heading back home. I still wave out of the car window like a child until they're completely out of sight as the car goes up the street away from their house.

Whilst I always look forward to seeing my parents, I was dreading this weekend's visit, due to having to explain to them that I was going to undergo bariatric surgery. I felt so nervous when we got there, I asked the PW not to push me into talking about it. I needed to do this in my own time when I was ready. I decided that this should be after lunch, I don't think anybody would have wanted a large roast meal after discussion of a sleeve gastrectomy. I waited until everyone was sitting in the living room, in post-lunch digestion relaxation mode, when I finally bit the bullet and confessed what was ahead of me. I began, "anyway, I need to tell you both something." The room went silent and I knew my mum and dad could immediately tell from my voice and face that this was going to be serious. "I don't want you to worry about me, but I'm going into hospital for a little operation" (I thought I'd play it down). "Don't worry, it's not a sex change." (I tried to lighten the mood). "I'm having an operation called a sleeve gastrectomy, it's basically weight-loss surgery, I'm going to have my stomach reduced so it will be about the size and shape of a banana." There was a stunned silence in the living room as my parents digested what I had just said, the PW looked at me really sympathetically. "I don't want you to worry about me though," I continued, "it's keyhole surgery, no big scars, and it's very low risk, I'll be fine and I need to do this, you know how much I'm struggling health-wise, and this will really help me." I paused and waited for a response, "we will worry though" my mum said, "of course we'll worry." Both of my parents looked shocked and a bit sad. I'd spoiled our Sunday together, but I needed them to know, and if I hadn't told them, they would have been upset.

The PW interjected, "he'll be fine, it's not a big operation where they open him up, it's done as keyhole surgery." I felt that I had to give more background. "I've been building up to this for years, I've been on a program with Leeds Weight Loss Service for about 4 years, I've had counselling, and had to keep my weight at a certain level to be considered, I've done everything that I was required to do, and now the countdown to the operation is finally on." "So when will you have the operation?" Dad asked. "Probably in the next couple of months," I replied, despite thinking that it could be in the next 3-4 weeks. "We had no idea that you'd been going through all of this," Mum said. "I know," I replied, "I've just not wanted to talk about it, but now the time is close, I knew that I had to tell you." The rest of the visit was then dominated by talk about my banana journey so far and what the future would likely look like for me in terms of eating and drinking. Later that evening I hugged my parents extra hard before as we were saying our goodbyes. My dad hugged me and quipped, "I'll be able to touch my fingers soon when I hug you then." As we left my parents' house that evening and drove up their street I waved frantically. I was so relieved that I'd finally told them. It was a huge weight taken from my mind, just as much as the operation would be a huge weight taken from my feet.

The six weeks following the pre-operation assessment passed, I was then in uncharted territory time-wise. Having now seen Mr Metha and being placed on the final countdown to surgery, I no longer saw Janine for my monthly appointments at LGI. Instead I saw another member of the team that Janine worked in, called Mary. Like Janine, Mary was very supportive and passionate about helping people who were overweight to improve their lives. Mary had a very matter-of-fact manner and told it exactly like it was. I imagined that she'd heard every excuse under the sun over the years from people who had strayed whilst on their weight loss journeys. I knew that honesty was the best policy, so when we met for a weight check and discussion, I was completely honest with her. I was concerned that the time was taking too long, I was worried about gaining weight the longer the time took for me to have the operation. We discussed my eating and drinking habits, which had in recent months vastly improved, and Mary told me that I needed to maintain the momentum, I needed to keep it up, and she was right. I needed to pull myself together and stay focused, which admittedly is sometimes easier said than done.

As the 6 weeks had passed, my pre-operative assessment had lapsed and I was called in for a second one, which was a briefer version of the first one. I didn't have to complete the questionnaire again, or have the ECG, but my bloods were taken again, I was weighed and I had a shorter interview with a nurse to establish that nothing had changed in my health. I asked the nurse if she had any idea when I might be having the operation. "I think it will be soon," she said, "as this is your second pre-op, I can't imagine it will be more than a few weeks now, who knows though, everywhere is stretched, but I don't think it will be long at all now." I really hoped that it would be soon, the operation felt like the sword of Damocles hanging over my head. I just wanted to get it over and done with now, I wanted to get my life back on track. I wanted my future.

Wednesday the 16th October, 2019 was quite a day for me. I had been to the dentist in the early afternoon for a double filling appointment. I had broken one filling and pulled out another completely. The culprit for me doing this was an after-dinner toffee given to me at a local restaurant. Toffees should either be banned or carry severe health warnings, this isn't my first toffee-tooth incident. The dentist persuaded me on a consultant visit a couple of weeks before my fillings to opt for a private treatment, which should have some longevity to it due to the extent of the work that he had to do. If I went with the cheaper NHS treatment it likely wouldn't last very long. I'd never gone private for any healthcare before in the UK, but I could see the sense in his proposal. I'm a bit soft when it comes to dentists and needles, so the 40-minute treatment was quite traumatic and left me feeling as though I'd had a stroke in the right side of my very numb face.

The bus journeys both to the dentist and back home again on the number 6 via Otley Road through Headingley was extremely slow and very boring. This is one of the UK's most congested roads at all times of day, and for large parts of the journey the bus was only moving at walking pace, that is when it was actually moving at all, as it spent a lot of time stationary. I alleviated the boredom of the ride by playing the game Pokémon Go on my iPhone. At the slow rate that the bus was travelling, my phone was fooled into thinking that I was actually walking, so this helped me hatch invaluable eggs and earn my buddy some candies (if you know you know, if you don't know, just trust me that this is a good thing). Pokémon Go is extremely battery intensive, so when I got home, I plugged my phone in to recharge in my office as the battery was very low, after which I settled down in the living room to work from my laptop.

The PW was working from home that afternoon also, so we both sat in the living room in the autumnal gloom, in silence apart from the clicking of keys and the occasional groan or exasperated exhalation with our faces illuminated by blue-white laptop screen light. I tried drinking a cup of tea, but with a numb face half of it dribbled down my chin and onto my T-shirt causing me to swear. The PW seeing me struggle (and without me asking), went into the kitchen and retrieved me a drinking straw; the PW really is a perfect wife. As I was sitting there sucking my tea up the straw, the PW's work phone rang. "This is work," she said, meaning don't swear while I'm on the phone, the PW is a professional woman.

The PW's phone call reminded me that my phone was still in my office, so I went into my office to retrieve it. As I unplugged the phone, the screen lit up and I could see that I had both a missed call and a voicemail. Whilst this isn't unusual, I don't get that many voicemails, probably less than one per month, so I played the voicemail through the speaker of my phone. "Hello, this is a message for Stuart Moss, I'm calling from

St. James's Hospital, Mr Mehta wants you to start your pre-operation diet and he's got a date for you of the 30th of October for your operation. Can you give me a ring back and let us know that you've got this message?" I couldn't believe what I had just heard, so I played the message a second time, and it hadn't changed. I could feel the blood draining from my face. I went cold. Finally, after all this time I had got a date through, but after getting reassurances that I would have 3 weeks' notice, I had only got 2 weeks' notice, in fact I'd got slightly less. I returned the call, but ended up speaking to an answering machine, I gave all of my details and let them know that I had received the message loud and clear, that I would be starting my pre-operation diet the day after and that I would be there for the operation on the 30th.

I was supposed to be on the 800 calories per day pre-operation liver reduction diet (LRD) for 14 days, it was already Wednesday afternoon, and I had eaten over 800 calories in the morning, so I could only realistically have 13 days for the LRD. I missed a day on the LRD, which isn't so bad, but what about my 'food funeral'? What about my last supper? It is a bit of a tradition for bariatric patients to go out with a bang. I knew where I wanted to go for my last big meal, and that was to my favourite Indian restaurant, 'The Jewel of India' in the nearby town of Otley. I even knew what I would order from the menu: two poppadoms and pickle tray; onion bhaji starter; Jewel Special Balti; boiled rice, and; a Peshwari naan bread. The portion sizes are decent at The Jewel of India, so I would share the rice and naan bread with the PW. She would likely order similarly to me, but instead of having two poppadoms she would have one, she would order meat samosa instead of onion bhaji, and her curry would likely be a fishy/seafood one, not that either of us are creatures of habit, you understand.

I went back into the living room to find the PW, who was no longer on her work phone and was staring intently at her laptop screen. I stood silently in the doorway, quite expressionless, looking at her; after a few seconds she glanced up at me and then looked back at her screen, she then looked back at me and said, "what's wrong?" I walked over to her slowly looking her in the eye. I bent over her as she sat in the chair and whispered in her ear, "I'm having the operation on the 30th of October, 2 weeks today." "What?" she said shocked, "oh my God, what about the diet?" "I'll have to start it tomorrow," I responded. "Oh my God," she said again and hugged me from the chair as I bent over her. "I can't believe it after all this time." "We're going to Otley tonight," I then said to her, envisioning a few pints of good real ale followed by our last big curry blow-out. "I can't," responded the PW, "I'm going out tonight for a meal with work colleagues." "Oh," I replied, "I'd forgotten." I had indeed forgotten, but after she had reminded me, I remembered that the PW's dinner engagement was a long-standing leaving do and that she could not miss it.

So on the Wednesday night, my last night of gastronomic freedom, I ended up sadly eating alone at home, my last supper being baked beans and mini pork sausages, cold straight out of the tin, followed by jam on toast. I was too despondent to order a takeaway or have anything more elaborate. Afterwards I took a taxi to Horsforth Town Street, where I had a couple of pints of ale in the Town Street Tavern, and some two for the price of one fancy gin and tonics in La Casita, which is a Wednesday evening favourite of the PW and me. We call Wednesdays at La Casita 'Gin Wednesdays'. The PW joined me at La Casita after her meal, for a last round of gins. I didn't know when I would be drinking alcohol again, and the shock of the news meant that I needed a drink, otherwise I wouldn't sleep that night. In the end I slept like a baby, with the PW cuddled reassuringly into me. Tomorrow the hill was set to get steeper on my banana journey.

Matt Simkin was a student whom I taught between 2008 and 2011 at the then Leeds Metropolitan University (now Leeds Beckett University). I remember him as being a genuinely nice guy, as well as funny and cynical. He was one of those people that just got along with anyone, whether he liked them or not. He is somebody who would go the extra mile and be motivated to put himself forward to do those little extra things, because he wanted to help and be a central part of the class, which he was. I have a photo of Matt along with classmates Gina, Laura, Bob, and Faith, all wearing identical T-shirts, selling tickets for a student charity event that we ran back in 2008. I remember this photo because Matt's overly happy, open-mouthed expression and 'jazz hands' are etched into my mind as the picture makes me chuckle every time I see it.

One of the really wonderful things about being an academic and working intensively on a small course (in terms of student numbers) is that you get to know each and every one of the students really well over 3 years. Whilst professional standards must be maintained in terms of familiarity and impartiality, it is impossible not to become friends with the cohort of students when you see them day in and day out. You get to know about them, their backgrounds, families, work, aspirations, hobbies, interests, and also when things go wrong in their lives and they need someone to turn to, their tutors are often the first port of call. To me the students are like extended family, and I'm very protective of them, but at the same time I will let them know very firmly when they are out of line. Being an academic in higher education (HE) these days is about so much more than subject knowledge and teaching, as student welfare, guidance and to a lesser extent discipline also takes up a significant amount of time.

After 3 years the students depart, their time at university ends and they are gone, gone from class, and most are gone from Leeds. Seemingly one minute you have people in your life who you are working with closely, who you are helping through difficult and stressful times, the next minute they are gone, and replaced with the next cohort. It is a plain fact that after graduation I will never ever see the majority of my ex-students face to face ever again, and this for me is the saddest part of life as an academic. I've led the BA (Hons) Entertainment Management for 15 years, I'm one of a core team of three as well as Course Leader and a Personal Tutor. It is impossible not to feel sadness at graduation knowing that this for the majority of graduating students is the final farewell, as well as of course immense pride in their fantastic achievements. Every year I give the final year students their last ever lecture, and every year I have a tear in my eye and a quiver in my voice whilst doing so.

My students leave university and go on to do a variety of incredible things. Many of them go straight into jobs, some are entrepreneurs and begin their own enterprises, some go travelling, some undertake further study, and some do a combination of the above. As an example, out of the aforementioned students that I mentioned above: Laura works in marketing and communications in Wakefield; Sammy has emigrated to Australia and started her own sustainable fashion enterprise in Melbourne, and Faith is working in digital marketing in Bath. I find out what the ex-students of mine are doing through LinkedIn, Instagram and Facebook, which is one of the nice things about social media, in that it allows me to see the paths that many of my graduates take beyond university. Unfortunately, I don't know what Gina and Bob are up to these days and social media isn't helping me.

Out of all of the above Entertainment Management alumni, I have only seen Sammy in person since leaving university. The PW and I went to visit our eldest daughter Hannah in Australia in 2016. Hannah lives in Brisbane and we spent 16 fantastic days with her, and afterwards the PW and I had 4 days in Melbourne before returning home. I messaged Sammy on a Friday afternoon to see if she fancied a drink with us that night. She came along with her fiancé Paul, and it's safe to say that we all got pretty smashed in the bars overlooking the Yarra River in the city centre. I'll add to this story, that we were also joined for drinks by another of my alumni, Jen, who graduated in 2015 and was backpacking in Melbourne at the time of our visit, which was a nice coincidence, I found out that Jen was in Melbourne through Facebook while we were there. Before we left Melbourne we met up with another of my graduates called Ellie whom we took for lunch. Melbourne seems to be a bit of a magnet for Entertainment Management alumni. This isn't surprising as it is such a vibrant and 'happening' creative city.

So to bring this particular story to a closure I need to talk once again about Matt Simkin. LinkedIn tells me that Matt is currently the Commercial Manager at Wembley Park in London, which is an impressive and prestigious employment position to hold. Why I'm discussing Matt though, isn't because of his excellent qualities as a student, and it isn't because of his job title, it is because like myself, Matt is an author...

It is Thursday 17th October, the first day of my liver reduction diet (LRD) and my alarm has just awoken me at 06:30, the PW is already up and in the shower. I'm lying in bed holding a book in my hand called *Food, Culture, Latin America*, the author of which is Matt Simkin. Matt is actually the second of my graduates to become a published author, the other being BA (Hons) Tourism Management alumnus David Hatton, who has (to date) had four fiction books published. It is really nice to know other authors, you get a real appreciation of the efforts that they have gone to in order to produce literature that can entertain other people.

Matt's book is about his travels around Central and South America, the people he encountered, the challenges he faced and all of the wonderful food and drink he consumed on his travels. At least that's what I'm interpreting from the back page and the first few pages of the foreword and first chapter. I have decided that my pre-operation preparation is going to be about my mind as well as body, so have decided to use my phone less for social media, avoid the news and read more books for pleasure during this period. I need my mind and body to be in the best possible condition with lower stress and blood pressure as well as lower weight, when I go in for the operation.

My phone is a major culprit in causing me stress, and I have found a useful way by which to use it less. I have simply switched off notifications for all of my apps, so no longer will my mobile phone act like a Tamagotchi in my pocket. No longer will it vibrate or ping to tell me that it needs my attention, that it needs me to look at it because somebody has 'liked' something, or because somebody else has made a comment, because an email has arrived or because there is breaking news on the BBC. I don't want to know, I don't care. I've decided to take back control of my life from my mobile phone, now I am the master, and I will decide if and when I want to look at my phone. Using my phone less, means that I will have more time for pleasurable and less stressful activities such as reading something for the sheer enjoyment and not because I have to. It also could potentially mean that the dopamine 'reward' centres in my brain that give me feelings of positivity as well as motivation may be stimulated less. When I receive a like or a positive comment for a social media post it makes me feel good, as does all positive feedback. The dopamine that is released in my brain stimulates me to do more. Maybe I will not be motivated to post as often across various social media platforms, I shall have to see.

A carefully crafted photo edit and Instagram post, or a heavily edited YouTube video with the correct tags and descriptions takes time. Apart from these being largely sedentary activities, they take up a sizeable amount of my leisure time, and whilst this is creative time, I am pushing my creativity rather than absorbing and being entertained by the creativity of others. I wish I had more time in my congested life to read books for pleasure more often. I suffer from 'reader's guilt', which is a condition that I've made up in my head. As an academic, reading is a major part of my life. I have to read for work every single day, mostly online articles related to my subject area, but also research papers, student work and emails, lots and lots of emails. As my teaching is around the entertainment industries, I need to keep up to date with a very large variety of sectors, from venues such as bars, pubs and clubs, to festivals of all nature, museums, theatre, the arts, the music industries, gaming, commercial gambling, television, film, visitor attractions…the list goes on and on. Besides this, there is a small matter of a PhD that I am currently writing, which also requires a plethora of academic articles to be read. When I find myself reading something that isn't related to either my teaching or my PhD, I feel guilty. I know that this is stupid, but it's true, I don't know if other academics also suffer from 'reader's guilt', or if I'm the outlier, but either way, I have a lovely and growing collection of books of all natures, that I keep putting back on the shelf to read another day. Not anymore, I'm determined to read a little each day for pleasure during the LRD, and hopefully this will become a habit that I'll continue beyond it.

I have also decided to avoid newspapers and online news sites during this period, which I find quite often to be toxic; they tell lies, which is unjust, which is stressful, this keeps me awake at night, and this toxicity is another part in the jigsaw, which has put me where I am today. There are numerous studies that show a relationship between poor sleep and obesity. Getting to sleep late means waking up tired and stressed, being last-minute, missing breakfast or I'll be late for work, which is the everyday reality of my life. It takes me hours to switch off sometimes. The stresses of media lies combined with the corrupt politics of Tories, Brexit, Farage, Johnson, Trump, Putin, Erdoğan, Bolsonaro and many, many more rattle around my brain like ball-bearings in a paint can. The worst possible thing to do before trying to sleep is to lie in bed reading the news on my phone, yet I have done this for years. I don't want the stay-awake gremlins in my head anymore and I need to get them out. My self-imposed media ban is designed to relax me and put me in the best possible mental state for my operation, and also for my recovery beyond. It is a cruel irony that my physical body is going to go through its greatest trauma, the day before what was meant to be 'Brexit Day' (31st October, 2019), and that my recovery period is fully in the midst of a UK general election campaign. If I was religious, I'd say that God works in very mysterious ways, but as I'm an atheist I'll just say bugger!

I read the first few pages of Matt's book and begin to walk in his shoes during his journey. Knowing Matt personally (even though I haven't seen him for 8 years) means that the shoes fit quite well and the reading is enjoyable. Whilst reading the first few pages about Matt's time in Belize, the penny drops. Why don't I do what Matt has done? Why don't I write about my journey both pre- and post-bariatric surgery? I've written books before, albeit academic textbooks. So why don't I write reflectively about how my life, body and mind changes as a result of the path that I have chosen? I could write something that is autobiographical and reflective, which frankly explains how I have got to be where I am, combined with the challenges that I face as they arise on my weight loss journey. Such a book may be of interest to the many thousands of other people in a similar position to myself, and it might help enlighten and educate the masses who are conditioned into seeing fat people as a stupid inconvenience in society. In Matt's book, he has his GBH (girl back home), whilst I have my PW (perfect wife). It all begins to make sense, this will work, this is achievable, I know that I can do this and it might even be a therapeutic process for me, helping me to come to terms with myself and why I am like what I am, in terms of food and health. Matt Simkin sir, you have inspired me. So dear reader, this is why from this chapter onwards, what you are reading is written in the present tense (as it happens) as I begin to journal my days, apart from where I am reflecting upon stories and events from the past.

After this enlightenment, I get out of bed and slowly head to the bathroom feeling inspired. The weather outside is very damp, and this has triggered stiffness in my legs, particularly my right knee. I use a crutch to assist my passage downstairs to the bathroom. As I perform my daily ablutions, clean my teeth and shower, I consider that I will need to keep a diary of my everyday thoughts and experiences in order for this to become an achievable task. I'll need to write somewhere between 80,000 and 100,000 words for the book to be of a decent publishable length (I end up writing 143,000 words), and if I write a little each day, then I should be able to do this within 6 months easily. Ironically, for this purpose I decide to use the 'notes' app on my mobile phone (despite my planned phone time reduction), to keep basic bullet points for my diary as I'll always have my phone by my side, and if my phone is lost, the diary will be backed up in 'the cloud'. The only time in my life that I have kept a diary previously was when I went backpacking around the world, between October 1994 and November 1995, In October 1994, I and some mates from Darfield (a village near Barnsley), Skip and Fruddy went backpacking in Australia (we were later joined by friends Paul and Col). It doesn't seem like much now, but 25 years ago in Barnsley, this was quite a thing. My old travel diary is currently downstairs in my office and after I've finished in the bathroom, I plan to dig it out for some inspiration.

After drying off, I get out the weighing scales and place them on an even part of the bathroom floor. I gingerly step onto them, first my left foot and then my right foot. The scales inform me that my weight at this point is 25 stone, 5.25 pounds (355.25 pounds/161.14 kilos). If all goes to plan, this will be the most that I will ever weigh again for the rest of my entire life, which is quite a poignant thought. In my head, I think I'd like to get down to 17 stone (238 pounds/108 kilos), but realistically, I'll be happy at anywhere between 18 and 19 stones.

The PW then arrives holding a tape measure, this is new to me. "Let's measure you then," she says. With the skill of a tailor, the PW applies the measuring tape around my body. These results are as follows:

Head 58 cm

Neck 50 cm

Chest 136 cm

Waist 169 cm

Hips 150 cm

Arms 37.5 cm

Thighs 67.5 cm

Ankles 29 cm

I haven't been so properly measured before, so at least this will give me a point of reference to refer back to.

I get dressed and head downstairs, my first port of call being my office. I retrieve my Australia travel diary from my bookshelf and have a read through it over breakfast. I look at my diary for this date 17th October, 1994 which happened to be a Monday, and the entry is below.

"Get up late after Sunday session, only just get to work in time. Shit day in the office. On way home buy 400 ISO film for panoramic camera, get bus home then pizza for dinner washed down with a couple of VBs (Victoria Bitters)"

My Mondays in Sydney were so often hungover, we really partied hard at weekends, Friday night I'd be home as quick as possible and be in the shower with a beer getting ready to hit Balmain's pubs. Saturday would often involve a few steady bottles at home before going to the pubs in the evening, and then hitting a rock, indie or Goth club in the city at night. Sundays were famous for the 'Sunday Sesh', basically decide a location, ring everyone and go there and drink until you're ready to stagger home. Work was repetitively mundane and sometimes stressful (but well paid), so the weekend drinking was a form of therapy that I could afford. I was working for Vodafone at the time as an agency contractor, connecting phones to SIM cards mostly, but also blocking phones and changing phone numbers. This was when digital mobile phones first took off in Australia and the days could be intense with fast turnarounds required. The office fax machines would spew out requests from service providers, which we needed to fulfil as quickly as possible, before faxing them back with a confirmation. It was fairly humdrum and repetitive stuff, but we had a great office and many laughs. There were also perks to the job including being able to phone home for free (the phones were blocked for international calls, but I would ring from the fax machines – ha ha). This job also gave me the opportunity to learn about emerging technologies and improve my IT skills.

I've always been a keen photographer, and the above diary entry is an insight into that also. I had a camera that took special long panoramic photographs; loads of people had them in the UK at this time, as one of the cigarette companies were giving them away if you collected and sent off 25 of their loyalty cards. As I worked in a hotel before going to Australia, the cards were very easy to find. I also note from this entry that my dinner was a typically ordered pizza, which would have been from the takeaway around the corner from our house. We had a buy one get one free pizza card (called a

'Granton Card') that we paid AU$50 per year for, which was all too tempting to use after a hard day in the office and a 2-hour commute home. Washing dinner down with beer is something that was also routine in those days. Great memories though. I sit on my sofa and browse through the diary for a little longer. The PW once found my old diary and sneakily read it, and she finally confessed to doing so some time later. I asked her what she thought of it and her response was, "didn't you eat a lot of pizza and drink a lot of beer," enough said.

My first day on the LRD needs to be spent carefully, I need to take note of all the calories as I only have 800 per day. I have a cup of tea with a dash of milk (30 calories). For breakfast I have a poached egg (70 calories) on a dry unbuttered slice of toast (120 calories), which is 220 calories for breakfast, leaving me 580 calories for the rest of the day, which isn't a lot for two meals. I'm working from home on this day as I am not teaching, which gives me access to plenty of food to read the calorific information about. Working from home means sitting at my computer in my office for most of the day, writing lectures and responding to email as well as reading some articles for my PhD. I drink a lot of water throughout the day to keep me from feeling hungry and to flush my system. I seem to be peeing very regularly. I take my lunch in the mid-afternoon. I have a tin of 'slimmer soup' (190 calories), and a cup of tea (30 calories) with nothing else, which leaves me 360 calories for dinner. My dinner consists of 2 Quorn sausages (125 calories), chopped up and mixed with a tin of chopped tomatoes (94 calories), which I season with black pepper and dried mixed herbs (negligible calories). I follow this with another cup of tea (30 calories), and a yoghurt (90 calories), giving me a grand calorie total for my first day on the LRD of 779 calories. I'm actually under the 800 calorie limit, which is great. I don't feel particularly hungry when I go to bed, but I do have quite an 'empty' tummy feeling inside. As a first day on the LRD goes, this really wasn't so bad.

The next day I am working on campus all day, so I decide to have an improved breakfast, forfeit lunch and have an improved dinner, with more drinks in-between that aren't just water. I know that skipping lunch possibly isn't the way to do it, but in my mindset, I'd rather have two 'bigger' meals than three smaller ones. My breakfast consists of two Quorn sausages (125 calories), which I halve lengthwise, so that on my plate they look like four sausages (you need to employ a little psychology on this diet). I present them in a very artistic way in a square frame shape on a bed of shredded lettuce leaves, rocket, some chopped cucumber and some halved cherry tomatoes (60 calories). In the centre of the Quorn sausage frame I put one poached egg (70 calories), and season with black pepper and some dried chilli flakes. My plate looks like something you might see in a poncey overpriced hipster veggie café, so like any good social media slave, I take a photo of it and put it on my Instagram. I have with it a cup of tea with milk (30 calories), which gives my very tasty and satisfying breakfast a total of 285 calories.

I go to work and grab an Americano from the campus coffee shop, in which I put a dash of cold milk (30 calories) before heading to the classroom. My day is typical, a lecture-seminar followed by some one-to-one tutorials with my dissertation tutees. After which I have another Americano with a dash of cold milk (30 calories). My afternoon is mostly spent responding to emails and doing small admin jobs. By the end of the working day, I am tired and have a banging headache. I am aware that the LRD can cause headaches, and that I just need to keep my fluids up and take some paracetamol, which I do when I get home.

Dinner consists of a soupy stew that I make from: 100 grams of chicken breast (165 calories); a tin of chopped tomatoes (94 calories), and; a tin of carrots (48 calories). I season this with an Oxo cube (18 calories), dried chilli flakes, dried mixed herbs and black pepper (negligible calories). My bowl of food looks huge, certainly greater than its calorific content of 325 calories would suggest. This leaves me room for a yoghurt (90 calories) and a final cup of tea (30 calories), making my total calorific intake for the day 790 calories. On my way to bed that night I actually feel lighter on my feet as I climb the stairs; maybe it's my imagination, maybe it's wishful thinking, but I'm feeling quite upbeat about the LRD so far, apart from the lingering residual headache.

I must add, that if you are reading this book and you yourself are contemplating or indeed scheduled to have bariatric surgery, that there are different kinds of LRD, and it seems to be down to your surgeon as to which one you will do. In Facebook support groups for bariatric surgery, I have come across people who have to stick to milk and yoghurt for two weeks, or SlimFast on their LRD, and the thought of that is pretty grim to me. At least I could actually eat food, although it was repetitive. If you're reading this looking for amazing ideas for LRD recipes you're going to be disappointed, there are no amazing recipes when you're capped at 800 calories per day, you need to get that in your head now. It's about making the best of it, smiling in the face of adversity, keeping at it and not being a whinging moaner who is going to bring themselves down. Suck it up, it's only 2 weeks out of your entire life, which really is nothing. That said, if your surgery gets postponed and you have to extend the LRD, now that would be a massive shitter (and that has happened to people).

The LRD goes on, calorie counting becomes routine and isn't that difficult to manage, you've just got to take the time and make the effort. I notice that most packaged food has a suggested portion size on the labelling, I've never really acknowledged this before and I don't think that many people do. The calories on many packages are also often per portion and not per package, so if for example a tin of tomatoes has two portions in it and the number of calories on the label is per portion, then this needs doubling to make it calories per tin. There is inconsistency between brands, and I can imagine that this would trip up those who don't read the labels properly, so if you're reading this – take note! I find that broccoli and cauliflower are tasty and versatile foods that have a low calorific content, and incorporate them into many meals. The size of their florets is good psychologically when I look at them on my plate. Tomatoes (tinned and fresh), lettuce and cucumber become regular meal ingredients that are easy to make tasty with the addition of herbs, chilli flakes, black pepper, soy sauce and balsamic vinegar. Some days I have a good breakfast and dinner and don't really bother with lunch, some days I have a yoghurt at lunchtime.

Quorn is like a miracle food for me on the LRD. It's not meat, but it tastes and looks meaty enough. It gives me the chance to have meaty flavours and a bit of a chew without the calories. It's very lean, and if you stick to the basic Quorn products of sausages, burgers and Quorn pieces, you can make all sorts with them. It can be a bit like Groundhog Day, when you're eating Quorn, tinned tomatoes, lettuce, carrots and cucumber nearly every day, but the trick is to vary the way you cook, present and flavour them. I have spicy days, then herby days then very spicy days. Maximum flavour gives heightened satisfaction, a hot and spicy bowl of Quorn and veg soupy-stew leaves a warm, full and satisfied belly. I find white fish, lean chicken breast and tins of tuna in brine (not oil), are all also good protein foods to have, but I must admit I enjoy the Quorn more than any of them. It's a funny thing, Quorn, the PW hates it, she thinks it tastes like cardboard, but to me it's a flavoursome LRD staple, not bad for something that is a fungus grown from mould in fermentation tanks. Whoever invented/discovered it is a genius. Did you know that it was originally made by Marlow Foods, which was formed by Rank Hovis McDougall (as in Hovis the bread people) and Imperial Chemical Industries (as in ICI the people who make paint and petrochemicals)? What an experimental marriage made in heaven! Quorn is named after the village of Quorn in Leicestershire, England. Interesting fact, the village of Quorn used to be called Quorndon, but there was another village in Derbyshire also called Quorndon and the postman got confused, so the Leicestershire village was renamed. I think Quorn sounds better than Quorndon, certainly from a marketing and brand perspective I'd rather eat a Quorn sausage than a Quorndon sausage, Quorndon sounds too posh. I wonder if any budding entrepreneurs in Quorndon have ever thought about releasing their own line of posh vegetarian or meat substitute foods under the brand Quorndon. Now there'd be a trademark fight with a historic backstory! "We had to rename our village because of you lot, now you're nicking our veggie sausage idea." I digress, let's get back to the LRD.

I keep my fluid intake high, with lots of water as well as three to four cups of tea or coffee per day. The caffeine is a welcome energy boost and is a good morning kick-starter. I completely avoid bread after the first day, as its calories are pretty empty when you consider its low nutritional value, it's just a bulker that I don't really need now. I also have to avoid all fizzy/carbonated drinks (including sparkling water) and definitely no alcohol. This is going to be my longest ever stretch without an alcoholic drink since my late teens, but the prospect of this bothers me less than I had thought it might. I get into the habit of going to bed either early or at a reasonable time, with 22:00 being the absolute latest that I stay up until, and my sleep is good, I'm averaging around 7 hours per night, which is probably around 90 minutes more than I would have slept before beginning the LRD. I maintain a night ban on reading the news or social media in bed and that helps my mind rest easier before closing my eyes.

After the first 11 days of the LRD, I have lost 9 pounds (4 kilos) in weight, the operation is 3 days away, and the PW and I are heading to my parents for Sunday lunch. I'm seriously going to have to moderate my eating behaviour. Sunday dinners at my parent's house are served buffet style, and as I've previously stated, I'm no shrinking violet at a buffet. My plate usually resembles a gravy-soaked Pennine mountain, and then there is always the temptation of seconds. Today will be very different for me eating-wise.

We arrive at my parents and I give them the good news that I have lost 9 pounds so far. They are both really pleased, but then my dad, quite out of character says emotionally, "well if you can do that, why do you need to have the operation? Why do you need to take the risk?" I can hear the worry in his voice, and I feel guilty for putting my parents through this. My mum is standing there silently, and they both look sad. I look him in the eye and say, "because I've done this before, and the weight will just go back on, it isn't sustainable, I really need to do this, please don't worry." The PW backs me up by reiterating that it is low-risk keyhole surgery. I can see my parents welling up and I hug them, and the PW also hugs them. After that unusually emotional opening, the day plays out like it usually does. We give thank you gifts, I pack the car with wood with the help of my dad, we talk about family and friends and we enjoy one of my mum's lovely Sunday lunches. I do indeed moderate my behaviour, by sticking to only boiled vegetables and roast beef, with just a little gravy. "Is that all you're having?" asks Mum. "It's all I can have," I reply, "this will be the size of a meal that I'll be able to manage after a few months, in the first few weeks I'll only be able to eat a very tiny amount." I had talked about this on my last visit, but I went over again the different dietary stages that follow bariatric surgery. Liquids, then purees, then eventually normal solid foods. At the end of the visit before we depart I hug them more tightly and for longer than I usually do. We are all thinking the same thing; "what if this is the final hug?" I mentally tell myself to pull myself together otherwise I'll well up and I don't want my parents to see that. "I'll call you the day before the operation," I tell them, and the PW adds that she'll call them as soon as I'm out of the operating theatre.

The drive back to Leeds is quiet and contemplative. The PW and I make small talk, but as the operation draws closer, my nerves are making me anxious. What if I do die? I don't want to die, I love being alive, it's great, I love my life and I don't want it to be over. We go up to bed not long after getting home, the PW goes to clean her teeth and I sit on the edge of the bed thinking about what would happen if things went wrong. By the time the PW has returned, I haven't moved, my head is down and tears are dripping from my nose onto the floor below making a 'pat...pat...pat' sound. "Oh baby," she says and sits beside me putting her arms around me. "What if I die?" I say. "You're not going to die, silly," replies the PW, "your heart is strong, you've already lost weight, and Mr Mehta is a great surgeon, you'll be fine." The PW is a pacifying wonder as well as a very good nurse, and in all matters medical she knows her stuff. We can be sitting watching any program on TV and as soon as somebody appears to be unwell, she'll make the diagnosis and she is always correct. I'm useless at things like that, so her insights give me confidence. She passes me a handkerchief and I wipe my eyes and blow my nose. I can count on one hand how many times I've cried in the past 20 years, all of which were related to the death of family or pets, and admittedly the climax to the *Avengers Endgame* movie, which was powerful stuff. Now I am crying at the prospect of my own death. Death makes me cry. I hate death and I hate crying, but there you go, there is a strong positive correlation between the two for me.

I lie in bed looking at the ceiling, holding the PW's left hand with my right hand, while she holds a book with her right hand, awkwardly turning the pages with the same hand that she is holding the book with. Eventually I let her have her hand back to make her nightly read an easier and less cumbersome task. I kiss her goodnight, and pull the straps from my CPAP mask around my face. I press the on button for the familiar rush of air, and I am sure that I won't sleep tonight for worrying. As it happens though I fall asleep almost immediately and sleep all the way through the night soundly. Perhaps I needed to have that cry and express my fears, perhaps I need to talk openly about how I felt, you know a burden shared is a burden halved and all that. I quite often see a graffiti tag around Headingley in Leeds that says 'talk more'; it's a scruffy and rubbish tag as nearly all graffiti tags are, but there is certainly some wisdom in those words.

Beyond this, the LRD continues until surgery day, it becomes routine, ordinary and no longer a burden, it becomes second nature to calorie count, make good choices and eat very healthily and cleanly. This would not be sustainable long-term, but I'm taking a project management approach to the weight loss process, and the 14 days of the LRD is just a period on a Gantt chart. I can feel my body shrinking, the LRD really is the ultimate 'shredding' diet, albeit one that leaves me with little energy at the end of each day. My bedtime is typically very welcome, another day down, another day closer to the operation. I don't like counting down my days, as I mentioned before, I love my life, but when it comes down to it, I just want to get the LRD over and done with, so I can move on to the next project stage, the truly scary project stage, where I'll be under anaesthetic, under the surgeon's knife and having part of my stomach cut out and removed. I need to do this, I need not to be afraid, I need not to be hungry. I need this operation, and I'm having it. I think of comedian Peter Kay in the John Smith's advert, the one where he kicks the football into the back of somebody's back garden; "have it." I imagine myself as Peter Kay (we have a similar body shape, although he probably weighs less than me). Instead of kicking a football though, I'm kicking my bloated stomach away to a place where it becomes irretrievable and will be lost forever, "have it." I'm having it, I'm having that operation and that's all there is to it, "having it."

5 – Op day

I am awoken at 05:10 on Wednesday the 30th of October by the beautiful and serene sounds of a harp being played up and down scales, which is one of the default alarm tones on my old iPhone 6. I have slept surprisingly well, but now it is time for action on this most important of days. With fingers fumbling into the dark cold air I locate my phone, open its wallet, and hit the alarm off button as my eyes wince at the piercing light emanating from the fully illuminated screen. I had set this alarm specifically, as today of all days I didn't want to play alarm bingo and risk being awoken by something sounding like a car alarm or worse. Today needs to go gently and relaxing, no loud noises, no sudden movements, no jolts, no shocks, just nice and comfortable. I am about to face the most traumatic experience that my body has been through since being born, and I don't want to do so with a racing heart.

I stretch my shoulders apart and lift my arms in front of me expressing a "yoweeeyow" sound as I stretch the night's sleep out of the upper part of my body. Besides me in our super king-sized 'American style' mega-bed my wife, the PW, rolls into me and gives me a welcoming kiss on the cheek. Welcome to the last day of my current life, and welcome to the first day of my new and improved one. She places her hand on my domed belly, and whispers in my ear, "it's going to be alright," I smile in the darkness and reply, "I know." Of course, I didn't know, but I don't want to express that. I might have 5 hours to live if things don't go according to plan, but I'd managed to kick my nerves of 10 days ago into touch and don't want those horrible little gremlins back in my brain. "Would you like a cuppa?" she says, "Yes," I reply, "250 ml of plain boiling water in a cup would go down lovely." We both laugh. I am not allowed a cup of tea, as would normally be the early morning routine, I have been nil by mouth since midnight, but I have instructions to drink 250ml of plain water at 06:00, so by the time I have showered the time to drink it will be almost right, and the boiling water will be of a drinkable temperature.

The bedroom lights go on and the PW disappears out of the door and down the first of two flights of stairs from our 'dorma' loft conversion bedroom. I pull the sticky CPAP machine mask from my mouth and nose, and place it on top of the CPAP machine by my bed. I press the 'off' button on the machine and its whirring and the sound of blowing air ceases. The CPAP mask is connected to the machine by a plastic hose, which has a life of its own and immediately pulls the mask off my machine and onto the floor. Hand over hand on the CPAP hose, I retrieve the mask and disassemble the machine's peripherals to go into my small hand-luggage sized rucksack to take to the hospital with me, as for me the CPAP is essential life-preserving kit. I don't go anywhere overnight without it. My machine is a Resmed S8, which is an old machine branded as being an 'Escape Travel CPAP'. Trust me, I travel a lot, I always take this machine with me, and in my budget-airline-sized hand luggage it feels like it weighs a bloody ton. I'm always both mildly bemused and slightly annoyed by the 'Escape Travel' tag. The weight of it certainly doesn't feel very escapist when travelling. I leave the bag by the bed for my wonderful PW to take down for me, as I will struggle on stairs with it more than she will, particularly as on a morning I very often need to use a crutch to take the pressure off my sore knee and ankle joints. I came to terms a long time ago, that a lot of the 'man-stuff' that I should be doing, is being done by her instead now, simply because she is more capable. My weight is a disabler.

We have a fantastic and very large bedroom, which covers a footprint almost the size of our entire house. We live in Cookridge, which is in northwest Leeds, and have panoramic bedroom views over a few streets, before the countryside of Horsforth, and on the horizon Leeds Bradford Airport, which is around 1 mile/1.6 kilometres away (as the crow flies). Our huge and comfortable bed is a plane-spotter's dream bed, as we can often lie there watching aircraft approach Runway 32 from the direction of Leeds city centre – no uncomfortable standing necessary! This morning was to be no such morning. The clocks have just gone back, it is dark outside, and a miserable wet mist hangs over the shallow valley that lies in-between Cookridge and Horsforth. If you didn't know there was an airport there, you wouldn't have known from this drab view.

The weather isn't helping my painfully arthritic right knee, and I have to use a crutch and a walking stick to get out of bed. I stumble around the bedroom grabbing bits of underwear and t-shirts, enough for a 2-night stay in hospital, as the PW returns, her cup of tea in hand. "I've left yours in your office," she says. My office is my Man Cave, my retreat into a world of screens, music and media. It also has an office chair and a comfy sofa, both of which I have spent far too many hours of my life on.

"Let's measure you," said the PW, "good idea," I reply, it will be good to see what a difference the LRD has made. I stand naked, supported by a crutch in all of my not-so-glory as the PW sets about measuring me with a tailor's accuracy. Pencil behind ear, and notepad by her side she goes from the top to bottom of my body with her tape measure. Whilst I do feel lighter, the physical pain of my arthritis isn't making me feel any better about myself. The PW does the big reveal and I am gobsmacked. I smile and say a victorious "yes" at every number she reads aloud. When she gets to my waist measurement I almost dance in joy. At first I question the number being correct, and she assures me that it is, she is after all a professional woman, as well as my perfect wife. The numbers and reductions in brackets are below.

Head 57 cm (-1 cm)

Neck 48 cm (-2 cm)

Chest 130 cm (-6 cm)

Waist 151 cm (-18 cm)

Hips 145 cm (-5 cm)

Arms 36.75 cm (-0.75 cm)

Thighs 65 cm (-2.5 cm)

Ankles 26 cm (-3 cm)

With an extra spring in my limp, I use a single crutch to painfully hobble down the first flight of stairs to the bathroom. I hate having arthritis, and my hope is that after surgery and significant weight loss my permanently sore knees and ankles will begin to recover, although my fear is that I'll suddenly become overactive on them with the newfound freedom of movement, and that might progress the wear and tear of my aching joints. Only time will tell, but I need to think positively towards the future, and the all-round health and lifestyle benefits that weight loss will bring. As I go down the stairs, I can see the marks on the staircase wall that the arm clasps on my crutches have made, as I've leaned into the wall for extra support. The PW only painted this wall a year ago, it looked perfect then, and now the ruts made from my crutches in the plasterboard resemble a pot-holed country lane after a winter thaw, which is an indication of how my arthritis has worsened in the past year. The journey downstairs is painful. Nil by mouth means no oral painkillers until I'm told otherwise, so I'll try rubbing ibuprofen gel into the joint after showering.

Before showering of course, there is the delicate matter of bowel movements, a subject that can't be sugar-coated (now there's an image) on a weight loss journey. The last thing that I want having abdominal surgery is a backed up colon and I'm hoping that I'll be able to go one last time before my operation. The news is good, it's a perfect splashdown, three good-sized sausages that would have been a 'Type 4' on the 'Bristol Stool Scale', described as being 'like a smooth, soft sausage or snake'. Lovely stuff. What goes in, invariably has to come out, and since beginning the LRD I've noticed how my poos have changed from being somewhere in-between 'Type 5' 'soft blobs with clear cut edges' and 'Type 6' 'mushy consistency with ragged edges' to a normal and healthy 'Type 4'. We don't talk about poo enough in Britain, and I think we should, it's a valid part of our body's eco-system, and can be a good indicator of digestive health. If you've never heard of the 'Bristol Stool Scale' before, then Google it, I find it fascinating!

After my morning ablutions I shower very thoroughly, behind my ears, in-between etc, I'm soon going to be naked in front of strangers, so would like to give a reasonably good impression. I shave and apply a generous splash of Brut aftershave. I'm 47 years old, so I'm allowed to wear Brut, and honestly, I like the smell of it, and if my surgical team like the smell of it, then hopefully they'll be happy in their work. I wear a small silver hooped earring in my left ear, the PW bought me this particular one, and I put it in over 10 year ago and have never removed it since. It was her way of saying "out with the old and in with the new" as she replaced a previous gold hoop earring bought by my previous girlfriend, thus eradicating any remnant of her from my body. All jewellery must be removed prior to surgery, so I fiddle with the back-clasp until it finally pops open, and out it comes. My left ear is now naked and will be for the first significant amount of time since I got it pierced on a cold and wet Barnsley Market in December 1991 to a soundtrack of Nirvana's 'Smells Like Teen Spirit'. I was working as a Christmas temp at Our Price Records in Barnsley town centre at the time, after having worked at Ardsley House hotel previously. The then boss at Ardsley House, Mr. Petherbridge, didn't allow male employees to have long hair or wear earrings. Something, which when you look back from 2019 seems completely ridiculous, but that was a sign of the times back then, at least in Barnsley anyway. So working in the record shop, I was free to grow my hair, wear an earring and be a rebel like my musical heroes, whilst working for an employer who was more focused on fashion and gender equality than my previous one. Incidentally, as I was a Christmas temp at Our Price I ended up back at Ardsley House by the beginning of February, with shorter hair and an earring that I did my utmost to keep hidden from 'Peth'.

Bathroom duties complete, I quickly put a wash-bag together to take to hospital with me. One final weigh-in reveals that my pre-surgery weight is 24 stone, and 1 pound (337 pounds/152.86 kilos), which means my total weight loss since the start of the LRD is 1 stone, 4 ¼ pounds (18.25 pounds/8.28 kilos). The LRD certainly has worked for me in terms of losing weight, although if I'm completely honest, I would have liked to have seen a bit more off, but hopefully I've done enough to shrink my liver sufficiently.

I leave the bathroom and get dressed into loose fitting clothing, a pair of trackie bottoms, a t-shirt and a fleece jacket. The PW has already brought my clothes down for me and placed them on one of the empty beds on the first floor of the house for me to sit on and get dressed (she really is perfect). Being physically bulky and unwieldly on my feet I can no longer do simple things like put on pants and socks standing, I need to sit down. I often marvel as the PW majestically and aerobically walks into her socks that she holds open in front of her as she gets out of bed, I don't think I've ever been able to do that. I then descend the second flight of stairs awkwardly with my crutch, making the odd profanity as I struggle with my crutch over some clothing left on the stairs.

At the bottom of the stairs is my Man Cave, within which the PW has placed my rucksack for the hospital and my 250ml of now warm water to drink before we leave. As I sip the water with a thousand-yard stare, thinking of the great life that I have lived so far, I spy my Australia travel diary from 1994-1995. I reach for the tattered notebook and thumb through it until I find the 30th October 1994, which happened to be a Sunday, curious to see what I had been up to a quarter of a century ago on that date.

"Came in from the club with Paul, pissed at 06:30am. See Fruddy as he is getting ready to go to work. Go to bed and get up at 1:30pm, have soup for breakfast/lunch. Go into the centre of Sydney, see movie 'The Power Rangers' being made outside of the Queen Victoria Building. Head to Darling Harbour and meet Denise for some beers. Head home, call in fish shop for fish and a fishcake and have these with sweetcorn and tinned potatoes for tea. In the evening I watch crap TV and make a bed settee from various cushions, quilts and blankets that we'd had donated. Skip comes in from the pub, and we talk and drink beer until 12:30am, when it's time for bed."

I think about all the things throughout my life that have led me to where I am now; too many late nights in clubs, too many beers, too many battered fried fish, too many sneaky extra fishcakes. Looking back I'm surprised that I didn't have chips as well, I can imagine at the time that I probably told myself, that if I had sweetcorn and tinned potatoes instead of chips that this wasn't technically an unhealthy tea. The extra fishcake was probably a spur of the moment last-minute decision in the fish shop, when the realisation of not having chips, and the thought of taking just a fish home would have made me feel sad. What an idiot I had been, and what an idiot I still was. I mentally punish myself for a few more seconds as I poke my toes into my flip-flops and kick them into place around my swollen feet. My Man Cave door opens and the PW puts her head around. "We'd better get off" she says. I smile at her and tell her that I love her, something that I do every single day without fail.

The drive to St. James's Hospital takes around 20 minutes on quiet dark suburban roads in the rain. The badly maintained yet slightly cheaper car park across the road from the hospital on Beckett Street is our destination. It is 6:53am, and I have 7 minutes to get to check-in and I am going to be late because the payment machine in the car park is swallowing coins and not giving out tickets. I will miss my operation and have to go to the back of the queue or worse still be struck off the list, fuck! My stress levels are rising on the day that I most need a calm heart. After wasting £3 in the machine and not getting anything for it, I tell the PW to go, and she snaps at me that she'll do no such thing. I can hear the stress in her voice, which is very rare; *deep breaths, Stuart, think.* I see another payment machine and we try that, bingo! The maximum stay is 4 hours, and the parking is free until 8am, so the ticket is valid until midday.

We leave the car park and cross the road to St. James's Hospital, where we are looking for Lincoln Wing. I think I know where I'm going and I clearly don't. The PW saves the day, and we enter the correct building with 2 minutes to spare as I hobble as fast as my arthritic legs will take me, walking stick in hand and bag on my back. We find a lift, go up two flights, get out, turn right, cross a bridge and then hit a crowd of people. I am confused, what are they all doing here? "All these people are waiting for operations too," says the PW. After all that stress, there are 20 plus people in front of us anyway. I don't really understand what the system here is, but PW knows the drill. She used to be a student nurse at this hospital and she has seen it all before. I am still confused, but happy that I wasn't going to get operation blacklisted, which incidentally I wouldn't have been anyway. After about 30 seconds a pair of double doors open, and like a herd of early morning zombies, the crowd of people shuffles in. This is when it gets interesting.

The system is highly efficient; people give their names and are quickly told whether to go and sit in the waiting room or get behind a blue curtain where empty assessment beds are waiting. A pack of medical staff are on hand and chomping at the bit to pounce on their prearranged quarry, take bloods, blood pressure, MRSA swabs, temperatures and all manner of other readings. Soon it is my turn at the front of the queue and I'm told that an emergency has come in, and that I should have been going to an assessment bed, but am now going to the waiting room, to await further instruction. I'm still confused. Does this mean that I'm not now having the operation? After the LRD and the mental build-up to Op Day, this is a possibility that I can't contemplate.

The waiting room is long and narrow with a door in the centre. Chairs surround the room against all of the four walls. The room was evidently once a ward, as the ceiling has bay-shaped curtain rails on it and the bank of plug sockets on the walls at regular intervals around the room is something that I'd love in the Man Cave. Mental note. Is the loss of these hospital beds down to Tory government spending cuts on health or something else? I'll blame the Tories as it fits my life narrative.

We sit there silently before exchanging distracted small talk in hushed tones. The room isn't big enough to have a private conversation and there are around ten other people also sat waiting in there, mostly middle-aged or elderly couples with the odd person who has come alone. I feel a bit sorry for the loners; although I nearly sent the PW home when the payment machine in the car park wouldn't work, I'm now glad that she stayed with me, in sickness and in health. The door bursts open, a young female member of staff cheerily calls out a name, and we all look around the room to see who the lucky winner is. An elderly lady who is there on her own gets up and walks to the door with a small old fashioned brown suitcase in her hand; it's probably not the first time she has won at bingo. She is the first one called out and we don't see her return.

Then somebody calls into the room, shouts out a name, and a chap sitting opposite us with his wife stands and leaves the room, leaving his bag with his wife. The PW smiles at his wife, who then tells us that this is their third time here, and every time they have been prior, they have been sent home as no beds were available in the high dependency unit (HDU). *Fuck.* I needed a bed in the HDU due to my sleep apnoea, an emergency had come in, and now I was going to get sent home and have to go back on the LRD until God knows when. "I need a HDU bed too," I say to his wife. "I hope you have better luck than us" she says back. *Double fuck.* I whisper to the PW that if my operation is cancelled and I have to go back onto the LRD that I'll probably not have the operation at all and just stay on the LRD for the rest of my life. I am talking bollocks, and the PW knows it and I know it too. Stress levels are rising, *be still my beating heart, calm blue oceans, tranquil skies*, I close my eyes and breathe deeply, in through my nose and out through my mouth, in through my nose and out through my mouth, and relax.

I open my eyes at the sound of the door opening as the chap sat opposite returns. He is wearing a medical wristband, which his wife expresses is a good sign as he's never got this far before. It transpires that he needs a HDU bed as he has a heart condition, but he is in for a prostate operation. When this information is volunteered to us, I feel the need to have to explain back why I am here and why I needed a HDU bed too. I tell them, "I've got to have most of my stomach removed, and I need a HDU bed as I have sleep apnoea," There is a moment's silence as the room digests what I've just said. "It's amazing what they can do these days," volunteers his wife. I nod and half smile in return.

In the corner of the room a mobile phone rings loudly, and I'm annoyed; this is a hospital, surely like a church this is somewhere where your phone should be on silent. The lack of mobile phone etiquette in society disturbs me. The woman who answers the phone speaks loudly, the person whom she is speaking to speaks loudly. They are having an inane conversation about nothing of any consequence at 07:20am. The woman whose phone it is has obviously no idea about the volume controls on her phone as everyone in the silent room can hear every word of the two-way conversation that they are having. They are talking about a remote control battery, I don't care about their stupid remote control or its battery, but I wince at the woman's pronunciation of battery, which is "ba-ery." This is a Leeds thing and I hate it. People in Leeds are seemingly incapable of pronouncing the letter t when it sits in the middle of a word, battery becomes ba-ery, computer becomes compu-er, tomato becomes toma-o, and my biggest pet hate tattoo becomes ta-oo. If you can say the first t, why can't you say the middle bloody two!? Stress levels are rising, I close my eyes and tilt my head back, again I think to myself *be still my beating heart, calm blue oceans, tranquil skies*, I breathe deeply, in through my nose and out through my mouth, in through my nose and out through my mouth. Then the door opens again and this time my name is called.

I leave the room with my bag and the PW comes with me; is this it? Am I having the operation? We are led back to the assessment room and I'm told to sit on the bed. Somehow I manage to misjudge the distance between my backside and the bed and end up hitting the bed too hard, too heavy, at an awkward angle and on the one percent of the bed that isn't fully padded. I take in a sharp intake of breath and the PW tells me to be careful. I'm such a fat lumbering idiot. A cheerful male doctor comes over with an understudy. I know that he's a doctor as he's dressed in 'civvies' rather than a medical uniform. I don't know why, maybe it's his physique, but he looks like he's played a bit of rugby in his life. He tells me his name and it immediately goes out of my head; *concentrate, Stuart*. I'll call him Gareth, because he looks like a Gareth, a rugby playing doctor Gareth. As he speaks, the PW is nodding and listening, she is acting on my behalf of my brain, as information isn't going into my head properly, and my own actual brain has seemingly gone for a walk. I'm presented with paperwork, which I agree is correct. I'm told that I could die for the second time, which I agree that I know, then I have to sign the paperwork, literally signing my life away. "So is the operation going to happen then?" I ask Doctor Gareth. "Hopefully," he replies, "but we can't say for sure, as Mr Mehta has to go in and do an emergency case." My surgeon Mr Mehta is a busy man, I'd already gathered that from my previous meeting with him. "I'll cross my fingers and everything else then," I tell Doctor Gareth, who smiles and leaves with paperwork in hand. Next comes a female medical member of staff, who wants to swab me for MRSA, take my temperature, and ask me some questions, all part of the pre-operation routine. She then presents me with not one, but two identical medical wristbands that contain a QR code, a bar code, my name, date of birth, NHS number, case note number and other information. The wristbands are placed on each wrist, before we are told to go back to the waiting room and await further instruction.

Back in the waiting room, the couple sitting opposite us are still there, but the noisy phone woman has thankfully gone. I proudly display my wristbands to the couple, who smile and tell me that it is a good sign. I cross my fingers and smile back at them. The PW has spotted a bookcase at the end of the room, so she goes to thumb through the books because she loves her books, but returns with a fashion magazine for herself, a gadget magazine for me and a copy of today's *Metro* newspaper. I take the gadget magazine but rebuff *the Metro*, I don't want to read more media lies about the EU or Corbyn. I hate the biased British news media for the damage that it does to our country, all to protect the selfish interests of billionaire tax-avoiding owners who live in foreign tax havens. I hate the lies that are told, the smears to any genuinely decent politician, and the fact that so many ordinary British people are either kept stupid or made more stupid by the newspapers. People believe what they read and that's a fact, which is why out of my 47 years on this earth the Tories have been in power for 29 of them, it feels like a lifetime. Yes I'm a leftie, I'm from very humble beginnings and I see true decency in Labour Party policies, which are designed to improve society, and make people's lives better. If it wasn't for the Labour Party, we wouldn't have a National Health Service, and I wouldn't be having this operation, and neither would most people in this room be having their operations either. I can guarantee that a fair few of the people sitting around me are Tories and they are the people who will miss the NHS the most when it is gone.

As I see it, Tory policy is about protecting the self-interests of the rich and keeping the majority of the population financially poor and uneducated enough not to question why they are poor. 'Boris' (his first name is actually Alexander) Johnson came to power giving tax breaks to millionaires. Jeremy Corbyn wants to give the UK four extra public holidays per year by properly celebrating the national holidays of England, Ireland, Scotland and Wales, which would put the UK into alignment with the rest of Europe, which has an average of 14 public holidays per year (the UK has only 10). Which of these examples is a benefit to the average British person? Yet I know for a fact that the Tories will win the next general election, and we will have to endure at least five more years of their selfish rule. The Union Jack flag-waving Tories don't even want to make our national days holidays, because it will cost their billionaire corporation owning friends money.

Trickle-down economics doesn't work, it's bollocks, the trickle just gets smaller as those pouring the bottle tilt it less. Britain used to have an Empire, it was the richest and most powerful country on the planet, it enslaved, exploited and 'owned' seemingly half the globe, yet poverty in Britain was rife, prostitution was one of the largest professions of females in cities and life expectancy for the average person was in their 30s. If British people were living in poverty in the days of Empire, then there's little hope for today.

Jump forward to today and the average life expectancy in Britain is now 80 years and 11 months, thanks to advances in health, social services, working conditions, homes and education, which were all post-war Labour Party initiatives. I'm not saying that the Labour Party are the only reason that we live longer, improvements in lifestyle, diet and a whole plethora of things have played their part, but I can say for a fact that Labour policies have certainly helped.

Tory austerity has for the first time ever led to life expectancy in the UK falling. In some economically deprived areas women are living on average 100 days less than they were doing. The picture is less clear for men, but altogether under the Tories in the 2010s, the growth rate in the life expectancy of British people has stalled. Did you know that the Tory party want you to work until you are 75 years old? Can you imagine a fire fighter working until they are 75 before they can draw a state pension? It is utterly ridiculous. The British people recently voted *Mrs Brown's Boys* the greatest comedy of all time, it does make me wonder if they should be allowed to vote on anything more important.

Note: you might not agree with my politics or opinions, but I hope that you will not let this put you off reading this book. I might not like Tory policy, but I don't let it stop me from enjoying the products of those who do support it. As a society, we need to agree to disagree more often. According to Evolve Politics, Samworth Brothers Director Mark Samworth has donated £585,000 to the Tories since 2010. Samworth Brothers own the brand Ginsters, whose cheese and onion pasties have provided me with a quick fix of lunchtime stodge on too many occasions over the years. With the benefit of hindsight I wish that I hadn't eaten quite so many of them now, another piece in the jigsaw puzzle of my banana journey identified.

RANT OVER

The gadget magazine is a year out of date and not that interesting. I can't concentrate anyway. The PW's phone vibrates as the ringer is on silent and because she has good mobile phone etiquette she leaves the room to answer it. I sit there silently, occasionally smiling in the direction of the couple opposite. The minutes roll by and everyone else in the room is either reading or looking at a phone screen, with the only sounds being of a wall clock ticking and the occasional page turning. Suddenly, there is action in the corridor outside as I see through the glass in the door the first of several beds on wheels with people lying on them rolled past the waiting room and back into the assessment room. After only a little more than an hour from arriving, the first operations have been completed, and patients are being returned to their awaiting loved ones who are sitting amongst the people awaiting operations in the room that I am in. A lady sitting three chairs to my left says in an unusually plummy English accent, "that's my husband," as she smiles, holding her hands together in front of her chest almost praying, with a tear in her eye. The aura of happiness and relief emanating from her seems to give the otherwise stark room a sunrise glow. She stands and walks to the door, looking through the glass towards the assessment room as another bed passes her, and another. I'm impressed by the process here, the system is evidently a finely tuned machine of efficiency, as the first round of operations are over and the next round commences. The man opposite me is called out; after missing his turn twice, it looks like third time lucky. "Good luck," I say as he leaves the room with his wife. The man says, "thanks," and the wife says, "you too," then the plummy-sounding lady is called to go and sit with her husband in the assessment room as he drifts back into consciousness from the general anaesthetic.

The PW returns into the room, phone in hand. "What's happened then?" I ask her. "That was Becky," she says. Becky is our youngest daughter, who in her early 20s is today moving with her boyfriend Brendon to Stevenage. Wrapped up in my own thoughts about what I'm facing today, I had lost sight of what the PW was facing. Not only does she have the stress of me going into hospital, she also had the stress of Becky moving, not just because of the worryingly long journey for them down the M1 in the rain, but because the PW was also dealing with the removal company, who were coming to collect all of Becky and Brendon's belongings from our house at 4pm. It was an unfortunate coincidence. A few days before, Becky and Brendon had brought almost all of their entire possessions to our house, so that they could clean the rental property that they were in, in order to get their deposit back. An efficient chain of Becky – Brendon – PW had taken boxes of belongings upstairs to Becky's former bedroom (now my morning dressing room). Whilst doing so, I sat silently in my Man Cave below not helping out because of my clumsy weight and arthritic joints. I struggled to climb stairs with empty hands, let alone with boxes in them, at times I was less than useless. None of them held a grudge or thought I was lazy for not helping out, they all knew that I would be more hindrance than help, and that it would be easier just to get the job done without me. I do look forward to being useful again.

The reason for Becky's phone call was that misfortune had thrown a spanner in the works on their way to Stevenage. Fortunately they were both fine, as was their travelling companion dog 'Hera', but on the M1, the clutch on their old car had decided to give up the ghost, and their car had broken down. I was very relieved that this wasn't on one of the sections of the 'smart motorway' (now there's an oxymoron for you) that didn't have a hard shoulder. It had been in the news only a week before that the widow of a man killed on a stretch of the M1 that had been converted to run as a smart motorway was suing Highways England for corporate manslaughter. Smart Motorways were now under review by the government, and I sincerely hope this costly smart white elephant is made dumb again. The hard shoulder has always been the sanctuary at the side of a motorway for broken down vehicles, but now it is being used to ease traffic congestion, something that simply encourages more people to drive cars instead of using underfunded public transport.

It's scary breaking down on a motorway, I know first-hand. Returning from the Reading 93 Festival in a hire van to Barnsley, we had a front right-side blow-out. With bits of tyre flying everywhere to the right of the vehicle, our skilful driver 'Scoff' safely got us onto the hard shoulder. Sitting next to him on the double front seat and almost porcelain white through shock was his girlfriend Christine. Along with me in the back of the van were Maria and Anne-Marie. We were all good friends that clubbed, raved, gigged and partied together. As the tyre blew, our post-Reading Festival exhaustion and hangovers were being slept off across heaps of tents, blankets and sleeping bags. Scoff did the hard work of keeping awake to drive us all home. Our slumber was rudely interrupted by the heavy juddering of the van as the tyre rubber flew. It was technically illegal for people to travel in the back of a hire van, as the vehicle was not for passenger transport. At 21 years old, we didn't care about that, but now we did as we slid open the side door and fell out onto the hard shoulder in a frightened daze.

After the initial shock wore off we laughed at our predicament as thundering juggernauts hurtled by at 70 miles per hour. This was before the days of mobile phones. This was when people only used landlines and telephone directories. None of us knew how to change a tyre, or even where the spare tyre was. Thankfully, in the days of dumb motorways there were orange emergency phones along the hard shoulder, roughly every half mile. It was decided that I would be the one who would have to walk along the hard shoulder to make the emergency call. I had been walking for around 5 minutes, being very careful of the traffic hurtling past to my right (it really was quite scary), when I looked down and saw a metal hoop on the hard shoulder. I presumed it was part of a tyre. As a daft 21-year old-raver, I thought it would make a fun fashion accessory to wear around my neck. I bent down to pick it up, and out of the corner of my left eye saw something in the grass next to the hard shoulder that looked like a £20 note. Upon closer inspection I saw that it was indeed a £20 note, albeit sun-bleached and weather-beaten, but it would definitely be spendable. I bent down to pick it up, and then saw another, and another, and another and then a £5 note. In seconds I had collected £85 as my fear of the hard shoulder dissipated. I did a hands and knees finger-tip search of the grass for a couple of minutes but found nothing else. In those days, a week's wage for me was around £90, so I was more than happy with this unexpected bonus.

I carried on to the emergency phone, made the call, and rescue was summoned. We were instructed to get out of the van and wait on the grass by the side of the hard shoulder. I was so happy with my find that I almost skipped along the hard shoulder back to the broken-down van. Passing drivers must have thought that I was a right nutter skipping along the hard shoulder with a metal hoop around my neck. Back at the van, everyone was laid out on blankets on the grass by the hard shoulder. The shock and fear of what had happened had dissipated and now everyone was just chilling out sunbathing, drinking pop and eating crisps. I regaled them with my story and showed them the money, and everyone was impressed and happy for me.

Eventually AA rescue arrived, but it wasn't good news. The hire van's spare tyre was missing! Fortunately, the hire company was AA certified, so the van could be carried back on top of the rescue lorry and there was room for four passengers in the driver's cab. However, there were five of us, and that meant that one of us had to walk 2 miles by the side of the motorway towards an exit and make our own way back to Barnsley from there. Naturally that person was going to have to be me, and with my newly found £85 of travel money in my pocket I couldn't complain either.

It took a while to get the van onto the back of the lorry, with all winches and levers in action. The other four had got into the lorry's cab and we had already said our farewells (at least I wouldn't have to help unpack the very full van anyway). With just me and the AA man standing by the lorry while he secured the last straps, I pulled out £20 and said, "might this get me a lift in the back of the van?" "What, up there?" he replied incredulously. I smiled and held out the money. He looked at it, grabbed it, pocketed it, turned around, looked away and said, "I haven't seen anything." I quickly climbed up the lorry's ramp, opened the sliding van door, leapt in, and slammed it close. I fell back into a star shape on all the blankets and sleeping bags. The AA man was completely breaking the law and would have been fired if he'd been found out, but he was happy with his £20 and I was happy with my £65 and ride home. I kicked off my army boots, got myself comfortable and proceeded to eat all of the packets of remaining crisps and biscuits, before opening somebody else's leftover cider. I drank all of that too. I was a greedy bugger, a bingeing greedy bugger. Yet more pieces in the jigsaw to what had got me where I am today.

On the journey north, I remember waking up from my slumber needing a pee. I kneeled up on the sleeping bags and saw Meadowhall out of the van window, so we were crossing Tinsley Viaduct. I had quite the vantage point and the view of the sprawling shopping centre below was impressive. I found an empty pop bottle to pee in, which wasn't quite big enough at the top to comfortably guarantee no spillage and peed away as the van swayed on the back of the lorry. I'm pretty sure a couple of sleeping bags got a bit of a shower, but hey ho. Still to this day I wonder how that £85 had ended up at the side of the motorway; had it been an accident? Had it been thrown out by drug dealers being pursued by the police? I'll never know, but fate can play a strange role in life's journey, something that I would go on to find out again and again.

Back to today and Becky's phone call had cost the PW £450 for a whole new clutch fitting. At least they were safe, it was also fortunate that the job could be done straight away so they would still be able to get to Stevenage today, to collect their new house keys and to be at their new home in time for the removal company arriving with their belongings. This was stress off both of our minds. All's well that ends well.

The waiting room door opens again, and standing in front of me is my surgeon, Mr Mehta. "Stuart," he says to me and smiles, "step this way, we need to have a chat." I ask the PW to stay in the waiting room with my bag; if this is going to be bad news, I want to face it alone. I follow Mr Mehta out through the door and into a small room across the corridor. I sink heavily into a chair and Mr Mehta sits opposite me. Besides Mr Mehta is a trainee or junior doctor. I don't look at him once, I only have eyes for Mr Mehta. This is going to be make or break time. My mouth is closed and I nose-breathe with my hands resting on my belly, fingers intertwined, as Mr Mehta goes over all the previous things that he had gone through when we last met, and all of the things that Doctor Gareth had gone through too. His voice is soft but very clear, I nod occasionally as he speaks, he asks me questions, I answer them. Then he asks me if I have any questions. "So is the operation on then?" I quietly say. "Hopefully," says Mr Mehta, "but I can't guarantee anything as an emergency has come in and I'm now going to theatre." "So what will I do if it's cancelled?" I reply. "You'll stay on the LRD," says Mr Mehta. This is something that I don't want to hear. I'm going out, drinking gin and having a curry tonight if the operation is cancelled, I'll then go back on the LRD tomorrow with a hangover and a full belly. "Is there anything else?" asks Mr Mehta? "Two things actually," I reply. "If the operation does go ahead, can I have a pillow under my knees when I'm laying down? It's for my arthritis." "That's nothing of a request," replies Mr Mehta, it was something of a request for me if he wanted me up and moving any time after the operation. "And also," I add, "I've got theatre tickets for tomorrow night, if I do have the operation today, what are the chances of me getting there?" Mr Mehta looks at me as though I've just asked him if I could date his daughter. "You're kidding aren't you?" he says, "this is major surgery, there'll be no theatre for you tomorrow or any time soon, you'll be exhausted." I nod my head, half smile and say, "I was kidding actually." As it happened, I had two tickets to see Jonathan Pie at Leeds Town Hall, so I wasn't kidding, and Mr Metha knew that I wasn't either. What an idiot I am. What an absolute thick, fat, clot. Mr Mehta heads out of the room pursued by his understudy. I go back into the waiting room and sit with the PW. "It's not definitely on, but it's not off yet either," I tell her. She puts her hand on top of mine.

The time rolls on, the clock ticks, pages turn, people come and go. It is now 11:15am, and the PW has 45 minutes left on the car park ticket. I am resigned to the likelihood that the operation isn't happening today, when the door opens and a female doctor calls out my name. "Would you like to come through," she says. Bloody hell, it looks like it's on. My heart starts to race as my breathing shallows. We are led to an empty bed in the assessment room, a curtain is pulled around the bed, and I'm asked a few questions about what I've brought with me. This needs to be written down. When this formality is complete, I'm told to strip, put on a pair of mesh underpants, a pair of anti-embolism stockings and a medical gown that is tied together at the back. My lumbering bulk of a disability is immediately a problem, as after stripping, I can't get my feet in the mesh underpants. Ever the medic, the PW assists, and I'm standing there in mesh pants that look like they should have satsumas in them. Next comes the stockings, thank God for the PW, as I would have had no chance of getting them on or off. They bite tightly and it doesn't feel very nice. Then the floral patterned medical gown, which doesn't fit me at all, there's a huge amount of open flesh visible behind. The PW goes and asks for a larger gown. I'm given a bariatric gown that drowns me. This gown is different to the other gown, it is a vibrant blue and a more papery material, very similar to the curtains drawn around the bed. Then I realise that this gown is actually a curtain, just with strings attached at the back. I'm so fat that I literally have to wear a hospital curtain to go to theatre in, the final insult before my new life begins. The PW takes a photo of me in my curtain. I have to laugh and give a double thumbs up, it might be the last photo she ever takes of me. "Loss of Dignity 1 – Stuart 0," I say.

Time passes, and the PW is going to have to go soon with the car parking ticket set to expire. It gets to 11:45am, and I tell her to go. She knows that the chances are now good for the operation happening, and it is going to take her 10 minutes to get back to the car. She knows that she has to go, and I don't think either of us want a tearful goodbye in front of the hospital staff, so we kiss behind the curtain (not the one that I am wearing), we both say, "goodbye," and we both say, "I love you." The PW leaves the assessment room and I sit on the assessment bed with tears in my eyes. I can hear the plummy-sounding lady from the waiting room speaking to her now conscious husband.

Minutes pass by, then at 12:07pm the curtain is pulled back and the female doctor and a porter are there. My time has come. I get down from the bed as the porter has a wheelchair for me. Not just any wheelchair, but a bariatric double-sized wheelchair, in essence a wheelchair for two. This is one last final indignation for me in my old life as I am wheeled through the corridors in a double-sized wheelchair, wearing my curtain. My possessions are left in the assessment room to later be taken to the HDU, apart from my CPAP machine, which is accompanying me to the operating theatre. Whilst I won't be wearing it during the operation, it needs to go on me afterwards.

The journey to the operating theatre takes a couple of minutes, and once there I am approached by a smiling female surgeon wearing a bandana. She asks me if I can transfer myself onto a trolley. I manage this OK and she advises me where to shuffle my bottom onto the trolley as I lie down. My curtain covers me well and I slide with ease. Satisfied that my position is suitable, the female surgeon pushes me through to the operating theatre. There are flowers of lights on shiny metallic stems, the lighting isn't too bright, and there seems to be a metallic blueness to the room. I am introduced to the anaesthetist. I was expecting to be given a 'pre-med' to calm me down before the anaesthetic, but instead he produces a cannula, which is a tube that is inserted into the vein on the back of my right hand. "Sharp scratch," he says, there is a moment of stinging pain, and then the cannula is inserted.

As the anaesthetist prepares the anaesthetic, I volunteer that I have lost 18 pounds on the LRD, so I hope that my liver has shrunk enough for the operation. I am congratulated by both members of the team. The female surgeon tells me that she has lost 3½ stone on Slimming World so far. I am genuinely happy for her and congratulate her, and beneath the flowing gown she is wearing I cannot see that she is overweight. I explain that I tried Slimming World, but ultimately it didn't work for me. The anaesthetist then says, "If you can lose that weight on the liver diet, why are you putting yourself through this?" I'm slightly sideswiped by the question. The last time I was asked this was by my worried parents, I really didn't expect to hear it again on the operating table. I offer a one-word answer, "unsustainable."

I think about the good life I have had led, and all of the mistakes that I have made that have put me here. I am breathing in through my nose and out through my mouth. There is no sign of Mr Mehta. I mention to them both about my CPAP and my request for a pillow beneath my knees. The anaesthetist tells me that I won't need a pillow as I will be tilted upwards, almost standing to be operated upon. I imagine myself suspended in mid-air beneath the operating theatre's flower-shaped stadium lights, my arms and legs outstretched like Michelangelo's 'Vitruvian Man' with an overhanging gut, wearing a curtain cape and satsuma netting underpants.

The anaesthetic is connected to the cannula and the plunger depressed, shooting pure fire into the vein of my right hand and into my arm. "That burns," I say. "I'll go easier," replied the anaesthetist as the fire begins to consume my entire body. I know that this is it, I have passed the point of no return. I count down in my head from ten, nine, eight, seven…I close my eyes and am enveloped by the darkness.

6 – The HDU

General anaesthetic tastes somewhere between how a mixture of burnt plastic and superglue might smell. It's very chemically, very powerful, very horrible. Although I hadn't drunk any general anaesthetic, I'd had enough of it pumped into me to feel like a sponge that had been soaked in it, and now it was oozing out of every pore. It was all that I could taste, all that I could smell and I was breathing it out like a chemical dragon. If I'd been a superhero my name would have been 'The Anesthetiser', a man with breath so powerful, the bad guys didn't stand a chance, one breath and they're all asleep. Lock 'em up, sheriff!

The trolley sways and I open my eyes to see a hospital porter and somebody in a surgical outfit. I think that I hear the words "everything went fine, and you're off to HDU," but to be completely honest, I'm so out of it, I could have been riding on a cloud with Ali Baba. I sense motion and open my eyes again looking forward. The trolley bed is moving steadily through hospital corridors, and I'm sure that I'm passing intricate floral collage artwork, either that or I'm so stoned that I'm in a Hieronymus Bosch painting. How I wish I'd brought my Go Pro to film this trip, thousands of people would watch this film, Google Adsense would pay me a fortune for advertising on it.

The lighting changes from bright white to a subtle metallic blue; oh no, am I back in the operating theatre? Through the blur a friendly young female nurse's face comes into focus. "Welcome to HDU, Mr Moss, I'm Hannah." It is nice having a Hannah around, my eldest daughter is called Hannah. "Can I have my CPAP on please?" I reply. Even though I'm whacked out on general anaesthetic, and as it turns out a good dose of morphine, my survival instinct of needing CPAP emerges to the fore. On my 'Maslow's Hierarchy of Needs' the CPAP is definitely in the base level. I can't let myself fall asleep without it. My CPAP is assembled by Hannah and plugged in, and she passes me the face mask. The face straps are twisted, they are always twisted.

Hannah helps me to get them straight. "These things always do that, she says. I nod in agreement, they really do. Hannah removes a very delicate oxygen pipe from beneath my nose, and between us we get the mask on my face and over my nose and mouth, with the elasticated strap placed behind my head securing it tightly. Now I feel safe. I think that I am then given some orientation from Hannah about my bed and morphine, but I'm so tired that the words bounce off me. I close my eyes, breathing in through my nose and out through my mouth. The air in my CPAP mask tastes of chemicals from the anaesthetic. Suddenly I go from almost asleep to very awake as I open my eyes, take a deep mouth breath and croak to Hannah, "can I have a pillow under my knees please?" The knee pillow is also base level on my Maslow's Hierarchy. Hannah obliges and I can feel the comfort of having slightly bent legs again. I feel safe now, safe to sleep and take the next steps as they happen. "Thank you," I say to Hannah as I close my eyes again, breathing deeply. I'm not conscious for much longer.

I have very little recollection of this, but at some point in the late afternoon, the PW visits me. I do remember seeing her face, I do remember her holding my hand, but trying to escape the clutches of sleep to partake in conversation is something that I'm not yet strong enough to do. The PW later told me that out of the 3 hours that she visited for, I had been awake for no more than 10 minutes. She had been shocked at how poorly I looked connected to all manner of machines and fluids. After both of us had previously downplayed the severity of the surgery as being 'only keyhole'. I think that was the moment of realisation for her how major the surgery I'd been in for had actually been.

I'm awoken at some point later by Hannah's voice saying, "just going to take your temperature." I feel something being pushed into my ear; at first I think I'm dreaming, it feels weird, I hope nothing is burrowing into me. I open my eyes to see Hannah stood over me smiling. "That's fine," she says, looking at a gadget in her hand that looks like a glue gun. She then proceeds to take my blood pressure through an inflatable arm cup and my oxygen saturation from a peg on my right index finger. "They're fine too," she adds. I don't have a clue what fine is, my medical knowledge is limited. I peel the sticky silicone of the CPAP seal from my nose and mouth, and the air continues to blow through it. I raise myself onto one elbow. "Can I have a drink of water please?" "Of course," she replies and hands me a small tumbler. I notice that the tumbler is on a trolley table next to the bed and besides it there is a jug with around 500ml of water in it. The water tastes like anaesthetic, but I drink the whole glass, my dry cracked tongue and throat like a desert gully after heavy rainfall. I do a prolonged, strangled gurgled burp. "Excuse me," I say. "You'll do a lot of that due to the trapped wind inside you," says Hannah. She isn't wrong, I find myself burping constantly after drinking. Then it strikes me, shouldn't I feel a restriction? If I can drink a full glass of water like that, how much will my appetite be suppressed? I put my ability to drink the water so quickly down to the fact that it is only water, so must pass through quickly. Besides this, I am so dry after not drinking since God knows when, that my body is probably sucking the moisture out of my gut to replenish its supplies everywhere else.

Hannah sets about reorienting me to my bed and its surroundings, I have a remote control to adjust the position of my bed, which is useful, and I press a button to put me in a slightly more upright position. The cannula on the back of my hand is now connected to a saline drip. I have morphine on tap at the press of a button. I'm not sure where the morphine is entering my body, I can't tell and I don't care. I've just had major surgery, and I can't feel any pain whatsoever, and besides this my painful arthritic knee feels just fine. My knee has been agonising for weeks, so this is very welcome relief. I give the morphine button a push for good luck. There is a beep. I can press the button whenever I like, and if I overdo it, the machine won't administer. I'm fine with that. On the other side of my bed I have a call button; this will summon a member of the HDU team to my bed, and emits a different beep, it also turns on a light above me to indicate that my bed is the one where a staff member needs to go. It reminds me of the post office or Argos; "order number 52 to the collection point please." Hannah explains to me that she will be with me all night and that her work partner is called Sunni. Her warmth and friendliness puts me at great ease and I know that I am in safe hands here. Hannah leaves my bed to go about her duties elsewhere in the room, but is reassuringly nearly always within eyesight, such is the layout of the

HDU. I pour another glass of water, and another, and another, drinking and burping until the jug is empty. I'm not gulping it down, I'm 'heavy sipping', its cool moisture is relief to the desert floor of my mouth.

It is then at this precise moment that the realisation finally hits me that I've not only gone through with it, but I've survived the operation. I'm alive, I'm going to be physically fitter, I'm going to be able to do things that I haven't done for years, and I'm going to live longer. I should be very happy about this. I am very happy about this, I am euphoric! A wide beaming smile breaks across my face. *I've only gone and bloody done it. I've done it, I went through with it, I've done it.* I take a double shot of morphine in celebration before affixing the CPAP mask over my nose and mouth, and put my head back on the very comfortable pillow. I press the bed button to go back into a reclined position and sink deeply into a very happy and refreshingly moist chemical cloud of sleep.

"Hello, Mr Moss, I'm just going to take your temperature." This time the voice is male and the accent distinctly East Asian. There is the now familiar feeling of the thermometer probe burrowing into my left ear. I look up and see a South East Asian man. He tells me that my temperature is fine, then puts a peg on my finger and a blood pressure sleeve around my arm. The sleeve is inflated and grips me tightly before deflating in stages. "All good," says the male nurse. He gathers his equipment and turns to leave. I pull off my mask. "Are you Sunni?" I say. He turns around, smiles and says, "yes." "Where are you from?" I ask. "The Philippines," he replies. "I wondered if you were." I proceed to tell Sunni that I had been to the Philippines. "Really, was it Manila you went to?" remarks Sunni. I imagine he hasn't come across too many people from Leeds who have been to his home country.

In October 1994 on our way to Australia, Skip, Fruddy and I called en route for 10 days to the Philippines. We were three clueless 22-year-olds from Barnsley, who had mostly only done bucket-and-spade holidays before in Europe. Worldly-wise we were not. We would soon learn very quickly though. On arrival in Manila, we had very little local currency, very little idea of what the hell to do and very little idea about where to stay. In the end we saw a hotel advertised in the airport and just got a taxi there hoping for the best. Leaving the airport into the piercing sticky heat with a sea of shouting faces and outstretched arms was terrifying. Everybody wanted our attention and I was very glad to find the sanctuary of a taxi. We were three young white guys, I had a camouflaged backpack and hat on, and everyone thought we were American soldiers, at least they thought that I was. "We're English, we're English," we kept repeating, "no US dollars." The roads in Manila were also terrifying and I was completely amazed at the chaos and how I never once saw an accident. The hotel we found was awful and very expensive, we didn't have much money, but we didn't have much choice. We thought the Philippines was meant to be cheap! Maybe we were just being ripped off for being stupid. Skip and Fruddy had to share a double bed, whilst I had to sleep on a bare stained mattress on the floor. It was grim, and it got worse that night when we went out for a beer, only to be ruthlessly pursued by drug dealers and pimps. We literally had a criminal entourage.

The next day we decided to get out of Dodge, nine more days of that hell was not what any of us wanted, so we took a bus south to the city of Batangas and then a ferry to a little place called Puerto Galera, a nice beachy seaside town on the island of Oriental Mindoro. From there we took a taxi boat, (which was a motorised canoe with stabilisers on either side) to what I can only describe as a tropical paradise resort. The resort looked incredible from the sea, golden sand and palm trees, with small wooden thatched huts dotted here and there in-between. The taxi boat pulled right up onto the sand to the beach itself. I'd seen this before on TV, I knew the drill, somebody had to jump off the front and pull the front of the taxi boat further into the sand to hold it steady. I pulled my 15kg backpack on and like Action Man jumped from the canoe onto the beach. Big mistake. As I think back now, the next few seconds felt like they lasted minutes, as I hit the sand I heard the crack of a rifle, it was definitely a gunshot and I took a bullet straight in the right knee. I, with my military backpack and camouflage hat, had been singled out, I fell to the beach screaming at the top of my lungs, my backpack holding me down on my back with exposed belly as my t-shirt rolled up Winnie the Pooh style, my face was in the air, contorted in agony, "aaarrrggghhhh" at an incredible volume coming out of my mouth. Then I was silenced, and drowning and choking as the waves of the sea washed up the beach and completely over me, soaking me from head to toe, goodbye sunglasses. The water drained back and I writhed in agony like a flipped turtle about to be dealt a final death blow. I could hear laughter. Laughter? Not just laughter, my friends' laughter. Skip and Fruddy were in hysterics at the sight of me half drowned and floundering on my back, held down by my backpack. "My knee," I screamed, "didn't you hear it?" The crack was so loud I was convinced that everyone must have heard it. Then they realised I was actually in genuine pain and jumped off the boat to pull me up the beach. I hadn't been shot but my right knee was buggered or more precisely, my anterior cruciate ligament was torn (I found this out sometime later) and I was in inconceivable pain.

I don't know how the lads managed to get me up and off the beach, and I don't know how I managed to end up in an accommodation hut, in stifling heat and searing pain, but my tropical paradise became for the next 48 hours my tropical hell hole as I lay on another bare mattress, unable to move and getting eaten alive by God knows what. It took me 2 days to get out of bed, ask the resort to call me a doctor, and the nearest one was all the way back across the water in Batangas. I had to pay her fare on the ferry and for her water taxi as well as the call-out fee and for medicine. She arrived several hours later, a little old lady with a black medical bag and a stethoscope. She listened to my chest, she listened to my belly and then she listened to my knee. Which I must admit, I thought was a bit weird. She scribbled away on a piece of paper, gave me a box of tablets, and told me to take four per day. With that she left the resort and headed back to Batangas. There was to be no follow-up. As she walked away I looked at the piece of paper she had given me; she had written 'triple heartbeat, peptic ulcers and knee injury'. Skip and Fruddy almost wet themselves laughing at her amazing 'diagnosis'. I took the pills anyway, and you know what? I was high as a kite for the next few days and the pain subsided remarkably, enough to allow me to hobble around with the help of a walking stick made by some local lads from a piece of bamboo.

I am now high as a kite on morphine in the HDU, at least I am pretty out of it, too out of it to regale Sunni with that full story, so I simply tell him the names of the places that I've been to. "They're north," says Sunni, "I'm from south." "I thought I was south," I reply. He smiles and shakes his head. "No, definitely north," he replies. He seems disappointed that I didn't go further south, so I throw him one more titbit. "I'm also a Visiting Professor in Employability at the Imus Institute of Science and Technology." This is indeed true, although I haven't yet been to fulfil my Visiting Professor role, hopefully soon I will be doing. This seems to impress Sunni more, even though Imus is also north. Sunni goes about his duties, and I put my head back and think about the places that I've been and the many experiences that I have had throughout my good life. The legacy of that knee injury in the Philippines is my very painful knee arthritis today, something which will stay with me for the rest of my life. If only I hadn't tried to be the Action Man hero, jumping off the boat with a 15-kilo backpack on when nobody had asked me to. What an idiot, but that continued leg pain, the regular flare-ups, having to spend prolonged amounts of time sitting down and inactive are all aspects of my banana journey.

The effects of the anaesthetic and the morphine are slowly wearing off and I am awake. I can feel some pain in my abdomen and right shoulder, but I put this down to being trapped wind, which I have read much about, prior to coming into hospital. It strikes me how noisy the HDU actually is. There is a symphony of beeps, bells, alarms, and machine noises that are constant. Besides this the patient to my left, whom I cannot see due to a dividing curtain, is making a lot of noise, he is evidently in pain and is groaning as well as sleep-talking. I cannot tell what he is saying, his words seem strangely echoing, maybe it is the effect of the cocktail of drugs that my body has ingested. I remove my CPAP mask, and this time switch off the machine. I want to take in my surroundings a little better, so I find the bed remote control and adjust my position into a slightly more upright one.

The HDU is an impressively designed space. From where I'm lying, the beds seem to be set out in a clock face arrangement, with a nurses' station in the centre. Everyone in a bed has eyesight of the nurses' station for reassurance, and the nurses can all see their patients. There is a good amount of floor space, almost dance-floor-sized between the beds and the nurses' station. The lighting is subtle, and there is an unmistakable metallic blueness to its hue. It reminds me a little of the bridge in the Starship Enterprise, albeit with a dance-floor and different uniformed staff, who carry glue-gun shaped thermometers instead of deadly fazers. There is no sign of Captain Kirk, but I'm sure he'll be around at some point to throw some shapes on the HDU dancefloor. I press the bed button to recline my posture once again, reaffix my CPAP mask, hit the on button and have one more shot of morphine for my warp speed trip into sleeping space.

"Morning," a different voice stirs me from my slumber. This voice is cheery and distinctly Midlands-ish, but not quite. I open my eyes to see a short female nurse. "I'm Sinead." "Stuart," I offer in return. The familiar routine of temperature, blood pressure and oxygen saturation readings are taken. "The doctors will be round soon," says Sinead, "so let's just get you ready a bit." I'm not sure what "ready a bit" is, but I fear that it involves movement. I'm comfortable in my sarcophagus of sheets and blankets. Sinead presses the button that puts my bed into more of a sitting position. "Have we to have a wash?" asks Sinead. The dreaded bed bath, another loss of dignity. "Is that a West Midlands accent?" I ask Sinead, trying to change the subject. "Everybody says that," says Sinead, "everybody thinks I'm a Brummie." "I was going to say Wolverhampton," I offer in an attempt to demonstrate that I know that the Midlands consists of more than Birmingham alone. "Other side," responds Sinead as she sets about unravelling me from my mummy-like sheeting. "Coventry," I respond, "nah Stamford," says Sinead, evidently bored at my attempts to prove my accent expertise, something which ordinarily I'm pretty good at. I wouldn't have guessed Lincolnshire in all honesty, although I have taught a student from Stamford before, and upon reflection, the accent is unmistakable. I'm not on my game, which is understandable considering the medication that I've ingested.

Sinead encourages me to sit up and rotate myself to the right, so that I'm sitting on the bed with my legs dangling over the side. I am connected to all manner of wiring via sticky pads, and these pull and some pop off as I move, triggering an alarm. "Don't worry, you're still alive" she says. "Are we going to try standing up then?" "Can I have my stick?" I respond. My stick is something familiar that I know will assist, and with stick in left hand on a count of three I creakily stand, wires and pipes flowing from me, including something large hanging from my left side. Sinead sees me looking at the thing hanging from me, as I stand there in all my glory in my satsuma netting underpants. "That's just your drain," she says "and there's not too much in it, so that looks fine to me." "Would you like a wee?" asks Sinead, I hadn't thought about going to the toilet at all up to this point, but the mere mention of having a wee made me think that I would like that very much indeed. Sinead passes me a cardboard pee bottle, and then closes the curtains around my bed, saying, "I'll just give you some privacy." I rummage around in the satsuma netting looking for the stray chipolata that is trapped in there, eventually finding it and pulling it out of the netting over the edge. I affix the pee bottle around it and relax. At first there is nothing, I breathe deeply and relax and then there is a jerk, followed by a drip, followed by a slow trickle, followed by a steady flow. The plumbing is still connected! I feel relief at this as well as the space being created by the urine that is exiting my body. Then there is pure panic, as the sound of the wee going into the bottle becomes more high-pitched. I've hit the neck, and if I don't stop soon, there will be a flood. "Sinead," I shout, "I need another bottle." Fortunately my prostate is in good working order as I manage to completely halt the flow. Sinead appears with an empty bottle, and we do a swap. "Blimey," she remarks at the weight of the full bottle, "it's like an elephant's." I fill around one third of the second bottle, and Sinead measures that I've done a 750ml wee. I feel quite proud of that, and much emptier.

Sinead passes me some damp paper towels and lets me wash myself whilst standing. I try and get into all the creases and places where skin touches skin. I don't want to be the smelly person on the ward. Sinead washes my legs and back. "I've just got to look at your bottom," she says, lovely stuff. I'm then passed my toothbrush and toothpaste and give my teeth a welcome clean. "What's this?" laughs Sinead holding aloft my tatty old razor. "Surplus to requirements," I reply. I have a full beard, but I've already made up my mind that when I get home from hospital I'm shaving it off. New life, new face and all that. Sinead rummages in my bag and produces a pair of boxer shorts, a pair of shorts and a T-shirt. "Have we to get you dressed?" she asks. "Yes please," I reply. I want to look my very best for doctor's rounds later. Sinead opens my boxers and shorts for me to step into and then hoists them up. Bending is still painful for me due to the drain and the trapped wind. I manage to get the T-shirt on myself, although the wires and pipes connected to me make this a more difficult task than it need be. Eventually I get back on the bed, and with Sinead's help put the bed into a comfortable reclined position, with knee pillow beneath my knees. "Who is your doctor?" asks Sinead as she gets me comfortable. "Mr Mehta," I reply. "Oh he's great," she says, "you're very lucky, we love him in here, he's so thorough." I was already very confident in Mr Mehta, but now with this glowing and very heartfelt appraisal I'm even more pleased that he is my surgeon. Sinead moves on to go about her duties and, feeling rather exhausted from the exertion, I lie back and take another shot of morphine, before affixing my CPAP mask in place, hitting the on button and closing my eyes for just a little longer.

When Mr Mehta and his entourage arrive at my bed, I am half-asleep. I use the bed remote to adjust myself into more of a sitting position and peel the CPAP mask from my face. "How are you feeling?" asks Mr Mehta. "OK, I think," I reply. I'm a little lost for words, suddenly facing three medical experts who between them have probably seen and heard it all. With Mr Mehta is the junior doctor who was with him yesterday and Doctor Gareth. "We need to get you up and moving today," says Doctor Gareth. This is something that I don't want to hear. I'm comfy in my bed and movement is painful, particularly with the trapped wind. "You haven't taken too much pain medication," notes Mr Mehta looking at the readings on my morphine drip. To be honest, I thought I'd taken plenty, but they didn't seem to think that I had been excessive. "Have you been out of bed?" asks Mr Mehta. "Yes, I've got washed, dressed and did a 750ml wee," I say very proudly. "That's good, I think we can move you to a ward then," says Mr Mehta. This is followed by some discussion about whether a ward will take me with a CPAP if I'm on both a drip and morphine on-demand, and it is decided that I'll lose the morphine. Nooooooooo, not my lovely morphine. "We'll prescribe you Oramorph instead," adds Mr Mehta. That's half a result at least, I'm familiar with Oramorph as my late mother-in-law (the PW's late Mum, Marge) used to be on it for chronic pain. She'd be swigging it out of the bottle! I knew that it was top of the pain-relief pyramid, so at least I'd be pain free. Before Mr Mehta leaves, he informs me that I'm now 'free fluids', and this is music to my ears. It means that I'm now allowed to drink anything apart from alcohol or carbonated drinks. Result! I'm dying for a cup of tea.

With that, the three of them leave to go about their duties, Doctor Gareth heading in a different direction. "Mr Mehta, Mr Mehta" a voice calls from the nurses' station in the middle of the HDU. Mr Mehta turns back, seemingly strutting across the HDU dancefloor in his crisp white shirt like John Travolta in *Saturday Night Fever*. "I'm so sorry for shouting across the room at you," said the nurse apologetically, almost bowing in reverence. "Oi, Mehta" replied Mr Mehta jokingly, causing his understudy to guffaw. Despite his status in the hospital, Mr Mehta is human, and as it turns out, funny too. Smart people are often funny. I like Mr Mehta, I should do too, he has saved my life. It saddens me that Leeds people would pronounce this great man's name as Mr Me-ha.

Sinead returns to my bedside to inform me that I should get my things together as I'll be moving this morning. She coaxes me out of bed, disassembles my CPAP and helps me pack it into my green backpack along with my toiletries and some bits of clothing. Soon there's just me, my bag and my stick next to the HDU bed. I'm ready to leave, but the porter who will take me to a ward will take a while to arrive. "Would you like to watch some TV?" asks Sinead. "Yes please," I reply, it's 09:50am and in 10 minutes' time on BBC1 *Homes Under the Hammer* will be on. It's a guilty pleasure. Sinead brings me a TV on a trolley and a chair, which bubbles and rolls under my buttocks so as to prevent pressure sores. She also brings me a cup of tea and an apple juice. This is better than the Ritz-Carlton.

I sip away, enjoying the flavours of the drinks, but being careful not to drink too quickly, as my buttocks are massaged from below. It's a typical episode of *Homes Under the Hammer*, two success stories, combined with one not quite as successful, as the buyer failed to do his homework. Always do your homework, kids. It still blows my mind how Dion Dublin went from Premier League footballer to daytime TV home-buying guru, but he's a natural and has taken to the program like it's something he has done all of his life. Maybe he has? I often wonder how his transition from one career to another was instigated. Did he apply? Was he approached? Was it a casual conversation down the pub? I'm actually genuinely interested to know. As I'm watching TV, I notice in the distance to my left the chap from the waiting room who had been sent home twice before. It turns out that this was indeed his third time lucky, I'm pleased for him that he has finally had his operation, and at the same time relieved that I didn't have to go through what he has been through in terms of stress and disappointment.

As the *Homes Under the Hammer* closing credits roll, a porter appears with a wheelchair, still a double-sized bariatric one, but hey-ho, I left my dignity in the assessment room yesterday. The porter is a cheerful chap, and proceeds to transfer my drip to the wheelchair, along with my bag and stick. Sinead comes along to make sure that I've got everything and joins us for the short ride to Ward J82, which is just next door to the HDU. All part of the service. As the porter manoeuvres me in the wheelchair, I catch a short glimpse of the man behind the curtain next to me, who is wearing what looks like a space suit over the top half of his body. No wonder his words and groans were so muffled. There is always somebody worse off than you.

7 – Ward J82

There is no time for emotional goodbyes, Sinead is a busy woman, and her handover of me to Ward J82 is short, courteous and professional, much like Sinead. I am allocated a bed in a side room, which is located directly in front of the nurses' station. The side room called a 'bay', and contains four beds. My bed is to the right by the window, so that is a good start. I do like a window seat, although today any view is obscured by heavy rain and thick dark cloud. The porter wheels me to my bed, and I delicately clamber out of the wheelchair, using my walking stick to steady myself. The porter hangs my drip on a mobile drip stand, and I put my green bag on the floor by my bed. I thank the porter who leaves to do his next job and sit down heavily into the chair next to my bed, holding my stick in one hand and the mobile drip stand in the other. The chair creaks ominously, I can tell that it isn't happy about the bulk that has just awkwardly settled into it.

I am slightly out of breath and very thirsty. There is a fresh jug of water and a clean glass on my bedside table, so I help myself and drink thirstily while surveying the room. All eyes are on me, I am the fresh fish on the block, and nobody knows what I am in for, except that I must look pretty poorly, being connected to a drip and with a blood drain hanging from my right side. There is a guy sitting fully clothed on the bed opposite me who is called John, and I would guess that he is in his forties, although he looks much older. I know his name, as above his bed is a whiteboard with his name on it. I am still anonymous, patient X. John acts disinterested and there is a certain arrogance about him. He is impatient and keeps looking at his watch, tutting for all the room to hear. First impressions and all that, I don't like him and I think the feeling is mutual. He is wearing a scruffy leather jacket, beanie hat, filthy oil-stained jeans and trainers so mudded up, they look like they've been taken from a scarecrow. He is sitting on the edge of the bed balancing on a pair of crutches, swaying backwards and forwards muttering to himself and occasionally swearing. I hope he isn't going to be here all night, I don't think I'll relax with him in the room.

Next to John is Harry, and I cannot tell if he is looking at me or just looking blankly ahead. Harry looks to be in his late 70s or early 80s. He has a good head of white hair, and an assortment of drinks and snacks on his trolley table, which is positioned over his bed. He is chewing on something silently as he looks blankly ahead. He is fully in bed, beneath the sheets and blankets, which are pulled tightly up beneath his chin. His bed is positioned so that he is sitting slightly upwards, rather than fully reclined.

To my right is a chap with two black eyes wearing a dirty orange hoodie, dirty blue jeans and remarkably clean trainers, who looks to be in his fifties. Like me, he is sitting on the chair besides his bed. Like Harry he is also staring into space. I can smell him from where I'm sitting, a combination of unwashed clothes and stale alcohol with a hint of vomit for good measure. It's like being downstairs on a double-decker bus in Leeds, which is why I don't catch buses in Leeds very often. The chap to my right sees me studying him and turns and smiles, revealing a mouthful of black teeth that look like a burnt fence. I can't see his name due to the angle of the whiteboard above his bed and the reflection on it. So I offer him mine. "Hello, I'm Stuart," I say, and "Jozef" the man responds in a thick Eastern European accent. He reaches to shake my hand, so I oblige. His hand is sticky, but there is anti-bacterial foam at the end of my bed, which I immediately feel drawn towards. I'll just have to try and not be too obvious. "Where are you from?" I ask Jozef. "Poland," he replies. "I love Poland" I say, I've been many times. "Where have you been?" asks Jozef in his thick Polish accent, and I begin to reel off place names. "Gdansk, Sopot, Poznan, Warsaw, Wrocław, Katowice, Krakow." "Wow, you've seen more of Poland than me," says Jozef, "and I like how you pronounce Wrocław correctly." I'm well trained in the pronunciation of Wrocław, I've been a few times, I have friends there, and whilst the average Brit pronounces Wrocław as 'Rocklov', I am aware that the correct pronunciation is 'Broshloff'. The Germans refer to Wrocław as 'Breslau', and the Polish hate that, which isn't surprising, history considered. "I am from Wrocław," announces Jozef. "Do you like it there?" he asks me. "Yes, very much," I reply, "there is a lot to see and do." "All for tourists," he comments in response, as his face suddenly saddens, "it's a bit shit." Jozef sinks back into his chair staring blankly ahead, and I look away not really knowing what to say to that, as I am one of those tourists.

The room is silent again, until John shuffles from his bed and hobbles to the nurses' station. "I'm not waiting any longer," he says to the duty nurse who tries to pacify him, "they won't be much longer now, pharmacy have been really busy." John is evidently waiting around for his medication. "I don't care, I'm off." "John, if you're self-discharging you'll need to sign some paperwork," says the nurse. "Fuck that," grumbles John in response before shuffling off down the corridor. With that we are a room of three.

Within 10 minutes of John's departure, his bed is completely stripped and wiped down, his trolley table is cleared and wiped and the cupboards next to his bed are inspected and wiped; a fresh jug of water and a clean glass are placed on the bed's trolley table, all ready for the next patient.

"Jozef, your taxi is on the way," says the nurse. "Ah good," replies Jozef. "We need your exact home address for them and for your discharge form," says the nurse. "I don't know it," replies Jozef. "You don't know your own address?" says the nurse, an eyebrow raised. "No, but I know where my house is," says Jozef. "I just don't know the street name or the number." I'm pretty surprised by this exchange, as I've never met anyone before who didn't know where they lived, unless of course Jozef is homeless. "I live with my friend," offers Jozef, "it is his house." "How will the taxi know where to take you?" says the nurse. "I can direct," responds Jozef, "It is near the Tesco where I was found on the floor, just 50 metres from there." Realising that she isn't going to get any more accurate information than this, the nurse goes about her other duties. Jozef puts his medication and the few possessions that he has into a white plastic carrier bag. He leaves the room and visits the bathroom, which is directly outside. Despite his bedraggled appearance and obvious odour, Jozef seems like a reasonable enough person (at least when sober anyway).

Finding out he is from Wrocław, reminds me of New Year 2019, when the PW and I did a twin-centred visit to Poland taking in both Wrocław and Katowice. It was my third time in Wrocław, and the PW's first time. We met up with one of my alumni Honorata and her husband Radek. Wrocław is a large built-up city with excellent infrastructure and plenty to see and do for the visitor. Particular favourites included: Kolejkowo, which is an extensive indoor miniature railway, which goes through different landscapes and cities, the detail and intricacy was incredible; the old town hall, with its gothic magnificence, which is located in the bustling market square, and the incredible Cathedral of St. John the Baptist, which offers visitors not only stunning internal architecture and décor, but also superb and unrivalled panoramic views over the city from a viewing platform at the top. My enjoyment of all of these attractions was impacted upon by my weight. I simply couldn't stand for long enough to truly appreciate them. The soles of my feet and my ankles would be on fire, and I would be popping Ibuprofen-like pills at a rave, whilst looking for any available flat surface to park my backside on. The only reason that I made it to the top of the Cathedral of St. John the Baptist, was because there was a lift. In-between attractions I would want to visit pubs for a welcome sit down and beer (Poland has an excellent craft beer scene, as well as pierogi – dumplings). So in the end it became a familiar vicious circle of walk – attraction – pain – pub – sitting – beer – calories – food – more calories – weight gain and repeat. All jigsaw pieces that have brought me where I am today, and all lessons in life not just to reflect upon, but to learn from.

Getting back to New Year 2019 celebrations in Wrocław, we began the evening with a nice beer and nibbles buffet in Honorata and Radek's apartment, before heading into the city centre to see the celebrations unfold. The free to watch headline act was the Village People (another band ticked from the bucket list), and the event was the most overcrowded, health-and-safety-devoid spectacle that I've ever experienced. It was completely insane, people stood packed like sardines, drunkenly letting fireworks off from beer bottles held above their heads, before dropping the bottles to the floor, which had become a carpet of deadly and slippery broken glass. Besides this, some people had scaled the baroque architecture of the buildings around the old town square and were shooting fireworks above the heads of the drunken crowd below. It resembled more of a war zone than a cultural celebration, how on earth there weren't deaths I'll never know. At some point the crowd lurched into two different directions simultaneously and I ended up being carried (no mean feat) with my feet scraping over the broken glass. The PW and my friends watched in anguish as I was led away by the unstoppable moving horde. I remember looking around at their horrified faces, I felt like I was in a riptide being carried away from shore, where I would drown in a sea of broken glass. When I eventually found the sanctity of a lamppost to hug as the horde scraped past me, I tried calling the PW, but all mobile networks were dead. There were just too many people phoning and texting *szczęśliwego Nowego Roku* (happy New Year). Eventually my friends found me and fortunately they were still with the PW. I don't think I've ever been hugged tighter than I was by Radek that night, happy New Year! Later in the pub (inevitably), conversation fluctuated from one topic to another, health, how bad Polish TV adverts are, Brexit, and real estate prices. I had been impressed by the sheer size of Honorata and Radek's apartment, as well as how well they had renovated it from what was evidently an old building into a very smart and modern living space. The suburb where they live is north of the city centre, across the River Oder. Radek informed me that real estate prices had been very reasonable there, as the area had a historic association with crime, anti-social behaviour, drugs and drunkenness. These aspects of urban life were very much in the past for this suburb now, and I asked Radek what had happened to the people who had lived there before, who caused such problems. With a smirk he answered, "they all went to Britain." Great.

As soon as Jozef is out of sight I stand and hobble to the end of my bed, where the anti-bacterial foam is located. Its sterile cool cleanness is refreshing on my hands as I rub them together vigorously, eradicating any signs of stickiness. Admittedly I am something of a germaphobe. I only ever use public toilets to pee, I always wash my hands, and when it comes to opening bathroom doors to vacate them, if I can't wrap a bit of tissue around the handle, I will open the door using the part of the handle least touched by others, and with the tiniest amount of skin contact from my little finger. Sometimes I'll just wait for somebody to push the door inwards from the outside; "cheers, mate." Now I'm in a hospital, where all kinds of germs may be lurking, so I will certainly make sure that the smorgasbord of antibacterial pumps located around the ward will get plenty of usage.

An Asian man in a smart black jumper and black trousers with an ID badge enters the room, and looks at me. "Jozef?" "He's in the bathroom," I say, pointing. The Asian man gives me a thumbs up, says, "cheers, boss," and goes to the nurses' station, where he gets some paperwork signed. Soon afterwards Jozef emerges, collects his bag, looks at me and says, "good luck." "*Dziękuję Ci,*" I reply (thank you), remembering one of the few Polish phrases that I know. I always find when travelling, that knowing the polite words such as please, thank you, sorry, excuse me, hello and goodbye, always seems to go a long way with my host community. Then Jozef is gone, and Harry and I are two. We still haven't spoken, in fact I haven't heard him speak at all since being there. Again, within 10 minutes of Jozef's departure his bed is completely stripped and wiped down, his trolley table is cleared and wiped and the cupboards next to his bed are inspected and wiped, a fresh jug of water and a clean glass are placed on the bed's trolley table, and all is ready for the next patient.

Like a ray of very welcome sunshine on a wet autumnal day, the PW appears at the entrance to the ward. Her welcoming smile of unconditional love is enough to make me feel fit and ready for home. "Come here," she says. I push myself out of the seat, and there is a loud cracking sound, as the back right part of the seat cannot take the strain of my push and becomes detached from the frame, so that it is now held only by fabric. Another one bites the dust. We kiss and she puts her arms around me as I steady myself on my stick and drip stand. The PW's visit is in the mid to late afternoon. Time seems to stand a little still in hospital, especially when it is so dark outside even in the middle of the day. With her nurse's head on, the PW inspects my blood drain, which she comments "has quite a bit in," followed by my bed area, cupboards, trolley table etc. She sets about unpacking my bag, taking my dirty laundry and setting up my CPAP for me, and she also presents me with two good wishes cards from my parents, sister and nephew, thus making my little corner of J82 more homely to me. I'm going home tomorrow, so I'm not sure why she's bothering, but she likes to fuss me, and I don't mind being spoiled. She presents me with a flask of peppermint tea, which should help ease my trapped wind, and a bottle of chocolate protein drink, which as well as being a welcome tasty treat, should promote recovery. The trapped wind is irksome, so I go for the peppermint tea first. I've never been a fan of fruit or herbal teas and I never will be. They all smell OK, but they all taste like something scraped off a beach shoreline that's been boiled with grass, and I mean boring grass that cows eat, not the exciting Amsterdam stuff. I sip the peppermint tea with a slightly pained expression, burping after every sip; "excuse me," "trapped wind," "better out than in." I repeat one of those lines after each and every expulsion of air, until I cannot face anymore peppermint tea. "No need to rush it all at once," says the PW. I do have a tendency to throw my drinks down like I'm swilling out a bath-tub with a bucket. That is now certainly going to have to change.

During the visit, hot drinks are brought around, and we both enjoy a cup of tea, as does Harry. When he asks for his, "tea with milk, and a sweetener," it is the first time that I've heard him speak. He is evidently a local man with a thick South Leeds accent. I'm going to guess Beeston, everyone from South Leeds seems to be from Beeston, and as a point of interest the mid-word letter 't' in Beeston is always fully pronounced by Leeds folk, which is something of a rarity. Don't get me started on nearby Middleton though, which borders Beeston. Middleton gets abbreviated to 'Miggy'. That makes no sense whatsoever to me, surely it should be 'Middy'?

The PW tells me that she got home yesterday in time for the removal company arriving to collect Becky and Brendon's things, and it only took them 40 minutes to load the van, which considering how much there was, is impressive. Besides this, and despite their car breakdown en route to Stevenage, Becky and Brendon got to their new home just fine in the end, the house is big and lovely and they were there in time to collect the keys before the removal van arrived. So all turned out perfectly well in the end. Becky's first impression of village life in rural Hertfordshire (just north of Stevenage) is very positive, and we are both happy about this. I'm pleased to see that this particular big stress for the PW has now reduced sharply. She has so much on her plate all of the time, and copes amazingly well.

Following drinks, the early evening meal service arrives. Harry has sausage and mashed potatoes, "bangers and mash, please, love." I decline the offer of food as I am on liquids only, but ask if there is any completely smooth soup with no lumps in. "We've got tomato cup-a-sup, love." "That will do nicely, thank you." I haven't felt a shred of hunger at all since the operation, and despite my love of bangers and mash (usually soaked in a tin of baked beans), I feel no compulsion towards the food whatsoever. Ordinarily I would have looked jealously at Harry's dinner, now I feel nothing at all. Not only am I not experiencing hunger, I'm not jealous, and at the same time I'm not repulsed. I had read that some people become repulsed by food following bariatric surgery, going from overeating to anorexic. I'm pretty sure that won't be the case with me. I appreciate the appeal of the food that I can see, and I know that I would enjoy the taste if I were allowed to eat it, but I feel nothing like of an emotional draw towards it. I have always maintained that in my brain there is a food switch that needed tripping, in order to reset how I appreciate food. I'm actually beginning to feel that this might have happened now. This excites me, and I share my thoughts with the PW, who is very happy for me and the brighter new future that we will share together. Incidentally, the cup-a-soup is delicious! Burp. "Excuse me."

The double doors into our bay are opened, and a trolley bed is pushed in. The empty trolley bed occupied by John is removed and replaced with a new one containing a new occupant. I'm no longer the new kid on the block. There is a swishing of curtains around the bed, some activity, and then the curtains are reopened to reveal another old chap, a similar age to Harry, who is sound asleep. Despite the fact that he is lying down, I can see that he is tall, and has a full head of thick white hair. His head is back, his mouth wide open and he has an oxygen tube beneath his nose. The nurse writes on the whiteboard above his bed, 'Eddie'. The PW and I both have a sly nosey at Eddie from where we are sat, but Harry remains motionless, staring blankly ahead. I'm not even sure if he has realised that we have a new roomie.

After around 2½ hours of the PW being there, I start to feel tired, and decide to go to the bathroom for a pee and to clean my teeth in preparation for an early bedtime. The PW offers to help, but I am determined to do this alone. I need to get moving more, and I need some normality. With the stick in my left hand, the drip stand in my right hand and my wash bag tucked under my right arm I hobble to the bathroom. Once in, I close and lock the door. The handle is sticky, which is pretty grim, but anti-bacterial foam is all-around. It is then that I see myself properly for the first time since my operation in the bathroom mirror, and I'm shocked at how much thinner my face looks already, it's only been a day! I also look very dishevelled with my beard seeming too long, too grey and too scruffy. My hair is a ridiculous mess somewhere between The Cure's Robert Smith and *The Simpsons'* Sideshow Bob. This is from being continuously backcombed by the elasticated CPAP mask straps going on and off. I actually look older, and I hope that the operation won't age me, not that I'm vain or anything! Maybe it's time for a fresh haircut and some hair dye, just for men. A bit of guyliner might bring out my eyes too, as they're currently bloodshot with small pupils due to the morphine. *OK stop it, Stuart,* you're being silly now, a shower and shave will make all the difference, but tonight I'll settle for a sink wash and teeth cleaning. I'll shower tomorrow when I'm home, and I can't wait for that.

After washing and teeth cleaning, I gingerly lift the toilet seat; however before peeing I feel the compulsion to wash my hands before touching little Stuart. When I finally retrieve my champion warrior, there isn't much action. Typical, this is no time for a shy bladder, but then within a few seconds, Iguazu Falls pour out of me; what a beautiful feeling, and just for good measure this is accompanied by a nice long gassy fart prrrrrrrrrrrrrrrp. This is my first fart since I was pumped full of air for the operation. I'd previously read on Facebook other bariatric patients saying how wonderful their first post-op fart was, and now I have experienced this symphonic gusty masterpiece for myself, I can concur that they weren't wrong. This is truly the sound of music and I feel ever so slightly deflated for it.

Before leaving the bathroom I use a piece of toilet paper to push the handle to flush the toilet, and using the same piece of toilet paper I put the seat back into the sitting position, because I have good toilet seat etiquette. I then use the toilet paper to unlock and open the bathroom door, before depositing the toilet paper into the toilet, giving my hands one final wash, collecting my toilet bag, stick and drip stand, and hobbling back to the PW, who is reading the notes at the base of my bed. "How did you get on?" she asks, as I press the anti-bacterial foam pump to coat both of my hands and my walking stick handle with germ-killing bubbles. Beaming, I whisper back to her, "I've just done my first fart." We both giggle. Farts are funny and I don't care what anyone says.

It isn't long after that, that the PW can see my attention is waning as I'm getting tired. "Have we to get you tucked up in bed then?" she asks in a high-pitched voice that a mother might say to a child. I used to absolutely hate going to bed as a child, I considered it a form of punishment; until I was around 9 years old, my sister Carla and I had a strictly regimented bedtime of 8:00pm, this was even in summer when the nights were short and the days long. The single worst sound in the world was the music accompanying the end credits to the TV programme *Coronation Street*, because that was the signal that Carla and I had to go upstairs, go to the toilet, clean our teeth, have a wash, get undressed, put on pyjamas, get in bed (to be tucked in tightly, no room for escape).

Up to around the age of 7, I used to enjoy a bedtime story in order to prolong the inevitable lights-off, Ladybird Books and the Mr Men were particular favourites, then the door would be closed (not fully), and finally the futile exercise in trying to sleep. It was Mum's 'job' to put us to bed, apart from on Wednesdays, when she and seemingly half the women from Darfield walked down to Low Valley School, for 'Women's Club', which was a more working class and fun version of the Women's Institute, minus the stuffiness and casual fascism. On Wednesdays it was Dad's duty to put us to bed, and he never detracted from the 8:00pm deadline either. I'd sometimes sit up in bed, peeping through my blinds at him gardening in the last hour of the day's golden sunshine. I had to make sure that he didn't see me though, otherwise he'd be straight in, putting me back into bed beneath even tighter tucked covers.

Our cousins Maxine and Andrew, who lived next door, would be allowed to play out in their back garden or the cul-de-sac street in front of our houses until 8:30pm. They had a more reasonable 9:00pm bedtime, as did our friend Pam, who lived next door but one and our other friends Michael and Jaqueline who lived at the bottom entrance to our street. Come to think of it, I'm not even sure that Michael and Jaqueline had a set bedtime. They were so lucky! As a parent now, of course I understand the importance of routine with children, the PW instilled this in me as she is a parenting wizard. From a child's perspective it was so unfair having to go to bed before everyone else did, particularly when you could still hear your friends outside laughing and playing in the summer sunshine or having one last final snowball fight in winter.

15 years later, when I became a university student in my mid-twenties and there was so much going on at night in my halls of residence (Sugarwell Court), I fought the urge to sleep with every inch of my body. An average bedtime would be well after 4am, irrespective of what time I had to get up (or not). Nights would be spent drinking beer, cider, vodka or my home brew, as well as smoking, listening to music, watching DVDs, playing PlayStation games and eating highly calorific takeaway food at 3am, something nice to go to bed on. I had a good bunch of mates from halls, I'm still in touch with many today. My best mate from halls was Chris, who ended up being the best man at my wedding to Linda, I could tell you a thousand funny stories about him, but I'll save some of those for the next book.

A small posse of us would all troop to the gates to meet the takeaway delivery driver at around 2:50am like clockwork. We always had some friendly banter with the security guard, Steve, who was himself very overweight, near retirement and from Rotherham.

He was a proper old-school Yorkshireman, and one day he asked me what the food was that we would order in the big boxes. "Pizza," I replied. "Pizzer," he said back to me in his thick Rotherham drawl, "is there different types?" He literally had no idea, here was a man that by day worked part-time as a gamekeeper, he hunted, shot, snared and ate everything from pigeons to rabbits from the estate woodlands near where he lived, but he'd never had a pizza! I was amazed. "Yes," I told him excitedly and went to retrieve a menu for him from my flat. He studied the menu for 'Pizza Milano' like he was swatting up on the Highway Code before a driving test, before finally asking me, "and which one do you get then?" "Large, deep pan vegetarian," was my reply. "Vegetarian!" exclaimed Steve, suddenly, losing faith in both 'pizzer' and my food choices. I'd actually been a vegetarian for around 10 years at the time, it was a bit of a Morrissey thing that stuck, until one drunken night too many, when I ordered a doner kebab with all the trimmings and ate the lot. The next day I awoke feeling like the blood running through my veins was ten degrees warmer. It felt great in my cold student room, so I tested whether or not I was truly a carnivore by having a bacon sandwich, which incidentally was pure heaven. I never looked back and would have one every day on my way to uni.

A few nights later I was having a romantic encounter in my flat at around 3am, after a Monday night of drunken debauchery at Brannigans and The Atrium, when the buzzer to my flat went. "Oh bollocks," I said, preferring my current horizontal position to answering the front door. Then there were three loud bangs on my bedroom window, which was a ground floor one. "Bloody hell, this better not be someone looking for Rizlas," I said to the half-dressed young-lady who told me to, "ignore them," and then there were another three loud bangs. "Fucking hell." I climbed off my bed and angrily tore back the bedroom curtains, standing only in my boxer shorts, as my female friend burrowed herself beneath the bed quilt like an escaping mole. Standing there was Steve, beaming in pride, rocking backwards and forwards on his security boots. In his left arm he proudly displayed to me his first-ever delivered 'pizzer' with box lid open, its contents steaming in the cold early morning air. His right hand was giving me an insanely positive thumbs-up. "I saw your light were on, does tha want a slice?" he asked, "it's vegetarian." I opened the window ajar and said, "Steve, I'm a bit busy," indicating towards the contracting quilt with my head. "Oh, oh, right, sorry, lad, crack on," he said, before scurrying off with a red face to devour his pizzer alone. As it turned out, there would be no 'crack on' that night, as the moment had been compromised, and my female friend headed back to her room under the cover of darkness, rather than having to do the next day 'walk of shame'.

Steve and I ribbed each other about that incident for months afterwards, but from that night onwards he was hooked, and every night, as well as his 'pack-up' lovingly prepared by his wife, he would also order a 3am 'pizzer', and you know what? He only ever ordered vegetarian!

Whilst my story weaves and digresses, these very obvious and sometimes familiar jigsaw pieces of a lack of sensible bedtime routine in adulthood, too many late nights drinking and smoking, 3am pizzas, and bacon sandwiches for breakfast aren't just jigsaw pieces that have put me where I am today. I didn't get morbidly obese overnight, it happened over a long period of my life. These jigsaw pieces are also stepping-stones of poor judgement and ill-discipline taken over a lifetime, the cumulative impacts of which have either directly led to or exacerbated all of the health problems that I face today. I have had a GREAT life, but I've also had too much of a good thing. As the PW, the plausible wordsmith regularly says to me, "less is more."

Tonight, 30 hours after my operation, I am exhausted, and ready for bed at 7pm. The thought of drinking, smoking, pizzas and even dear old Security Steve couldn't be further from my mind, and I'm more than happy for the PW to draw my bed curtains, help me undress, get me into bed and tuck me in tightly. There is no bedtime story tonight, but the goodnight kiss that she gives me is adoring, before she affixes my CPAP mask firmly in place. I love her more than I could ever express in simple words alone, and when she is gone, I drift off into a happy slumber; goodnight, my perfect wife, goodnight, Harry and Eddie.

I'm disturbed and awoken at some point not long afterwards, as a patient in a wheelchair along with two porters, (one carrying the patient's old-fashioned leather suitcase) arrive to occupy the bed to the left of me, previously taken by Jozef. The patient is male, and I would guess in his early 70s. He wears spectacles balanced on the tip of his nose and has similarly wild white hair to the character 'Emmett "Doc" Brown' from the film *Back to the Future*. Our little room will be a full house again. The familiar procedure of drawing curtains around the bed takes place as the porters and a nurse go about transferring the patient from chair to bed. "Are you comfortable, Tim?" I can hear the nurse asking, "would you like the bed adjusting?" The nurse's voice is very loud, too loud. I was asleep, we were ALL asleep, the pitfalls of communal living. Tim doesn't respond, so the nurse repeats her questions again even louder, until Tim finally answers in a hugely loud voice. "Yeees I'iiim fiiiine thaaaaankyoooou," says the hugely loud voice of Tim, except Tim's voice isn't just hugely loud, it is quite plummy, it elongates the middle vowels in words, and wavers up and down octaves as he speaks, in what is essentially a hugely loud plummy warble. Tim is a greater warbler, a hugely loud plummy greater warbler, and he's right next to me. I'm sure that David Attenborough would be fascinated to hear his mating calls. I put his high volume down to the theory that he's probably hard of hearing and over-compensates his own voice volume so he can hear himself. I used to have clogged ears as a kid and did the same, often getting chastised for shouting across the dinner table. There are the sounds of further shuffling and adjustment, before the curtains are opened for the big reveal. Ladies and gentlemen, tonight for your listening pleasure is hugely loud, plummy greater warbling Tim. I have to blink to stop myself seeing Tim doing Roy Orbison at the karaoke.

Harry and Eddie are both awake staring blankly ahead, mouths open. At least I think they are awake, Eddie seems to have perfected the art of sleeping with his eyes open, just like my elderly cat (who also happens to be stone cold deaf and extremely loud). As the nurse and porters begin to leave the room, Tim calls out in his hugely loud warble, "I like your crucifix." The comment seems slightly out of place, and all three stop and turn to Tim, before the porter with the wheelchair, a young man in his twenties, pulls out a cross on a chain from his open shirt-top. "You mean this?" he says in an Irish accent. Tim then asks "where are you from?" "Ireland," replies the porter, looking slightly uncomfortable at the attention. "Where?" shouts Tim. "Ireland," says the porter, this time louder. "Oh," responds Tim, "which bit of Ireland?" This is going on too long now, even I feel discomfort at the questioning of the uncomfortable looking porter. "Belfast," he replies in a very loud voice, which Tim hears first time. "Oh, you're one of them then?" say Tim. Where on earth is this going? Alarm bells are ringing. The porter looks at Tim and says loudly, "I'm not sure what you mean," and he is going slightly red around his neck. "A Proddy!" shouts Tim. Wow, just wow, the alarm bells have just rung right off the wall, The Good Friday Agreement is in tatters. I'm gobsmacked, this man has just pushed Tim in a wheelchair from God knows where, to where he is now, and instead of a thank you, he gets that! "I'm Catholic," the porter responds before turning and leaving, thereby ending the most painful of conversations. The departing porter looks not only embarrassed but a little narked and very confused. I'm sure that he is looking forward to being anywhere other than where he is right now. I'm puzzled by Tim's questioning. I don't think that he intentionally meant to be rude, but it was certainly a classic lesson in how not to make friends and influence people. In the end, I put it down to Tim being a blunderer, a hugely loud, greater warbling, plummy blunderer. I survey Harry and Eddie for a reaction to Tim's opening moments. There is nothing, not even a raised eyebrow.

The room is in silence now, the lights are on, but seemingly nobody is home. Annoyingly I'm no longer tired. I have a book and my mobile phone, but I don't want to look at either, I'm completely disinterested. I look at the ceiling before glancing towards Eddie. His mouth and eyes are wide open. I can't see him breathing and wonder if he is alive. I hope that he is, it's very hard to tell sometimes. Harry is sound asleep, breathing heavily. I glance towards Tim, and he is lying back reading a book by David Baldacci. I can't see his face for the curtain. A nurse enters the room and takes the usual measurements from me, temperature, blood pressure and oxygen saturation. This routine is repeated every four hours from this point onwards. A little later comes medication for everyone in the room, waking up Harry momentarily. My Oramorph with liquid paracetamol makes me feel drowsy fairly quickly. I put my head back and stare at the ceiling, before affixing my CPAP mask in place, closing my eyes, and eventually falling asleep.

The bright overhead bay lights are switched off around an hour later, leaving just the dim emergency lights on in the room. This sudden change in lighting stirs me momentarily. I'm not fully awake, but I'm not fully asleep either. I begin to drift deeper and deeper, positive thoughts about going home tomorrow occupy my mind. Then something strange begins to happen.

I've only ever been in a 'jungle' once. It was in The Gambia, and I use the term jungle loosely as it was actually a forest, called Makasutu Culture Forest, which happened to be in Africa, so I guess that would qualify as being a jungle, but I'm no expert here. I wasn't sleeping in the jungle, but I was enjoying an evening of local food, which happened to be beef domada with boiled rice. Domada is a rich peanut stew (The Gambia is a major grower of peanuts), and my portion was of course very large. The wonderful food was washed down with many Julbrews, which is a Gambian beer (no surprises there), whilst watching Gambian dancers, singers, musicians and performers in the early evening as the sun began to set. The transition from daylight to dusk to the total blackness of night, triggered another wave of jungle musicians to come to life, including insects, bats, mammals, birds, frogs, monkeys and an assortment of other beasties. A symphony of animal noises turned the night-time jungle into a distinctly more eerie and louder place than it was during the daytime.

The dimming of the lights in our bay room triggers a jungle operatic performance of a different kind. At first it's Eddie, who has been silent so far up to this point, then Harry, and finally Tim. All three of them are sleep-talkers. Predictably Tim is a hugely loud, greater warbling sleep-talker. Sometimes it is a single word, a name, or a question, there is the occasional rambling sentence from each of them. Sometimes words are coherent and abstract, other times they are incoherent and continuous as if

143

the three of them are zombies communicating in a language that the living aren't meant to understand. I hope that they aren't all biters too, I've seen enough episodes of *The Walking Dead* to know that it probably wouldn't end well for me, I'm definitely a good-sized meal for any zombie. I look around the room to see if any of my roommates are looking for a piece of me. Alarmingly, despite having the sides of his bed raised, Eddie has almost an entire leg between the bars and is moving and wriggling with a certain energy that he hasn't displayed since his arrival. It is at this point from a perspective of concern for Eddie, and not my living flesh, that I press my call alarm.

A few moments later, a nurse arrives and puts Eddie back in bed properly, swaddling him in his blankets, then she thanks me for alerting her and turns off my alarm light. Like naughty schoolchildren behaving in front of the teacher, the three of them are silent while the nurse is in the room. The second she is gone, the talking starts again. I lie there awake, wishing the blowing sound of my CPAP machine would drown out their voices. At some point shortly afterwards, the nurse re-enters the room to take my temperature, blood pressure and oxygen saturation, waking me up even further. During my time on Ward J82, I later find out that Eddie is in hospital after falling down his stairs at home at night, because he is what is known as a 'sun-downer', which is somebody who is unusually active after dark.

I lie there awake for what feels like hours, I think again of David Attenborough and what he might say to narrate the current scene in Ward J82, before finally being beaten by exhaustion into a rough, and bumpy night's sleep amongst the jungle talkers. Thank God that I'm going home tomorrow.

8 – Stir crazy

The night has been torturous and my attempts at sleeping were an exercise in futility. It is now approaching dawn, and I feel physically and mentally drained. The conversations amongst the undead have died down, Eddie hasn't yet escaped from Alcatraz and even better, nobody has bitten me. Finally, exhaustion plays its role in forcing my body to accept that I need to have some sleep and with that I painfully drift off.

"Hello, hello, Caroline." I'm dreaming of Tim shouting, maybe he's going to do a karaoke warble of 'Sweet Caroline'. "Hello, hello, yes it's me, Tim." My eyes painfully open and I realise that this isn't a dream, it is a living, waking nightmare. Tim isn't even sleep-talking. He is sitting up in bed on his phone, having an extremely loud warbling conversation with a woman, who it turns out is his sister. It is 6:40am, and for the second time in less than 12 hours, Tim has woken up everybody in the room. This time not just because Tim is a hugely loud, greater warbling, plummy blunderer, but because Tim is a thoughtless, ignorant prick with absolutely shit mobile phone etiquette. It fits my political narrative to assume from his selfish behaviour that Tim is probably a Tory, in fact Tory Tim is who he will be from this point onwards. Even his sister sounds dazed and confused to be getting a phone-call so early in the morning. I am absolutely furious, and have to severely fight the urge not to shout, "get the fuck off of your phone, you Tory prick." I'm so tempted. Instead, I angrily pull the CPAP mask from my face and put my bed into a sitting position. I gingerly step down from the bed and poke my toes into my flip-flops, before angrily limping to the bathroom with my walking stick and drip stand.

As I pass Tory Tim's bed, I very disapprovingly scowl at him. I can give a good scowl, I was taught by the best scowlers I know, the Germans. In order to scowl effectively, one must bring the eyebrows down into a good elongated 'v' shape, whilst narrowing the eyes. The nostrils must be flared, and the mouth and lips bent downwards into a wide frown, with the bottom lip protruding outwards. All of the above must be accompanied by a side-to-side shaking of the head. Tim got the full maximum scowl, or as the Germans would say, *maximales finsteres Gesicht*. I'm not on this ward for much longer, so I don't need to be friends with all of my roomies. Not that I've spoken to any of them yet.

Upon entering the bathroom, I go through my usual routine of constant hand washing and skin to handle avoidance where possible. I have an angry forced pee, no waiting on ceremony here this morning, get out! The force of the pee releases an equally angry fart, which rips out painfully. At least that's some trapped wind released. "Anger is an energy." I think of John Lydon chanting this line from the song 'Rise' by Public Image Limited. After stopping to compose myself for a few seconds in front of the mirror, I take note of how much my face shape has already changed in less than 48 hours. It doesn't seem real. It feels weird, and is very unexpected. I look down at my blood drain, and notice how full it is, this dangling bag has certainly filled up overnight, it is doing a very effective job.

I leave the bathroom, as usual using a piece of toilet paper to coat the handle, before hobbling back towards my bed. This time I ignore Tory Tim; that fucker certainly isn't getting a "good morning" from me, not a chance. Harry and Eddie are both lying in bed staring at the ceiling, I'm not sure that a "good morning" would register with either of them, so I just shuffle to my bed. I coat my hands and walking stick handle with anti-bacterial spray, before heftily sitting down into the already damaged chair by my bed, which again creaks disapprovingly at me. I retrieve my mobile phone from my pocket. I've had this on me since yesterday, when the PW brought it in for me, as she is also my phone warden. I have had no urge or interest to look at my phone, I'm not one of those people who has to share every minute of their waking life on social media. I still use social media too much for other purposes, but I'm not a 'look at me, look at me' type of user. I am certainly not the type of person who shares vague social media health updates from hospital, such as an abstract image of my foot in a hospital bed with the caption "today's view." Those people can fuck off equally as much as the people who respond to such images with "U ok hun x." I'm definitely in a bad mood this morning, thanks to Tory Tim.

I look at my inflated blood drain bag and decide to snap a photo of it. This isn't for social media, instead I text it to the PW, as she will appreciate the medical value of the image, with the accompanying words: "Good morning, beautiful, I'm awake early and can't wait to come home today. The drain has filled up nicely, there's probably 500ml in it, love you and can't wait to see you x." I sit there looking at the apps on my phone-screen. I'm generally disinterested in most of them. I don't want to read the news, I don't need that stress. Social media can get lost, I'm bored with it. What's left? I look at the weather forecast. It is rain, rain, rain. Everything is depressing. I put my phone back in my pocket, but then after a few seconds it vibrates. This must be a reply from the PW, and indeed it is a reply from the PW, something nice at last, her reply reads: "Hi, have you told the nurse, if not press your buzzer, don't wait, this is not a good sign x." What? That wasn't nice. Not a good sign? Why? I thought that blood drains were supposed to drain blood? Now I'm worried, for the PW to say that alarms me slightly. I press my call buzzer, and shortly afterwards the duty nurse enters the room. She is a young very chirpy personality wise, definitely a morning person. I show her my bag and recount the text messages between myself and the PW and she concurs that, "there is more fluid there than would normally be expected." I note that the nurse uses the word fluid instead of blood, I wonder if this word substitution is a pacifier, a technical term, or just to avoid using the word blood in front of a frightened patient. She leaves the room and returns with a cardboard bowl that looks like a trilby hat. She places the bowl beneath the drain, undoes the clip on the bottom of the drain and gradually releases the fluid into the bowl. I can't feel anything, but it still isn't very nice. The bowl fills up with a very dark sticky looking liquid, which in layman's terms is blood.

Once emptied, the nurse re-clips the drain bag, and raises the bowl, looking for internal measurement lines. "Just over 500 mil," she says to me. "Is that bad?" I reply. "I'm sure it's nothing to worry about, we'll make sure your doctor knows when he does his rounds." "Do you know when that will be?" I ask her, and she tells me that it will probably be between 8:15am and 9:30am. With that, she leaves and I am sitting there wondering if there is really a problem with this amount of blood or not. I don't have time to think for very long, as then an alarm sounds next to me; oh no is this it? The nurse re-enters the room. "Nothing to worry about," she says to me for the second time in a couple of minutes, "your drip has finished and can now be disconnected." At least that is some good news. The nurse disconnects the drip from the cannula in the back of my hand, before putting a plug into the cannula. She then removes the wires, pipes and bag from the machine on the drain stand, before finally disconnecting the machine itself, and taking the lot out of the room with her. Now I feel a little freer at least, not being permanently connected to the drip stand, so if I go for a wander from this point, I'll only need my stick with me.

As I sit there looking around the room, counting down the seconds to doctor's rounds, I distinctly hear my name being said by a male member of staff at the nurses' station outside. I lean forward and can see a man in a different kind of uniform, not a nurse as such, I'm not sure what or who he is, but I don't think that he is a doctor either. I then see him having a conversation with the nurse who was in the room earlier. They both look towards me and see me looking back at them. Oh no, is this going to be bad news for me? The nurse comes into the room and informs me that the PW has been on the phone to the registrar of the ward after seeing my blood bag picture. She has rung up to find out what is going on, so the PW is evidently pretty worried. The nurse explains the call from the PW to me and then adds, "we've explained to her that at this point, it isn't anything to worry about, and that we can't say any more until your doctor has been to see you." I thank the nurse for the update and retrieve my phone to text the PW not to worry, but as I do so, a text arrives from her. "I've rang the ward, but we've got to wait until after your doctor has been, how do you feel? x." I smile at the message. It takes a lot to get the PW flapping, so I think that a phone-call would be nicer. In terms of mobile etiquette, everyone in the room is awake, Tory Tim is deaf, not that I care about him anymore, and the other two are just staring into space, mouths open. I'm not even sure if they're fully conscious or not. I make the call with a hushed voice, I don't want the whole room to listen to my conversation with my most loved one. I reassure the PW that everything is fine and dandy with me, just that there was a bit more 'fluid' than expected, and that it's probably nothing, but I need to wait and see what the doctor says. I tell her that I feel totally fine in myself, and that I'm just a bit tired from not sleeping well, nothing more serious. I tell the PW that I'll call her after doctor's rounds. We end the call, with an exchange of "I love you," and I feel much better for hearing her voice.

The morning ward routine rolls on, temperature, blood pressure, oxygen saturation, meds, cup of tea. I see Harry and Eddie activated at the mention of a cuppa. Tory Tim is lying on his bed in a dressing gown reading his book, everything the staff say to him has to be repeated twice at a double volume. I hear Eddie speak for the first time too, and just like Harry he likes his tea with milk and a sweetener. I like how old people say sweetener. Eddie is evidently a Leeds man by his accent, I'd guess South Leeds too, but I'm not sure where, maybe Bramley? He looks like somebody that I might have seen nursing a pint in The Old Unicorn pub there. My cup of tea goes down well, although it doesn't taste as nice as the Yorkshire Tea that we have at home. Outside the sky is grey, and whilst the twinkling of lights on the drizzly panoramic cityscape before me is fairly pretty, I can't help but feel that a lovely sunny day would have lifted my mood a lot more.

A group of medics confidently enter the room in a variety of surgical outfits and uniforms. They head towards me; should I be happy or alarmed? A man of South East Asian appearance spearheads the pack and smiles broadly with an outstretched hand, which I shake. He tells me that they are Mr Mehta's surgical team. I'm quite overwhelmed all at once and have difficulty processing everything that is going on right now. I think that there are possibly five of them, but there might be as few as three, I'm not sure if the lady with the bandana is amongst them, I think she is, but then I'm unsure. They all look warmly at me, as though they've found an old friend. I don't know any of them, apart from possibly bandana lady if she is there, but this team of medical superheroes have seen me naked, outstretched like a fat Michelangelo's

Vitruvian Man wearing satsuma netting underpants. I have nothing to hide from them. I imagine that to them I am 'their work' and they've come to see how 'their work' is progressing. They certainly give a very positive vibe, which puts me at ease and makes me feel better. I'm never usually lost for words, but my mind is all over the place. Then I remember the blood drain and immediately ask about it. They are aware of the amount of 'fluid', and they're awaiting Mr Mehta's decision, he really is the main man. There are so many questions that I want to ask: How long was the operation? Were there any complications? What percentage of my stomach was removed? Should I be in more pain than I am? When will the trapped wind go away? Did you really operate with me in a standing position? I ask none of these questions, I feel like an illiterate fool who is unable to think for himself, and as 'their work', I feel that I must be quite a disappointment to this expert team of life-saving heroes.

Then the magic happens, the lights go down low, the disco ball in the room ceiling that I'd never seen before twinkles and turns, a white spotlight hits the entrance door and Mr Mehta strides into the room. Before him on a medical trolley are not two turntables, that's for your average DJ, Mr Mehta has three, because his hands are quicker than the eye.

"You say

You say

You say

You say

You say

You say one for the trouble

Two for the time

Come on girls let rock that"

Mr. Mehta transforms into Grandmaster Flash, playing his signature track "The Adventures Of Grandmaster Flash On The Wheels Of Steel"; this is one of my most favourite tracks from my teenage years, and Grandmaster Mehta knows it. As he cuts and scratches, his surgical team transform into The Furious Five: Melle Mel, Rahiem, Scorpio, Kid Creole and Keith Cowboy, body-popping and rapping for pure unadulterated hip-hop entertainment. Our room becomes a 70s New York club, and this is an exclusive performance just for us, call it a post-op celebration. I am overwhelmed with emotion, Harry and Eddie are throwing their hands in the air and waving them like they just don't care. Tory Tim can't hear anything but is filming the gig with his phone, the tosser. This is one of the greatest gig experiences that I have ever had and it will live with me until the day I die.

"Stuart…Stuart." Grandmaster erm Mr Mehta is standing directly in front of me and looking into my eyes. "Yo," I reply, before pulling myself from this sleep deprived, morphine infused daze. "Are you OK?" asks Mr Mehta. I nod slowly like a lunatic with an open mouth and wide eyes. I know at this second that I don't look OK and realise the need to very quickly pull myself together. "I'm fine, how are you?" I respond, immediately realising that this interaction could be going a whole lot better. "I'm fine, thank you," says Mr Mehta peering into my soul, which he can see is currently troubled. "What about the blood in the drain?" I ask. Mr Mehta looks me in the eye and nods before replying, "there's definitely a bit more there than what we would have liked to see, at the minute I can't say why, so we're going to send you for a scan and see what that shows us." "But do I get to go home today, still?" I ask. Mr Mehta shakes his head while giving a sympathetic smile. "I'm sorry, but we can't discharge you until we know what's happening, worse-case scenario is that it's a leak. I don't think it is, but we won't know until after the scan, and you're in the best place to be, considering." I know that Mr Mehta is absolutely right, and I know that I would be stupid to question his knowledge, diligence or authority. I don't want to spoil the post-op party, so I agree and thank Mr Mehta and his team for everything that they've done for me. One final sting in the tail is that I'm now restricted to clear liquids only (effectively water) and put back on my ball and chain drip for the next 24 hours. With that, Grandmaster Mehta and The Surgical Five leave the room and I'm sitting once again in the silent disco.

I climb onto my bed and ring the PW to give her the news, and she tells me that she will be over to visit this afternoon. I'm feeling a bit fed up at my current predicament. I study the blood drain, the bloody blood drain. Why did it have to work so effectively? There's nothing I can do, so I make the best of it by taking advantage of the free to view morning television (8am until midday), which is on an extendable arm over my bed, and it will soon be time for *Homes Under The Hammer*, my guiltiest of guilty pleasures. As I lie there, playing with the controls, I overhear Tory Tim telling a nurse at the nurses' station that he is "going for a naughty cigarette" and that he'll back in a little while.

I'm fed up, and not even Martel, Dion and Martin's tales of real estate shenanigans can lift my spirits. I decide to take myself back to bed to claw back some sleep. Before I do, I pull the dividing curtain between my bed and Tory Tim's, in a feeble attempt to block out any sounds he might make. I get myself into position in bed, pulling the covers up around me, pull my CPAP mask into place, turn the machine on and close my eyes. Sleep encapsulates me much quicker than I had thought that it would. My dreams are wild, abstract, colourful and vivid. I'm watching a classic detective series in which a Sherlock Holmes type figure, an English monocle wearing and pipe smoking gent played by Martin Roberts complete with deerstalker hat, is looking for clues in a house as to where his colleague Martel Maxwell might be. She has disappeared in a house that needs renovating. Upstairs in the same house Dion Dublin is dancing wildly in huge baggy parachute looking trousers that are tapered at the ankle, Dion looks at the camera, stops and points to a dividing wall that needs knocking down in order to make the bedroom that he is in big enough to be made en-suite. "Hammer time," he says, before producing a hammer and wildly dancing and striking the flimsy plasterboard wall that needs to come down. "Oh oh oh oh here comes the hammer," chants Dion. Downstairs there is still no sign of Martell, and Martin 'Sherlock Holmes' Roberts is getting frustrated at the banging from Dion 'MC Hammer' Dublin, which isn't helping him in his hunt for clues for the missing Martell. *Bang, bang, bang* goes the sound, I can feel it vibrating through me. I take a sharp intake of breath and open my eyes, realising that I've just invented a new TV series called *Holmes under the Hammer*. I look around groggily at a cleaner who is mopping vigorously around my bed, realising the motion of the mop hitting around the bed must have been the banging. I have no clue what time it is or how long I have been asleep for, but I close my eyes and try to squeeze out just a little more slumber.

I'm interrupted at some point for the usual measurements of temperature, blood pressure and oxygen saturation, which I don't even bother opening my eyes for, merely extending my left arm and tilting my head sideways for the thermometer. Then I hear Tim's name called. I open my left eye and see a doctor standing over Tim's empty bed. This is interesting and a small chance for revenge, so I pull my CPAP mask down and tell the doctor that Tim has gone for a "naughty cigarette." The doctor looks puzzled and goes to the nurses' station. Ha ha, that's Tim dobbed in with his doctor. I can see shoulders shrugging and heads shaking as well as a clipboard being pointed at. I look at my phone and see that Tory Tim has been gone nearly an hour. What on earth is he playing at? I close my eyes and reaffix my CPAP mask.

I'm catching up on much needed sleep, I can't eat or drink, and I don't want to read or look at my phone. I don't want to take the ball and chain drip stand for a walk either, so sleep seems like the best option. I fall out of consciousness again for what must be a couple of hours, as the next time that I'm awoken is by the lunch trolley arriving. Harry, Eddie and Tim are all having sausage sandwiches for lunch. Whilst I don't feel hunger, I feel a pang of jealousy. I love a sausage sandwich (always with tomato sauce, brown sauce is for bacon), a good quality, hearty sausage sandwich is my regular Saturday morning breakfast, but not anymore. Whilst I can't say I'll never eat a sausage again, I'm sure that I will, I am doubtful that very much bread will pass my lips from this point onwards due to its propensity to expand when moistened, and the potential pain this might cause to a banana-shaped stomach. I remove my CPAP mask, switch off the machine and drink my very exciting water, imagining that it is sausage flavoured. It doesn't really help. Whist I sip, a nurse enters the room and gently but loudly chastises Tim for disappearing; his doctor might have discharged him today, but now the doctor has gone, and he won't be back until Monday. Part of me wants to say that the idiot deserves this for going for a smoke, but it also means I'll have to put up with Tory Tim for even longer. There are no winners here.

I spend most of the rest of the afternoon lying on my bed reading. After a couple of hours, I finish Matt Simkin's book, *Food, Culture, Latin America*, which I'm very impressed by. For a debut novel, this is excellent stuff and I feel no reader's guilt at completing it while I'm recovering. The book is educational and discusses two of my favourite topics at length (food and travel). It makes me wonder how my relationships and habits with food will change when I'm travelling in future. I always want to try new local foods, as well as old favourites (when in Germany I'll happily eat a schnitzel every day). I'll certainly have that ability physically curtailed, but will my desire to keep trying new foods be lessened also? I guess only time will tell, and whilst a future travelling without trying as many new foods as possible does elicit a tinge of sadness and disappointment from within me, I also need to consider how frequently I travel, and how frequently I try new foods, and how a life of travel and gastronomic discovery is also part of the puzzle that has put me where I am today. I suspect in future that I'll still be trying new foods as well as old favourites when travelling, just less of them, and that's the key, moderation as well (of course) as making better and healthier choices.

It's now late afternoon and the PW arrives, bringing warmth with her into the fairly cool room. I'm so happy to see her and be distracted from my current predicament, apart from that being what the topic of conversation inevitably begins with. She gives me news from home, kids, cat, garden, neighbours, which helps to neutralise the medical talk. Not long after her arrival, I'm approached by a nurse who is holding a 1 ½ pint (0.85 litre) bottle of water. The nurse explains to me that I need to drink as much of this water as I can over the next 90 minutes, as I'll then be going for my CT scan and the water contains a 'dye' that will be visible on the scan. This seems like a big drink in the allotted time, but I'll certainly try my best. The water smells plasticky and tastes dirty. It is like something I might have drunk as a child from a bucket in the garden, when playing army or a survival game with our Andrew from next door and

Michael from down the street. The scenario might have been that we were behind enemy lines without rations, and that the water would give life and strength. We'd probably dare each other to take bigger gulps of what was essentially muddy rainwater in a bucket. Come to think of it, we did used to get upset tummies and diarrhoea a lot as kids.

The CT scan water goes down slowly at first, but then I pick up the pace and begin to see it as a challenge. It tastes awful, it makes me burp, but it's for the greater good, so I just need to man-up and down it. The number of occasions where I've 'downed it' over the years for fun, is an irony that isn't lost on me in my current situation. After an hour, I've managed to get rid of the lot, and get a "well done, love" from the PW, who incidentally is enjoying a hot chocolate. Earlier than expected, the porter arrives to take me for the CT scan. I am to be transported there in a wheelchair, and the porter has arrived not with a double sized wheelchair for two, but with a standard sized-one. News must be spreading of my slimming figure. I clamber (and fit) into the chair, whilst the porter transfers my drip equipment to the chair, I'm then led away. I'm really sad to lose sight of the PW so soon after her arrival, but she says that she will wait by my bed for me. I leave my phone with her as I don't know if I'm allowed it in the scan room.

The journey to the CT scan is quite long. I pass the abstract flower pictures that I saw on the wall after the operation, and I'm relieved to see that they were real. We go down a few floors in a lift and along several corridors. I have absolutely no idea where I am now in St. James's Hospital, and there's no way I'd easily be able to find my way back. I ask the porter how many steps per day he walks, and he tells me at least 10 miles (16 Km), he says he used to count the steps but now he doesn't bother. That's a pretty impressive daily step count though, I imagine what a difference such a level of activity would make to me instead of sitting at a desk nearly all day long. I'm deposited in the chair in a waiting room near the CT scan room. The waiting room is full and my chair takes the last piece of floor space. The waiting room is quite dark, but I can see that the majority of occupants are elderly and female. I guess there is going to be a queue for scans, but fortunately I guess wrong, as after only a couple of minutes my name is called at the entrance to the room. I raise my hand and say, "here," and a young female assistant comes forward and takes control of my wheelchair. She pushes me forward a short distance and into the CT scan room.

The CT scan machine is in front of me. I've seen these before on TV, but never before in real life. I am helped from the wheelchair onto a platform. I am expecting to hear whirring and bangs, as well as a cold breeze. There is nothing so dramatic. I lie there supine, while the platform enters the machine, and it moves me back and forth a little. There are some sounds, and then within a minute or two, the scan is over. "Is that it?" I bewilderedly ask the assistant. "That's it," she responds to me, before helping me back to my chair. In all honesty, the CT scan was a bit of an anti-climax, I really thought that it was going to be much more of an experience. I will have to wait until tomorrow before I find out the results of the scan and cross my fingers in anticipation. The CT scan assistant pushes me back to the waiting room, but it is now completely full, so I am parked outside in the corridor alone.

I am staring down a long empty corridor into perspective. I have been sitting for 20 minutes and have seen nobody collected from the waiting room, I am getting concerned that I might be here for hours, and that by the time I get back to my room, the PW will have gone. Why didn't I bring my phone with me? I think of newspaper headlines about people being left in hospital corridors. It won't happen to me, it can't, I need to keep the faith. Down the corridor I see a man in a porter's uniform approaching; he walks towards me and then turns to the left into the scan waiting room. He calls a name, it isn't mine. He enters the room and emerges with a patient in a wheelchair, I watch them disappear down the long corridor until they become a dot in the distance and then disappear around the corner. Again, I'm left staring down a long empty corridor into perspective.

A tall man appears to the side of me, he is wearing a uniform of some sort, but I'm unsure what, and on top of it he has a plastic apron of sorts. He seems disinterested, he paces around a little as though he is waiting for something to happen, he then looks at me and moves slightly defensively. "Have they put you here because you're contagious?" he asks. I motion with my head to the waiting room. "No room at the inn." "Oh," he says, "have you had a scan then?" I tell him "yes," and then there is an empty silence that goes on for a little too long. The man paces a little more, so I begin to tell him my story, and at the mere mention of bariatric surgery, he stops and looks at me. "My brother is 30 stone and he's killing himself," the man blurts out, "I wish so much that he'd do what you've done." He asks me about the procedure, so I explain about the different ones, and my reasons for choosing the sleeve gastrectomy. The man is genuinely interested in what I am saying and we spend the next 15 minutes talking about the difficulties of being overweight in terms of lifestyle as well as health. He tells me things such as; his brother got his mother a disabled parking badge for the car, just so that he can use it; his brother's leisure choices have to include venues where he can sit down and spectate rather than participate in what is happening; his brother uses a shopping trolley like a walking frame in the supermarket, and his brother struggles so much doing everyday things, like putting on shoes, getting dressed and just "normal stuff." It is all far too familiar to me. I can see the pain in the man's eyes, and it is very evident in his voice how much his heart is hurting for his brother, whom he tells me will not discuss the topic of his weight, and at any mention of it changes the subject.

When you are a patient in a hospital, it is easy to assume that all staff whom you will encounter will 'just know about medical stuff'. This simply isn't true, of course some staff will know more than others, but if you consider the sheer size of a general hospital, as well as the multitude of health issues that people can have, there must be very few all-rounders. In the 15 minutes that this man and I spoke, he has learned more from me about bariatric surgery and the Leeds pathways to surgery than he has ever known before. I hope that equipped with this minutiae of information, perhaps he might be able to help his brother a little towards a longer life and a better future.

Our exchange also impresses upon me how 'selfish' it can be to be so overweight, when it is hurting those around you who love you. I know my own parents have worried about my health for years, and whilst the PW is largely unflappable, I recall an occasion where she did break down in tears once in a hotel in Spain, after seeing how much I struggled getting out of a chair in the bar earlier that evening. It is far too easy to be wrapped up in your own problems, without considering how they are affecting others, and the stress and worry that you might be causing those around you. I know that putting myself through this isn't a whim, it's taken 4 years, I am committed. I also know that it isn't a magic fix either, mindfulness and effort on my part are going to be needed for the rest of my life.

A door down the corridor opens and I see somebody make a hand gesture in my general direction. "That's me," says the tall man, and he looks me in the eye. "Good luck with what you do, I hope it works for you," he says. "Thank you," I reply, "good luck with your brother." The man smiles and leaves. What an absolutely chance encounter that was, and how very thoughtful and reflective I feel for it. I think for both of us, two middle-aged men unbeknown to each other who rarely discuss our burdens, that it was a positively therapeutic experience.

I can see down the long corridor in front of me a figure in a porter's uniform approaching, and for me it's second time lucky. 90 minutes after leaving my ward room, I'm back in there with the PW and I couldn't be happier. I spend the next few minutes telling her everything that has just happened to me. The rest of the PW's visit seems to go too quickly, but her car-parking ticket is set to expire, so I get into bed and let her tuck me in tightly, hopefully I'll be going home tomorrow. Sleep comes to visit me quickly, but unfortunately it is interrupted by a liquid reflux of the CT scan dye water that I drank earlier. A valuable lesson is learnt, don't drink too much before going to bed from this point onwards. I'm certainly going to need to reform some drinking habits in future, but I'm committed to this life change, I cannot be afraid of it. With a slight burn in my throat but determination in my heart, I let sleep return and take me.

9 – Positivity & friendships

I awake early morning naturally. Before opening my eyes, I inhale deeply through my nose and hold the breath for a second before exhaling through my mouth. When I open my eyes, I turn instinctively to the right, towards the large panoramic window to attempt to guess the time of morning by the daylight. I am very pleasantly surprised by the cityscape in front of me; the clouds have gone, which means the rain has gone. The sky is a very deep blue, as behind me the sun is inching its way above the horizon. I'm guessing it's around 6:45am. I have no watch on to verify this and I can't be bothered with my phone. I've still got a slight burning sensation in my throat from last night's reflux, but it isn't enough to dampen my spirits, as I have woken up feeling well rested after a good sleep that was much needed. I'm in a good mood already, and I'm glad about that, after yesterday's rude awakening and subsequent problems. Today is a new day, and I'm feeling positive and motivated. I turn off the CPAP machine and remove the mask from my face resting it on my bedside cabinet.

The cityscape before me from right to left includes parts of Harehills, Burmantofts, Sheepscar, Woodhouse, Little London and Leeds city centre. Some of these areas might not necessarily be at the top of everyone's list in terms of desirability, but as I lie here watching lights twinkle on buildings set against a navy-blue sky, I think that the architecture and structures in these suburbs look magnificent. Leeds is a big city, in fact it covers 213 square miles (551 square kilometres) and has a population of 789,000 people (known as Loiners). Leeds like any other major city has 'good bits' and 'less good bits'. The 'less good bits' are areas where poverty, anti-social behaviour and crime are higher than they should be, and the areas that I'm looking at would largely fit that description. It's easy to point fingers at the people who live in these areas, typically people who are less fortunate than yourself and say that it's 'their fault'. The fact is however, that if you erode education, social services, access to welfare, public services and policing, then problems will and do arise, and not just in Leeds, these problems can exist anywhere. As I look at the cityscape, I wish I had a decent camera in my possession, in order to be able to capture a permanent reminder of what I'm looking at, and I consider how I may return to do this in future. There is a multi-storey car park behind St. James's Hospital, and it is likely to be getting a visit from me at some point, as from the top storey of it, the view will be just as good, if not better.

I watch the sky gradually lighten and then the magic unfolds. The first fingertips of sunshine begin to caress the tops of the tallest buildings, before gradually dragging golden orange light down the building façades, hitting glass windows, steel beams and other reflective surfaces that glisten and beam the sunlight back at me. The panorama before me makes Leeds look like a fairy-tale city, it is quite extraordinary and I'm completely captivated by this evolving spectacle of twinkling lights. I glance around our room and see that the other three occupants are all asleep, and for this moment have let me enjoy the magic in complete silence. Thanks, fellas, it's appreciated. Eventually the sun is high and bright enough to neutralise its own magic as the sky turns a pale blue with the dawning of a new day, and the reflections become diluted in the brightening daylight. I lie on my back and look at the ceiling above me, smiling for no particular reason other than the fact that I'm alive and today is going to be a good day, whatever happens.

The serenity of the emerging morning is broken by an alarm. It is the alarm on my drip, and in a repetition of yesterday, a young nurse emerges and frees me from my saline shackle. "You're all done now," she says. I certainly hope so, it would be wonderful to be able to go home today, but deep down inside, I suspect that I might be spending the weekend here. I'm not going to let that realistic possibility spoil my mood though. As the nurse is leaving the ward, Eddie calls out to her, "is the rugby on, love?" I wonder if he's dreaming, as the nurse looks puzzled at him and asks, "what rugby?" "England and South Africa," replies Eddie quite feistily. Of course, today is Saturday 2nd November, 2019, the day of the 2019 Rugby Union World Cup final game between finalists England and South Africa. "It's on at 9am," I chip in, and all eyes are then on me. I explain that due to the time difference between Japan (where the game is being held) and the UK, the game will start at 9am, and that the coverage will probably begin an hour before that. The nurse doesn't seem that interested and slowly nods. "Right," she says. "I'll sort it out on the TVs, don't worry," I announce to the room, which the nurse seems happy to hear and leaves with my now ex-drip paraphernalia.

I peel myself out of bed and into my flip-flops, grab my walking stick and head over to Eddie's bed. "Would you like me to put your TV on when it's time?" I ask Eddie. "Yes please, you're a gentleman," he replies. "No problem." We smile at each other, and I head back to my bed, grab my washbag and then head to the bathroom for the usual morning routine of pee, wash and brush teeth. I haven't pooed since being in hospital, and I don't care either. I haven't eaten anything solid since the day before I was admitted and I know that the morphine can have costive effects, so I'm really not concerned, as in many respects it is a relief not having to sit with my bare bottom on a communal surface.

The time is broken up with the usual measurements of temperature, blood pressure and oxygen saturation, as well as a blood test for me. I must be lucky, "sharp scratch," yes I've had plenty of those now. My blood drain bag has significantly less in it this morning, around 200ml, so that is a positive. Soon 8am arrives and our daily 4-hour ration of free TV is upon us. After switching my own screen on and navigating the menus, I head over to Eddie's bed and do the same, pulling the screen down so that he can view it comfortably from his lying position. I head towards Harry. "Would you like your screen on?" I ask. "No it's OK, I'll do it myself for kick-off time rather than watch all the guff," responds Harry, who is evidently more aware and capable than I had realised. I turn towards my bed and make eye contact with Tim whilst turning. I can't stay mad at him forever, he might not even be a Tory. "Would you like me to put the rugby on for you?" I ask Tim loudly. "Is it time?" he replies loudly. "The pre-match build up is on now," I say loudly. Tim nods his head and says, "yes, can you put it on for me, please," loudly. I oblige, and with that, yesterday's negativity vanishes. Drinks arrive, and whilst the other three can tuck into their teas with milk and a sweetener (coffee in Tim's case, still with milk and a sweetener), I'm still on water only until Mr Mehta returns.

We lie in our beds, all with our TVs on the same channel. My volume is fairly low, Harry and Eddie have their TVs on a bit louder than mine and Tim is wearing a pair of foamy headphones, presumably at a loud volume. Apart from Eddie we all have our glasses on. 9am arrives, the game kicks off, and then little cries of "go on," "get stuck in," "get in at him lad," "what the bloody hell," "wrong way," "that's not out," "come on, England," "oh bloody hell," "for crying out loud," "what you playing at?" and many more clichés fill the air for around the next 90 minutes. The cries get lesser in volume and more infrequent as the game progresses until they become replaced by tuts and groans as England are walloped 12-32 by the Springboks. I'm slightly disappointed for England not to win, but at the same time, I can't help but feel a little happiness for South Africa whom I feel are more deserving victors.

I switch off my TV and push the long extension arm away over to the other side of my bed. Harry and Eddie are still watching their TVs, so I leave them in peace, Tim has switched his TV off and is now reading his book. I notice activity by the nurses' station outside and see the familiar tall and slim figure of Mr Mehta, with a couple of his team. Spearheaded by their leader, the trio enter the room. "Good morning, Stuart," says Mr Mehta cheerily. "The scan results are largely good," he begins. I note the use of the word 'largely'. "There isn't a leak," Mr Mehta continues, "but there is a slight haematoma outside of the stomach on the staple line." I ask what a haematoma is, because I've only ever heard that word used before to describe a blood blister, and the response is that it is a pool of blood that has collected, effectively an internal blood blister. I'm assured that it isn't anything to be too worried about, however when I went for my scan last night the haematoma was around 350ml (that is some blister). With what has drained out overnight, it should now be less. Despite the positivity of Mr Mehta's message overall, I can detect a cloud on the horizon. "I'm staying another day, aren't I?" I say. Mr Mehta nods his head and says, "yes, just to be on the safe side, we'd like to keep an eye on you for another day." I am mentally prepared for this and am less disappointed with this news today, than I was yesterday. "The good news is though, you're now free fluids again, so you can drink what you like as long as there are no lumps in it." Every cloud has a silver lining, this is great news. Before leaving, Mr Mehta reaches forward and shakes my hand, wow. A Mr Mehta handshake is probably more exclusive than a Paul Hollywood handshake, it is indeed an honour and leaves me feeling very proud. There is no need for anti-bacterial foam following this hand-to-hand contact, in fact I ought to take a DNA swab for posterity. If I could grow an army of Mr Mehta's, the world would be a better and healthier place. Mr Mehta informs me that he'll see me tomorrow, and with that he leaves, as I dream of a day of free fluids including tea, coffee, cup-a-soup, Bovril, smooth yoghurt, custard, fruit juice and milkshakes. The world is literally my smooth liquid oyster, and I decide to smarten myself up and go for a walk around the hospital. I am aware that there is a coffee shop on the ground-floor; a change of scenery will do my mind some good, also getting a few steps in won't hurt me either.

I send a text message to the PW to tell her that I'll not be coming home today. I don't get a reply straight away so I presume that she is at the gym, she is a bit of a physical warrior. After a wash, I change from my shorts into jogging bottoms and put on a fresh t-shirt. I feel ready to face the world, albeit slowly and with my walking stick. I grab a few stray pound coins from the bottom of my bag and put my phone in my pocket and with that I leave the room. Before leaving the ward, I go to the nurses' station and check that it's OK that I go for a wander. "I'm going a little stir crazy in there," I say, and "that's fine, love, you go and stretch your legs," I'm told. I'm sure that's a Barnsley accent I can hear, it's quite unmistakeable, but I'm too eager to leave to ask, so with that, I hobble along the corridors and out of the ward.

As the ward doors close and lock behind me, I feel a combination of relief and fear. I'm happy to have 'escaped' but I haven't got health care staff watching over me now, I don't have my alarm button anymore and I'm not really sure where I'm going either. Eventually I find a lift. It arrives quickly and thankfully is empty, allowing me time to study the options. I press '0'. I mentally take note of the fact that I'm on the second floor as the lift descends, the doors open and I emerge wide-eyed and open-mouthed from a quiet hospital corridor into a bustling wide-open atrium, that is more akin to a resort hotel or shopping mall than a hospital. The sheer number of people milling around or walking with a purpose quite takes me back. People in flowing surgical gowns are mixed with a range of hospital uniforms as well as people in suits, and then just regular people in 'civvies', such as me in my 'Public Enemy' t-shirt, jogging pants and flip-flops. I feel like a bit of a scruff in such a bright, vibrant and dynamic space, but I hope that my very visible bright-orange patient bracelet and walking stick will identify me as being a resident here, so perhaps my scruffy look can be forgiven.

I stand there balancing with my stick, head back, taking in the sheer size, the sleek architecture and the bright light of the cavernous space before me. It feels futuristic, even scientific, as though I've got out of the lift onto a film set. I slowly amble around the atrium taking in all sights, sounds and even smells. After the relative calmness of the small ward-room where I am resident, the open space before me is a sensory overload. I notice a range of artwork around the atrium, including free-standing sculptures, functional sculptures that have been designed to be benches and wall-hung paintings and photographs. I look intently at every single one of them, as though I were in an art gallery and not a hospital. In the relatively short amount of time that I've been 'incarcerated' here, my mind has been starved of creative input. Now my eyes are feeding my very hungry brain cells with neurons of information relating to what is in front of me. I spend minutes in front of each and every painting and photograph absorbing their content, focusing on their shapes, colours, moods and perspectives. I read the small plaques of information about the artist and the names of the pieces. I decide that my favourite overall is an oil painting on canvas by Amy Charlesworth, called 'Books, a jar and a bulb'. It is a dark and simple image of books on a shelf, alongside a lit lightbulb in a jar. I like books and I like the beauty and functionality of shelves, and I think that this is why this particular painting spoke to me.

I move along the wall of art, not letting those hustling and bustling in front of me, in-between me and the artworks bother me. I don't feel like I'm in a hospital anymore, and that has brought a calmness to my soul and some much needed nourishment for my mind. I reach the end of the artworks, and then spot the coffee shop, it is a 'Costa Coffee', just like we have at my work. I head towards it, but then see some words on a wall above me, the words are as follows:

"The effect in sickness of beautiful objects, of variety of objects, and especially of brilliancy of colours is hardly at all appreciated...People say the effect is on the mind. It is no such thing. The effect is on the body, too. Little as we know about the way in which we are affected by form, colour, by light, we do know this, that they have a physical effect. Variety of form and brilliancy of colour in the objects presented to patients are actual means of recovery"
Florence Nightingale, Notes on Nursing, 1859.

I am moved by these words as everything that they say rings true with me. Times might have changed, but the fundamentals of providing a caring environment that inspires as well as heals certainly hasn't, so well done St. James's Hospital.

The coffee shop is quiet, and its visibly low ceiling makes it feel like a hobbit hole. It feels very strange indeed being in there and a world away from my 'sick bed'. Now I am a customer and not a patient. Firstly I look in a tall fridge to the left. There is a good range of sandwiches and sweet and savoury snacks, and there are also many sweet treats behind the glass counter. Before the operation I would have immediately felt a compulsion to buy something to eat, even though I was only going in there for a coffee, but now I'm looking at the food as though it were exhibits in a museum. It is nice to look at, but I feel no attraction towards it whatsoever. I'm certainly not repulsed by it, but I do not feel drawn to it in any way at all. I have become impervious to temptation marketing, the invitation to sin with a tasty snack treat is lost on me. Now this is a huge change in me, and it makes me feel very positive about the operation and my future. I approach the counter and ask for an Americano with a dash of cold milk in the top. This is my regular coffee order, even fat me appreciated the empty calories were pointless in full-milk coffees and cappuccinos. The assistant asks me what size cup I would like; fat me would have definitely gone large, I liked a big drink, but now as I gaze at the sheer size of the large cup, it seems more like a gallon bucket to me than a coffee cup. I opt for a regular sized coffee instead and even that feels huge in my hand.

I take a seat in the coffee shop with my mini-bucket of coffee and survey the room. There isn't a great deal of people-watching to do, so I get out my phone and send a message to the PW to tell her that I've gone for a coffee. I think that she will find this pretty wondrous, and indeed she does with a reply saying "wow, that's great, well done you." I sit there sipping my coffee and looking at my phone; I still don't want to read the news or look at social media, what is there left to do? Then it strikes me, why don't I find out some information about my saviour, Mr Mehta? The first thing I decide to do, is to understand where the name 'Mehta' comes from. After a quick Google, it turns out that the name 'Mehta' is of Indian origin and literally means 'chief'. It all makes sense now, the top man, the boss man, Grandmaster Mehta, of course he's the chief, he oozes chief, Mr Mehta AKA Mr Bossman. It's amazing how a name can shape a person; my surname means soggy bog dweller, but at least it's short and easy to spell.

I then wonder why Mr Mehta is Mr and not Dr Mehta? I guess in terms of medical pre-nominal titles that Mr must be top of the title tree. You spend years at medical school, you get awarded the title Dr, then you carry on rising, until the Dr title becomes an unrealistic constraint on the superhuman person that you have become, the reward being the allowed use of a civilian title in a medical sphere, or that's my guess anyway. I find myself on the Royal College of Surgeons website. There is an explanation, and it is a fairly long-winded one, but nevertheless very informative and interesting, so here it is:

"In most other parts of the world all medical practitioners, physicians and surgeons alike, are referred to as Dr while in the UK surgeons are usually referred to as Mr/Miss/Ms/Mrs. This is because, from the Middle Ages physicians had to embark on

formal university training to gain possession of a degree in medicine before they could enter practice. The possession of this degree, a doctorate, entitled them to the title of 'Doctor of Medicine' or doctor.

The training of surgeons until the mid-19th century was different. They did not have to go to university to gain a degree; instead they usually served as an apprentice to a surgeon. Afterwards they took an examination. In London, after 1745, this was conducted by the Surgeons' Company and after 1800 by The Royal College of Surgeons. If successful they were awarded a diploma, not a degree, therefore they were unable to call themselves 'Doctor', and stayed instead with the title 'Mr'.

Today all medical practitioners, whether physicians or surgeons have to undertake training at medical school to obtain a qualifying degree. Thereafter a further period of postgraduate study and training through junior posts is required before full consultant surgeon status is achieved. Thus the tradition of a surgeon being referred to as Mr/Miss/Ms/Mrs has continued, meaning that in effect a person starts as Mr/Miss/Ms/Mrs, becomes a Dr and then goes back to being a Mr/Miss/Ms/Mrs again!"

(Royal College of Surgeons, 2019, available from: https://www.rcseng.ac.uk/patient-care/surgical-staff-and-regulation/qualifications-of-a-surgeon/).

My next move is to look for Mr Mehta himself. Surely I can't just Google search 'Mr Mehta Leeds', there must be hundreds of results. There are actually 1.6 million hits on this search term, but like the cream on the milk, the big chief rises to the top and is the first result returned. Mr Mehta has his own website, and along with it, a first name, which is Sam. We share initials! I would never have picked him as a Sam, but there he is, Sam Mehta, my saviour and chief. His website is succinct and impressive, much like the great man himself. It states that Mr Mehta's *"expertise within the NHS is Oesophageal Cancer surgery, however he is also a leading general Upper GI and Bariatric surgeon, providing weight loss surgery with excellent outcomes."* The last two words in that sentence fill me with joy. I have absolute faith in the work that Mr Mehta has done. I go on to look through Mr Mehta's publications, which go back to 1994, when I was little more than a daft lad going travelling with my daft mates. Oxford University educated Mr Mehta's publications are predominantly journal articles based upon his medical research with a handful of papers related to socio-legal issues in healthcare. I am impressed. I appreciate the work and value of academic publications, having a few of them myself, however my own research into various aspects of the entertainment industries and popular culture seems insignificant when put next to research into obesity and cancer including oesophageal adenocarcinoma.

I flit from Mr Mehta's website to LinkedIn, the professional networking tool for well, erm professionals. I find Sam Mehta straight away and hover my finger over the 'Follow' button. However, it's too soon and I tell myself that I'm becoming a stalker, so I put my phone away and carry on sipping my now cold coffee. I could leave the coffee and go, but I'm not going to do that as I've paid for it. Upon reflection, that Yorkshireman's mentality hasn't really helped me a lot over the years, yet another piece in the pavement on my banana journey.

I leave the coffee shop and slowly make my way back to Ward J82. I have a good navigational head and find my way back quite easily. I chat with the nurse at the nurses' station and ask where her accent is from, and find my earlier suspicion of Barnsley was indeed correct. We share a few Barnsleyisms and Barnsley anecdotes between us, before I head back into my bay. Upon entering the room the unmistakable whiff of slightly unwashed old man hits my nostrils. I can't blame anyone individually, I have three to choose from, it's probably a collective odour, and one that you don't notice when you're in there, but when you come into the room from a different environment, the smell certainly registers. I try and breathe more shallowly whilst I head to my bed, hoping that the air over there might be clearer. Instead of getting into bed I sit in my creaky bedside chair.

I look around my bed, when a voice pipes up from across the room. "My lad lives in Wrocław." I look across to see Harry looking at me. "It's a nice place," I reply. What a coincidence, out of the four of us who were originally in this room, three of use (Jozef, Harry and myself) all have a knowledge of Wrocław. Tim is on his bed reading, and Eddie seems to be asleep with his mouth wide open and his eyes slightly peeping; both are unaware of the conversation that is beginning to happen. "I heard you talking about Wrocław yesterday to that fella," says Harry, pointing towards Tim's bed. "Have you been?" I ask Harry. "No," he replies. I proceed to tell Harry about the city of Wrocław, including some of the cultural sites and attractions as well as the very good public transport. Harry goes on to tell me that his lad has worked all over the world, and his granddaughter has become fluent in several languages as a result of living in different places, including Polish, Russian and even Swahili, after she spent time living in South Africa. Harry seems extremely proud of all of his family, which also includes high ranking police officers and children/grandchildren working in high ranking legal positions as well as in pharmaceuticals. Prior to this moment, Harry and I had barely exchanged a word between us, and now I feel as though I've known him for a while. I ask Harry where in Leeds he lives, and his reply of, "Beeston," confirms my previous suspicion. He tells me where he lives in relation to Elland Road Stadium, and I know the exact street, having walked up it in the summer, on a long walk around South Leeds that the PW and I did together.

On a good day I can walk for miles, and on this particular day we had walked from Leeds Railway Station, out to Elland Road Stadium via Holbeck, up through Beeston to Dewsbury Road where the legendary Tommy Wass pub is located, and then from there back towards the city centre via Hunslet Carr, the Middleton Railway and Hunslet. It was a 10 mile (16 km) walk in total and took all day (also calling in several pubs for refreshment and a welcome sit down). I was filming along the journey for a film that I am making called *Leeds the Movie*, which if all goes to plan will be online and free to view by 2023 – watch this space. The PW patiently walked alongside me. My snail's pace must have been frustrating for someone who strides with confidence like the PW does, particularly when I was constantly stopping to film another shot.

"I'll not be a minute, love," must have come out of my mouth about 200 times that day. The PW simply patiently waited for me, she's such a star.

Harry and I talk about Beeston, Leeds and the places I walked through, we talk about the boundary between Beeston and Hunslet Carr and how this geographical line on a map is often not considered realistic by the people who live there. "It's all Beeston to most people," adds Harry. Harry tells me about a farm that used to be located near where the Tommy Wass pub currently is; it is all real Leeds history, and Harry's words are of true educational value.

With sadness in his voice Harry then tells me that his wife left him last year, and at first I think that Harry is telling me that she had actually left him, as in separated from Harry. But then I realise that he meant that she had passed away. The room goes silent and I can see that Harry's eyes are glistening, so this is evidently still very raw and difficult for him, and I don't know whether to pursue this conversation, or whether I should change it. I don't get the opportunity as Harry continues, "60 years we were married, she was German, I met her in the war."

Harry proceeds to tell me a series of fascinating stories, including how he had lied on some paperwork to join the army at 15 years of age. He wanted to go and fight, but the war was over. He was still sent to Germany though at the end of the Second World War. "There was nowt left," he said. He was stationed in Goslar, which is in Lower Saxony, and his job was to help reconstruct and rebuild. The British weren't particularly liked, Harry explained, after all we were an invading and occupying force and the Germans had just lost a war to the British and their allies. There were a lot of American service personnel in the area too, and they weren't liked either, but they earned friends with chocolate and cigarettes, products that were in short supply.

Harry told me about an American unit that had rolled into a half-destroyed town in a convoy spearheaded by tanks. As the tanks rolled down a derelict main road in the town centre a young boy ran across the road and pointed a pistol at the tank commander who was sitting at the top of the leading tank with his upper body and head exposed through the turret. "The lad ran across the road, he wasn't even looking or aiming properly, but he pulled that trigger, and by God it was a one in a million shot, but that bullet went straight through the tank commander's head killing him instantly." Soldiers from the unit pursued the boy through the town on foot until they finally cornered and captured him, and he was frogmarched back to the section commander and beaten severely for what he had done. Despite the unit wanting his blood, the commander stopped short of having him executed after the boy (through an interpreter) sobbed that his father had been killed by an Allied bombing the month before, and he had shot the American with his late father's pistol. The unit still wanted revenge, so the commander ordered the evacuation of the entire town; every man, woman, child and animal was made to leave. Then the town which was already half demolished was completely raised to the ground as the tanks in the unit used it for target practice for the next hour. "It was senseless," said Harry, "there were no winners, there were just losers on all sides, but at least the boy lived, I often wonder to this day if he's still alive and what he did with his life since." Harry has a thousand yard stare as his mind takes him back 65 years.

"Course, when I say that nobody liked the British, that wasn't strictly true, because the young girls did, they couldn't get enough of us, but I was shy and didn't push myself forward enough. There were barely any young men left in Goslar, a whole generation wiped out by the war, either fighting on the frontlines or bombed in their homes, the girls were looking for husbands, and we were conveniently in the right place at the right time for them. Then I met her, I met Ruth." Harry stops speaking momentarily and I can see him reliving that precious moment, something which I'm certain that he has done over and over again throughout his life. "I thought she was beautiful, I spoke terrible German and she spoke terrible English, but we got on nicely, we spent a bit of time together when I was off duty, but I wasn't sure if she was really interested in me romantically. I was a bit thick like that to be honest, until an officer warned me that if I wasn't careful she'd be marrying me." Harry smiles and looks at me. "Those words were music to my ears, so I asked her outright if she were interested, which was very brave of me at the time, and she told me that she was. So when my time in Germany was coming to an end, I asked her if she would move to England with me and get married, and she did. We got married at Leeds Town Hall 3 weeks after arriving back in Leeds, we were the second English-German couple to get married in Leeds after the end of the Second World War and there were a few more afterwards too." Harry stops to take a drink of water. He has spoken for quite a while, more than he has done in all the time that I have known him. "It was hard for her though, she couldn't speak the language very well, and the Leeds accent was confusing for her, but she managed."

Harry sits back, folds his arms and smiles. "She met Hitler, you know." That isn't a sentence that you hear every day, and even a now awake Eddie turns towards Harry to listen in. "Oh aye," says Harry, "he patted her on the head, told her she was a good Nazi." "When was that?" I ask. "Before the war, in the build-up, she became a member of the Hitler Youth, they all did, it was no different to joining the Boy Scouts or the Girl Guides to them. Oh Hitler was adored, he was like a messiah to them, a god, a cult leader, they couldn't get enough of him, and they did these huge coordinated parades in front of him." I was aware of the rallies at Nuremberg, I've actually been to what was the Nazi rally parade ground, and it's now a slightly dilapidated car park. Hitler, like Mussolini and all good Nazis liked a parade, he liked to address the masses, and he did so very animatedly, arm movements, fists banging, shouts, rants, and he did it well. The people listened, they had to or they'd get shot. Harry continues, "aye, they did this parade in front of Hitler and afterwards he walked up and down the ranks of them, inspecting them. He stopped at Ruth and patted her on the head, she adored Hitler from that moment onwards." I've never ever heard Hitler be admired by anyone, should I feel shocked? I don't know, it was just interesting hearing this perspective. Our conversation about Germany, Ruth and Hitler gets interrupted by the arrival of a Catholic priest, in what can only be described as a divine intervention.

The priest surveys the room with unfriendly eyes and a frown, maybe he didn't like the Nazi talk. He then spies a sleeping Tim whom he goes over to. "Hello, Tim," says the priest in a strong Irish accent, Tim stirs and opens his eyes like an old bear coming out of hibernation. "Faaarrrther," croaks Tim in his drawn out wavering voice. "How are you today?" says the priest as he makes his way around the bed and begins to draw the curtains to give them some privacy, which was fairly futile as we can still hear everything. "I'm goooooood," wavers Tim in response. I wonder if the priest has come to give Tim his last rites, but it turns out that he has come to deliver Holy Communion. As an atheist, this is a slightly surreal experience to me, I've only ever seen this done on TV, now I was a captive audience to it. Before the priest begins his communion prayer I say out loud "would you like us all to be quiet?" I do this out of a sense of respect, I can't help being respectful sometimes. "No that's fine, you all just carry on with what you were doing," says the priest.

And with that, to my left behind a curtain, the priest delivers communion, and in front of me Harry carries on talking about Hitler and the Nazis. To say that this is a surreal experience is a massive understatement, it's bloody bonkers! "I'd love to read his speeches, you know," says Harry, "those words that carried so much power, that persuaded so many people that what he was doing was the right thing, you can't imagine the power of those words." I pick up my phone. "I'm sure that they must all be online, you know, there must be some kind of historic archive." I begin googling 'Hitler's speeches', which I'm sure must have confused the Google advert bots, although thankfully no Nazi memorabilia appeared in my Google Adsense adverts afterwards. Can you imagine 'Suggested for you, an authentic iron cross emblazoned on a swooping eagle, just 5 monthly payments of £29.99'. No thanks. Sure enough, Hitler's speeches are online, and translated into English in a convenient PDF file, which is about 300 pages long. "Erm, I've found them," I tell Harry. I take my phone over, and he puts on his glasses and pulls them down the bridge of his nose to try and read from my screen. "It's too small," he says and looks disappointed. "Well I'll hopefully be out of here tomorrow," I say to Harry, "and I'll be back next week, I could bring them if you like, I can print them out." What on earth have I just offered to do? Not only have I offered to print out the speeches of history's greatest villain, a complete and utter monster, but I'd just offered to print out 300 pages worth of his

Nazi bile. Maybe it was a moment of insanity, or maybe it was me being caught up in a moment and wanting to help someone, but I said it. "Well I won't be going anywhere," replies Harry, "this is my final countdown, when I leave here it will be to be back with my Ruth." The stark realisation of the fact that I was sitting talking to a man who knew that he was dying and had only at most a few weeks left to live, hit me like a knife in the heart. Can you imagine being in a position where you know that every day might be your last, and that death is a way out of having to live a life of pain? "Could you print me something out about Goslar too?" asks Harry, "I'd like to read about what has become of the place." "Of course I can, no problem," I reply, knowing that Wikipedia exists for just such purposes.

"It's been really interesting, all this," pipes up Eddie suddenly from the corner of the room. He had sat there silently throughout, occasionally nodding, and I never fully knew if he was really listening or not. Harry looks at Eddie and asks, "do you remember the war years?" "Oh aye," replies Eddie, "I was just a nipper really, but I remember the air raids and I remember the rationing, we were all happy though." Harry replies to Eddie, "I sometimes look at the mess of the world that we live in today, and I have to admit, I do wonder if the right side won." OK that is going a bit far for me, so I make an excuse to leave the room that I need to stretch my legs and leave the two of them to continue their conversation, whilst the priest continues his communion with Tim.

I decide to walk circuits of the ward, which isn't difficult and I actually manage to walk five complete circuits before I feel like I need to return to my bed for rest. Exercise makes me hot and my mouth gets incredibly dry. This is something that I know will take some getting used to. I re-enter our little room. It still has that old man smell. Tim's curtains are now open, the priest has gone, Tim has been communed, if that's the right term, and now he rests again, eyes closed, snoring slightly. This image is repeated opposite him with Harry and next to Harry with Eddie. *Oh well*, I think to myself, *if you can't beat them, join them*. I have a drink of water and then climb into bed, adjust the mattress position, and put on my CPAP mask. The cold dry air blows into my already drying mouth. I try not to think about mouth dryness as that will keep me awake, so I lie back and close my eyes, thinking about my new life, and also thinking back to the story that Harry told me about the young boy shooting the American tank commander. I wonder if the tank commander's family ever got the full story about what had happened? It doesn't take long before my thoughts become dreams as sleep takes over.

10 – Home

I'm in the car, and I'm going home; the ride is very smooth, the road looks like glass and twinkles under the vanilla street-lights. As we proceed into Harehills, along Barnsley Road (I kid you not), suddenly the road beneath our wheels becomes extremely bumpy as the glass-like surface begins to break up leaving sharp edges, which cut into the car tyres, causing the vehicle to violently judder. The PW is sitting in the driver's seat (of course), and she looks perplexed. In the back seat a voice says, "this is what it was like in Goslar, no roads left." Why on earth is Harry coming home with me? I mean I like the guy, but I don't know if I want him at home, that's a lot of responsibility. Suddenly the car bangs and then flips forward, it's happening in slow motion and I can see the broken road beneath me through the windscreen as the car flips over with a forward roly-poly momentum. This isn't going to end well. I close my eyes and then open them with a sharp intake of breath. The CPAP machine is blowing hard, there is a side leak from my mask and I'm no longer in the car. I'm in Ward J82, which apart from my blowing wind machine is silent. I adjust my sleeping position in bed, which causes a little abdominal pain, and a sharp pain in my right knee that has set quite stiff and straight. I fumble for the off button on my CPAP, then peel the silicone seal of the mask off my face with one hand and pull the elasticated straps over my head with the other one.

CPAP off, I adjust my bed using the controls into a nice comfortable wavy shape with my back slightly raised and my knees slightly bent. I look around the room, Tim isn't in his bed, Eddie is cat-napping with one eye closed and the other eye half open, Harry is sitting in his bed with his arms folded looking directly at me.

"They wanted me to take down a picture I've got at home of her," says Harry. It takes my brain a few seconds to catch up and realise that Harry is picking up exactly where we left off several hours ago. Old people are brilliant at doing that, it's as though the time period in-between never actually happened, probably because he slept through it, just like I did. Harry continues, "I told them to get lost," indignantly nodding his head and frowning. "Who did what?" I yawn, before continuing, "sorry, Harry, I'm not fully awake yet." "The kids," replies Harry, "they said that I ought to take down the picture of my Ruth, now that I've got carers, coming in." "Why would they do that?" I ask, as it seemed like a strange request from them. "Well because there's all kinds of people coming in, you know different races and nationalities." I frown as I strain my brain to understand, which makes Harry realise that I am pretty lost in this conversation. "The picture," says Harry, "it's a photo in my lounge on the wall of when my Ruth was in the Hitler Youth, she was so proud of that photo, you know with Hitler patting her on the head and that, she's wearing a swastika broach on it." Ahhh now the penny drops. I can see why that might be an issue in Britain, 2019. "That picture stays exactly where it is," said Harry, emphasising the word exactly and at the same time pointing physically to the picture that he is seeing in his mind's eye. "People get too easily offended these days," continues Harry, "you can't change history, and my Ruth will stay exactly where she is." Harry once again emphasises the word exactly. Tim re-enters the room looking confused like he usually does, climbs into his bed and grabs his book. I nod silently looking towards Harry. It would be completely pointless for me to try to explain or debate an alternate viewpoint with regards to swastika imagery. Harry is grieving, Harry is dying, Harry is going to get the last word here.

The room becomes silent again, and not long afterwards Harry is asleep, along with Eddie and Tim, who has his book balanced on his chin and his glasses balanced halfway down his face at a peculiar angle, a bit like a Benny Hill character.

The rest of the evening plays out along routine lines. The PW comes to visit. We go for a coffee downstairs, which is the highlight of my day. My legs are sore and stiff, from the lack of usage I presume, I just want out of here now, a bit of normality. That night I sleep remarkably well, considering that I had a decent siesta in the afternoon. My body is still very much in recovery mode, and sleep is a great healer.

The next morning my drain is inspected, and there is much less liquid in there, somewhere between 150ml and 200ml after 36 hours, which the nurse thinks that this is a good sign, and if she's happy, then I'm ecstatic. A little while later Mr Mehta enters the room, but it's not good news, it's GREAT news. On his rounds, my saviour gives me the green light to go home. I could literally hug and kiss that man, but I settle for another Mr Mehta handshake, that awesome all-encompassing healing handshake. I feel blessed. Before leaving, Mr Mehta instructs one of his team to make me an appointment to return in 3 days' time as a day patient for a review and my drain removing.

I cannot wait to leave and as soon as he is out of the room, I set about gathering my belongings and packing. I cannot leave straight away as there are various procedures that need to happen first including the delivery of some medication from the hospital chemist and I also need to have another MRSA swab before I go and collect a sick note for work. I'm excited at the prospect of being home though and have a slight spring in my stiff and painful step. "Do you think you'll change your behaviour now?" asks Eddie as I unplug charging cables from besides my bed. I hadn't realised that Eddie was awake, it's difficult to tell sometimes, but his question takes me by surprise. I'd never really discussed my reason for being in hospital with Harry and Eddie, but I'm sure they must have picked up snippets of conversation between the doctors and myself. My reply is a short, "definitely," as I try and formulate an answer in my head. I consider the people around me, people who are genuinely ill and dying and feel guilty about coming into a NHS hospital because I couldn't stop getting fatter. "I'll never go back to how I was before, especially after going through this, it's going to be…it's already…life changing for me…definitely." I say the words with reflection and conviction as I stare at the ground, before looking Eddie in the eye and nodding. I can see that Eddie believes what I say as he nods back at me and smiles. "Good lad," he says. I'd never really considered before what the other patients in the ward might think of me, I hope that they don't think that I am a fat waste of resources. I'm pretty sure they don't, but a feeling of remorse and guilt does creep in. Why couldn't I do this by myself? Why can other people successfully lose weight by dieting but not me?

I suppose the answer lies somewhere in how my brain is wired, I think the psychologist that I saw got closest to the answer, with my addictive personality and binge eating disorder. The fact is that I needed help, and thankfully the NHS have given it to me. I'll be forever grateful, and I won't let them down by going back to my old ways.

My final day in hospital passes slowly. I ring the PW and tell her that I'm coming home, but I can't say exactly when as I'm waiting for the pharmacy to deliver my medication. I prepare myself for my home departure, by having a good scrub and wash in the shared bathroom. I even have a shave and put some aftershave on. My face tingles as the aftershave irritates my newly exposed skin. I'd let myself get beyond a bit 'stubbly' during my hospital stay. Truthfully, I was beginning to look like a bit of a scruff with my unkempt facial hair, sloppy tracksuit trousers, baggy t-shirts and flip-flops. I get dressed into a half-smart pair of shorts, half-smart in the sense that they look a bit like 'dress shorts', albeit with a fat-man's elasticated waist. I daren't wear anything other than an elasticated waste in case it hurts my stomach, although now my abdominal pain is only very slight, just a bit of tightness. I'm more concerned about my knees, both of which are quite sore. My limp seems to be getting worse and I'm definitely going to be using my walking stick today through necessity rather than caution. My shorts are complemented by a clean and fresh (albeit still baggy) t-shirt and flip-flops as I can't presently get socks or shoes on by myself. Not that I ever wear shoes, if I'm not wearing flip-flops or rocking my Crocs with socks, I tend to wear trainers or sturdy boots. Trainers offer my sore ankles a bit of respite with their cushion, and sturdy boots, whilst lacking a soft cushion, offer a good degree of ankle support. I bought a pair of boots in Dresden, Germany about 12 years ago, and they are a very well-worn but firm favourite. They do stink though! Too much information, Stuart.

I lie in my hospital bed browsing through the news on my phone, and it's depressing. I turn it off, I'm about to put the phone down, but decide to have a quick trawl through social media. Just a quick one. Is there ever a quick one when you fall down the rabbit hole? I need to continue being disciplined with my screen time. I open up Facebook, and there are nine notifications, all of which are nothingness. Twitter, nothing just lots of political arguing. Instagram, lots of nice pictures mixed with irritating 'look at me I'm great' pictures. Facebook Messenger, there's one message from my cousin Maxine. I open it and it reads "Hi Stu, I'd kind of figured out you've been in hospital for an operation, hope you're doing OK and well on the way to recovery, sending get well wishes xx." I'm quite taken aback by this message, whilst I definitely welcome the good wishes of my cousin, I hadn't actually publicised my hospital visit to more than just a very few people. I had intended to wait until I'd got out (alive) before slowly revealing the news about my operation. I feel a little cheated at the power to reveal the news myself being taken away from me and truthfully a bit annoyed. Somebody must have blabbed, and now my paranoia starts to kick in. Is there chatter on social media about my sleeve gastrectomy? I don't want to become the next Vanessa Feltz with her famous gastric band, I'm just plain old Stuart Moss that had two thirds of his over-sized stomach removed, no biggie.

I ponder how this might have happened, and if Maxine knows, who else might know, am I suddenly the talk of Darfield, the village where I grew up? I eventually reply to Maxine, thanking her for her message and I explain that I hadn't publicised it, but was going to talk about it further down the line, once I'd got through the other side of it all. I put my phone down and stare into space, thinking, always thinking, always overthinking, a terrible habit of mine. I close my eyes and try to clear my mind, thinking of home, thinking of the PW and thinking of a brighter and lighter future.

My thoughts are interrupted by a male nurse who enters the ward and comes over to my bed to inform me that he has come to do my MRSA swab. Not a problem, "swab away, my good man," I say chirpily, as a dab from his cotton bud is one more step towards my freedom. But then he begins to draw the curtains around my bed, and as he does so I raise an eyebrow. "Can you stand?" the nurse asks. "Erm yeah," I reply, shuffling to the edge of my bed before gingerly putting both feet on terra firma. "Where exactly is this swab taken?" I ask, wondering why he has pulled the curtains around the bed. "Inside your anus," is his reply. Let me tell you something, dear reader, I've got no idea what salary that poor bugger is on, but it needs doubling if his daily routine involves sweeping the chocolate chimney pipes of soon to be ex-patients. Fortunately for him I hadn't been for a poo since the day I came into hospital. "Can you drop your shorts?" he asks. I do, and part my cheeks as he says, "you might feel a little uncomfortable." That was an understatement, my bottom is only for one-way traffic and the twisting and rotating swab felt more like a toilet brush going around my u-bend. After what was probably 5 seconds, but felt like 5 painful minutes, the final indignity is over, and now I'm just left to wait for my medication, albeit with a slight chafing feeling in my sphincter.

Some-time later a junior doctor enters the room and comes over to my bed. He looks around 25-26 years old, very young, but very smart, polite and well-mannered with quite a gentle voice. He explains that he has come to issue me with a letter for my employer about taking time off for recovery before returning to work, in layman's terms, a sick note. He asks me about my job and I explain what I do, and he asks me how long I feel I might need off work. In all honesty I don't feel that ill. I know that I've had major surgery, but my mind seems clear and whilst I'm a bit achy, I don't feel incapable, I ask for 4 weeks. The doctor looks slightly taken aback and explains to me that he thought I was going to ask for much longer, he also adds to this that I am actually the first patient that he has written a sick note for. I imagine that he thought I might be looking for a ticket for a good skive off work, but that's not me. The doctor suggests to me that maybe 8 weeks might be more realistic considering the extent of my surgery. It's strange how I don't feel as though I've been through major surgery, just a bit of an operation, but I don't want to be a martyr, although 8 weeks does seem like a long time. In the end we settle on 6 weeks and I explain that if I feel I need longer, nearer the time I can ask my GP to write me a note. With that, the junior doctor completes his paperwork, and I now have a 6-week ticket for some serious rest and down-time, which in reality I envisage will be 6 weeks of creative writing time on this book.

Eventually, after what feels like an eternity away from Mr Mehta green-lighting my departure, my meds arrive from the pharmacy. I'm overjoyed, as this is the final hurdle to me making my departure. I am given a multi-vitamin medicine, soluble paracetamol, lansoprazole chewy tablets and a small bottle of Oramorph. The likelihood is that I'll be taking tablets for the rest of my life. The lansoprazole is to protect my stomach and is supposed to be swallowed, but I've been instructed to chew it for the next two weeks at least. When I was first told that I would need to be on medication for the rest of my life after the operation, I was quite upset, it almost put me off having the operation, but now I feel quite unbothered at the prospect of a daily pill-pop. In point of fact, I'm already used to doing it with my daily vitamins and statins, a couple more tablets will hardly break me, although I may need to get a larger dosset box.

Once the pharmacist has gone, I call the PW and tell her that I'm ready to go, and on the phone she sounds as excited as I feel. I get the rest of my belongings together and then sit by my bed waiting for her to arrive. My knees are really quite sore, and under normal circumstances I would have taken ibuprofen and paracetamol but now I'm unable to take ibuprofen as my stomach won't tolerate it, but at least I have the soluble paracetamol and Oramorph for the pain and I'll take some once I am home, although the Oramorph is meant to be for abdominal pain. The PW is insistent on coming to the ward and walking with me to the car, rather than me meeting her outside. I look across at Harry and Eddie; both are asleep. I hope they wake before I go as I would like to say goodbye to them. Tim is nowhere to be seen, he is off on one of his many wanders.

The PW eventually arrives and brings with her a happy glow. She is positively warm and her smile radiates around the room, seemingly bringing Harry and Eddie out of their slumbers, and who wouldn't want to wake when a beautiful 6 foot blonde enters the room? Along with her happiness, the PW brings a tin of chocolates to give to the ward staff. "Nurses love chocolate," the PW tells me, and she brought the correct ones, that's for sure – Cadbury's Heroes! A truly sweet metaphor for the heroes who had been looking after me. I say my goodbyes to Harry and Eddie, shaking both of their hands. I tell them that I'll be back next week. Harry reminds me to "print me that stuff out." "Of course," I reply, feeling a little reticent at the prospect of printing out 300 pages of Hitler's shouty speeches (why oh why did I offer to do that)? With that, we leave the ward and with the PW supporting my wobbly unbalanced and quite painful steps, we head down the maze of corridors and lifts to the car park, and home.

I'm 47 years old, but I still think I'm a Jedi when it comes to doors that open automatically. As we approach the exit to freedom and the outside world, I raise my hand like Luke Skywalker as if the power of the force emanates from me parting the glass doors from the centre, with one sliding left and the other right. "I haven't lost my powers," I say to the PW who rolls her eyes at my lack of maturity.

The outside air is cold, very cold. "Oh my God," I say, "it's freezing out here," and the PW tells me that it was 5 degrees in the car on the way here. I never feel the cold, being from Barnsley, I'm quite used to going on a winter night out in just jeans and a T-shirt, but tonight, even though I'm fairly-well covered, the cold penetrates my skin and into my bones. I wonder if this is a sign of things to come, I wonder if this is what weight loss does, after all that nice layer of blubber beneath my skin must surely have some reasonable insulation value to it. I've been in the hospital for 6 days, and the temperature inside the hospital was regulated and constant, it felt neither warm nor cold to me, just comfortable, which I guess is the intention.

The inside of the car feels like a fridge, the seat is cold on my still slightly tingling backside, and I can even see my breath slightly. The drive home isn't dramatic, my premonition of the road breaking up, Harry on the back seat and the car flipping over thankfully doesn't come to fruition. We arrive home 20 minutes after leaving the hospital car park and I've never ever been happier to stand on our driveway. It's amazing how being in a hospital for such a short amount of time feels like so much longer. I take in the sight of our home and garden, the sounds and the smells of the cold night air, which is tinged with the smoke from secret wood-burners dotted around our estate (which is meant to be smokeless, but really who cares)? Standing on the driveway is a sensory feast, I feel elated.

We head indoors, and the cold is making my legs really ache quite badly, now it is my left knee joint, which historically has given me the most pain, particularly in autumn and winter. I take in the smells of the house, cooking and the unmistakable odour of a freshly cleaned kitchen. "I've cleaned all the house," the PW says excitedly before throwing her arms around me and hugging me tightly. "Oh I should be careful," she says, looking at my stomach. "It doesn't hurt much," I reply, lifting my t-shirt to show my white flabby and bruised belly, which in all honesty doesn't look that bad at all to say it's been punctured in various places.

I make my way to the living room and sit in my chair, the killer chair, the chair in which I've spent far too many hours of my life. "Are you alright having a drink?" the PW asks. "I'd love a cuppa," I reply and let me tell you, dear reader, that first cup of tea made by the PW in our house, was the best cup of tea that I have ever tasted. I'd had plenty of drinks in hospital, but you literally cannot beat a good cuppa made by the PW, which of course HAS to be made with Yorkshire Tea. The PW gives me a small cup, what I would call a child size cup. "I didn't want to overface you," she says nodding towards the cup. Overface is a northern English term associated with consuming too much. "I'm fine actually with drinks," I tell her. I stayed well hydrated in hospital and drinks seem to pass through easily without over-filling me. I'm not sure if this is a good or bad thing or even a thing at all, but I learn very quickly that I can drink out of a big mug quite easily. I have a delicious supper of half a tin of custard before heading to bed satisfied and very, very happy.

The next day I weigh myself as soon as I get out of bed. I would usually wait until I'd had a poo, but I don't need a poo and I can't wait. I'm disappointed to see that I've only lost another 4 pounds (1.8 Kilos) since entering hospital. I have to keep reminding myself that this is a marathon and not a sprint. I call my parents and speak to them to reassure them that I'm fine and that the operation was a great success. I had been giving them regular text updates from hospital, and the PW had spoken to my parents each day that I was in the hospital. I didn't like making phone calls from the ward as everyone could easily listen in, even though they likely wouldn't have been that interested. I'm the same on trains and buses, I rarely make or answer phone calls when I'm sitting amongst strangers.

I have an easy and relaxing day at home. I throw myself into writing this book, easily writing over a thousand words, something that would continue almost daily for several weeks. It's a good mental distraction to keep my mind active and me off mindless social media. It also allows me to be creative, which is something that I really enjoy being.

The PW doesn't let me do anything around the house apart from make the odd drink. I'm totally fine with the liquid post-operative diet, which I have another 8 days of before I can go onto purees, which I will be on for 2 weeks before finally moving to solids. The two weeks prior to the operation and the month after it, are by far the most disciplined that it is necessary to be in terms of following the rules to the letter. This is particularly the case after coming out of hospital as this is now such a delicate time for my banana stomach as it begins to heal. I must admit that I have had barely any stomach pain since leaving hospital. There is a slight soreness in my shoulder, which is trapped wind, and my left knee hasn't stopped aching, which I suspect is partly due to me not being able to take ibuprofen anymore, something which I used to eat like sweets to keep the pain at bay. It probably wasn't doing my stomach a lot of good, so maybe it's a good thing. I'm drinking peppermint tea three times per day to try and ease the trapped wind soreness, but it's a bit of an unpleasant tasting ordeal.

At the end of my second day home I am going a little stir-crazy, I had been advised to exercise as much as my body would allow, and the furthest I had walked was from our bedroom on the second floor to our living room on the ground floor, as well as a couple of unsuccessful trips to the toilet, followed finally by one modest success, which is a couple of tiny chipolatas, somewhere between type 1 and type 2 on the

Bristol stool chart, indicating severe constipation. My bowels haven't opened since before my surgery and whilst I've barely eaten anything to excrete, this is the longest that I'd ever been without pooing. I'm hoping that more liquids in will soften things up and increase bowel production.

In the evening I decide to walk up the street to our local mini-supermarket, a Tesco Express, somewhere that I used to call into regularly for a naughty sausage roll, pasty or yellow stickered bargain. I'm well wrapped up, but it feels cold outside. The distance that I have to walk to the shop is approximately 150 metres, it's slightly uphill on the way there and slightly downhill on the way back. I'm not totally confident about my stability as I do feel a little wobbly and particularly with my knee ache, I decide to take and use my walking stick to support me on what should be a 5-7 minute round trip (including shopping time).

I have walked about 40 steps up my street and already I'm breathless and light-headed, thank God that I brought the walking stick as I genuinely need it. The incline of my street is very slight, but it feels like I'm climbing a mountain. I'm sweating profusely and panting like someone who has just finished a marathon, so this is not good. I had no idea that my body was so weak and that such a small walk would take so much effort.

By the time I get to the shop I'm a mess. Outside of the shop there is a metal fence, and I spend two minutes leaning against it catching my breath. I'm panting, shaking, sweating and shivering at the same time. All I need now is for my bowels to open, as I look like a junkie that is going cold turkey, and apparently that's what happens to them; maybe I'm having morphine withdrawals? I look at clouds of my breath as I pant into the cold crisp night air until I eventually begin to calm down and relax. My legs feel like jelly, but at least I feel capable of now entering the shop and interacting with people. Upon entering the shop, I instinctively head to the back where the fridges are. I know that this is where the yellow stickered bargains will be and sure enough, there they are: sandwiches, pasties, sausage rolls, and onion bhajis. I used to love all of them, but now I'm just looking at them like fatty carbohydrate relics from my past. I can't physically eat solid foods right now, but they all look so huge. How on earth could I devour so much before my operation? I could easily have eaten one of all of the above with crisps and a pudding afterwards.

Before coming to the shop, I had asked the PW if she wanted me to bring her anything back, but she said "no." I think truthfully, that she didn't want to eat anything naughty in front of me that might have given me temptation. As I stand there staring at the food, I feel nothing at all, it's as if I'm in a food museum that isn't that interesting to me. I raise my head and see something though that I would very much enjoy right now, and that is a milkshake. I had been encouraged to drink these as the calcium would be good for my bones and as my food intake is so little at present, something fatty and sweet would help to boost me. Maybe that's what I need to make me feel better after the effort of walking to the shop. I grab a fudge flavoured milkshake from the fridge and suddenly the lights go out, or at least it feels like the lights have gone out.

I find myself leaning sideways against the fridge with my head slumped forward into my chest. I must have looked drunk, I was so glad that I had the walking stick on me. A concerned member of staff approaches me. "Are you alright, pal?" "Yeah," I mutter in reply, "I've not been well, think I need to get some fresh air." I hope that the member of staff didn't think that I was drunk, I don't think that I'm slurring my words. I can see him looking at me and mentally considering where to go from that point. So I right myself from the fridge and slowly head towards the counter, sweat pouring from me. As I limp down the aisle I can feel his eyes burning into my back, I really hope that I don't fall into the chocolate bars that are on the shelves to my right. I can feel myself tilting towards them, that would be a nightmare. Those lovely naughty chocolate bars, actually they're all bastards, complete and utter sweet, delicious bastards.

I make it to the counter, and even manage a smile at the young lass standing at the till. I put my milkshake on the counter and say, "it brings all the boys to my yard." Even feeling delirious, I still make terrible jokes. She laughs, probably in sympathy for the pathetic shabby mess stood before her. "Is that everything?" she asks. "Actually no," I reply, "I'll have a lucky dip for tomorrow too." It's the midweek National Lottery draw tomorrow. Surely surviving the operation must be a good omen and besides that you've got to be in it to win it.

I limp out of the shop into the cold night air, once again exhaling clouds of breath like Puff the Magic Dragon, except I don't live by the sea. Although I did use to live by the sea in Great Yarmouth back in the late 1990s. I used to live above a pub and work at a theme park. Doughnuts and fast-food by day and beer by night. It was yet another unhealthy year of my life, another step on the path of my banana journey.

I arrive home around 20 minutes after I left the house, and the PW is standing in the doorway waiting for me with a concerned look on her face, "I was about to come looking for you," she says in a caring tone that at the same time feels like a slight telling off. She can see the pain in my face, my whole body is hurting, my left knee is absolutely throbbing, I am sweating, breathless and in a bad way. "You've done too much," she says, and as usual she is right, the PW is permanently watchful, nothing gets by her, and she makes sure that I know it. I can't hide anything from her, so there's no point in me trying to brush this off. I confess and tell her the story of my painful and surreal journey as soon as I'm sitting back down in my killer chair sipping my sweet and very flavoursome fudgy drink.

The following day, the PW takes me back to Jimmy's for my drain removing;' she is working so today just drops me off and will collect me later. She takes me there early as I know it will take me time to make my way up to Ward J82. I'm limping and using a walking-stick for support. I've printed out and brought Harry the Wikipedia entry for Goslar, which is quite a few pages long. In the end I decided against printing out Hitler's speeches. Firstly, they were over 300 pages long and I didn't think that I had enough ink or paper for that, and secondly, as grim a thought as it is, I was a bit concerned that if Harry passes while in St. James's Hospital, that it might raise a few eyebrows if amongst the very few possessions he had with him, was over 300 pages of Hitler's racist diatribe. I feel like I should have brought Eddie something, but I haven't. I decide to buy them both a fancy hot chocolate from the Costa on the ground floor of St. James's after I've had my appointment.

I've been away from Ward J82 for less than 72 hours, but it feels like it's been much longer. I am told to wait in a side room, and shortly Mr Mehta arrives with a female nurse who looks younger than my daughters. He asks how I am, and I tell him all good, I see no need to mention my near-mishap in Tesco yesterday. Mr Mehta is a busy man, and after our initial exchange, he instructs the nurse to remove my drain and he'll pop back shortly to see me. I am required to lie on a bed and half strip for the drain removing. The nurse explains that it might feel "a little uncomfortable," which seems to be medical speak for "this will hurt." The removal of the drain takes seconds, and in actual fact, peeling back the tape holding the drain in place on my skin hurts more than the drain removal, which did feel a bit weird, but wasn't painful. "50 millilitres," says the nurse, inspecting my dark red blood in a cardboard bowl. "Is that good?" I ask her. "Fine," the nurse replies as she applies a dressing to the drain site on my stomach. Mr Mehta returns a few minutes later and gives his seal of approval to the amount of blood in my drain being low enough and then he's gone and I'm free to go, just like that. I had expected to be there for much longer, but this is an efficiently project-managed machine. I imagine Mr Mehta will have numerous appointments as well as operations and surgical procedures throughout his carefully project managed day.

I approach the nurses' station outside of the bay I was in on the ward, I recognise the nurse who is there and although I don't know her name, she recognises me also and gives me a friendly "hello." We exchange pleasantries and then I ask her if it would be OK if I visited Harry and Eddie, it's outside of visiting times, so technically I shouldn't. "Of course it is," she tells me, and with that I pop back into the four-bed room, where I had previously been an occupant. The familiar smell of slightly unwashed old men immediately registers as I enter, and I'd already forgotten about that smell. I scan the room; my old bed is occupied by someone who is sleeping, Tim's old bed is now occupied by another elderly chap, who is sitting on the bed reading, and he doesn't look up as I enter, just as Tim wouldn't have.

Harry and Eddie are to my left, the curtain between their beds is closed and I wouldn't be surprised if they hadn't spoken to each other since I left, as I had been a catalyst for conversation in the room. Harry is asleep, but Eddie is sitting up in bed wearing glasses and reading a book about the Crimean War. I'd never seen Eddie reading before, in fact I'd never seen him wearing glasses before either. Eddie looks up as I enter the room. "Hello," he beams, and I can tell that he is genuinely pleased to see me, which is a nice feeling. We shake hands and I tell him why I'm back in the hospital. Eddie tells me that the food is still terrible and that he can't eat anything, I notice a range of open and probably half consumed vitamin-drinks by his bed. I ask Eddie if he'd like a hot chocolate from downstairs, but he doesn't want one. "No thank you," he says, wrinkling his nose and shaking his head "I just can't get anything down." I give him a business card with my contact details on. "What's that?" Eddie asks. "It's me, it's who I am, my contact details," I reply. "Oh" says, Eddie, "I'll write you down my phone number." Eddie starts to rummage on his bedside table. "Don't worry," I say, "I can put it into my phone." Eddie gives me his landline phone number. "I've got a mobile phone too," says Eddie, "but I never bloody use it." I tell Eddie that I'll call him in a few weeks to see how he's getting on. I shake his hand again and go over to Harry who is still sleeping, leaving Eddie to find the page in his book which he has put down without a bookmark.

I decide not to wake Harry, truthfully I'm a little relieved that he's asleep as I do feel a bit bad about not printing out Hitler's speeches for him. I put the Goslar papers and my business card next to his bed, but as I'm turning to leave, I hear his familiar South Leeds voice growl, "is that Stuart?" I turn back around and reply, "it is, how are you doing?" Harry smiles and says, "no different." I explain to Harry that I've brought him some information about Goslar. "Goslar?" Harry replies, "that's where I was in Germany." "I know," I respond, "I told you I'd look it up for you after you'd told me about it." Harry gives a long "ohhhh," as he seems to have forgotten our conversations of a few days ago, relief. "Goslar," Harry says again, before adjusting himself to a sitting position and putting on his glasses "Goslar, oh aye, Goslar." Harry starts to look at the papers. "Aye that's right," he says out loud as he reads, "It's good this, thank you." I offer to buy Harry a hot chocolate but he also tells me that he doesn't want one. We chat for ten minutes or so, mostly about Germany and Harry's war memories, much of which he has told me before. Harry also tells me that he was supposed to go to Palestine but that got cancelled, which I hadn't heard previously. The conversation begins to dry up and I feel that it's time for me to say my goodbyes. I actually spent 30 minutes in there with the pair of them, time has flown, but standing for so long was painful to my legs, and the pain in my left knee is getting much worse, despite me having my walking-stick to lean on.

I shake Harry's hand and wave to Eddie as I leave the ward feeling quite sad, I know that I'll probably never see Harry or Eddie again. I know that Harry's clock was running down and I know that the prospect of death didn't bother him, as he'd get to be back with his Ruth. As for Eddie I think he'll go on for a bit longer, I imagine he'll probably need to move to somewhere warden controlled in case he takes another tumble. I vow to call Eddie in a few weeks. In actual fact, I do call Eddie some weeks later, but there is no answer. Some months later in July 2020, I was going for a walk around Pudsey, the town where Eddie was from, so I called Eddie again, unaware if he'd remember me or not. Again there was no answer, I haven't called him back since.

As I wait for the PW to return, I struggle to find a chair that I can easily lower myself into whilst waiting for her, so painfully hobble around the main ground floor atrium of the Bexley Wing looking at the artwork on the walls. Whilst doing so, I see an enormous man, very smartly dressed in a suit, browsing his mobile phone, whilst sprawled across half of a bench. This man is easily one and a half times the size of me, I estimate that he must be around 35-40 stone (222 – 254 kilos) in weight. I feel the urge to tell him about my journey, but I don't. I once had a weight-loss evangelist stranger come up to me out of the blue and tell me that he was once my size, but he had "seen the light" and had strictly dieted whilst becoming a gym addict, urging me to do the same for the good of my health, life and future. I politely acknowledged the man's great success story, but I did not in the slightest appreciate him approaching me like that; whilst I'm sure that his intentions were good, his approach out-of-the-blue just made me feel a little bit more shit about myself. I wouldn't want to do that to somebody else.

The journey home in the car with the PW is a quiet one as I contemplate Harry and Eddie, as well as my own life, my own journey, the overweight man in the hospital, the weight-loss evangelist stranger and what would hopefully be a more positive future for myself. I guess writing this book is my way of broadcasting my journey and telling my story, and I hope that if just one person reads it, and it helps them to achieve something more positive in life for themselves, then it will be worth the effort writing it. What I certainly won't be doing though, is going up to an overweight stranger in the street and pushing my book into their hands, in the hope that they will read and follow my gospel, chapter and verse.

The next couple of days are largely spent supine in my killer chair. I spend a lot of time writing and I stick quite well to avoiding the stresses of both news and social media. The liquid diet isn't a problem, just like with the LRD, I've adjusted well to it, I'm enjoying my cups of tea and coffee more than ever, and they have in effect become meals as well as drinks. My legs are really quite aching and I'm a bit unsteady without my walking stick and I have been taking the Oramorph before bedtime to help me sleep, as my knee pain is quite distracting. In terms of abdominal pain, I've hardly had any at all.

Following my previous near-disaster expedition to Tesco Express, I'm not sure how the PW will feel about me going out for a walk alone again, but I assure her that I'm feeling much stronger and that I really NEED the exercise to aid my recovery, as movement might also help my knees. The PW is a big advocate of exercise, doing yoga, swimming, walking, gym and running herself, so it is less difficult than I imagined it would be to convince her to let me walk down to a local café for a coffee. The café is about 1 km from our house, which is a huge walk compared to the journey that I had undertaken to the shop previously, but the walk to the café is mostly downhill.

Mentally undertaking a risk assessment, the PW ensures that before I leave the house; I must be wearing comfortable walking shoes; I must be properly wrapped up to protect me from the cold; I must have my walking stick; I must have a fully-charged mobile phone; I must have a power-bank should my fully-charged mobile phone suddenly run out of battery; I also must have the charging cable to connect my power-bank to my phone; I must send the PW a text-message once I'm at the café; I must have my spending money; I must have soluble paracetamol with me; I must have some sweets in my pocket to suck if I feel like my sugars are dropping; I must carry a bottle of water on my person; I need to take a small bag as my pockets aren't big enough; I must have a business card on me (so if I collapse I can be identified), and probably I must have my name written on the ticket in the back of my boxer shorts.

After being inspected in the hallway, I am allowed to leave. "Just be careful," the PW says to me, "don't overdo it, and ring me if you need me to pick you up." I smile. "I'll be fine, I feel much better today." Just in case I don't make it back alive though, I tell the PW that I love her and we kiss on the doorstep like love-sick teenagers about to separate as one of them has to go home for tea. It's a bit sloppy, but we are a bit sloppy, our love has always stayed strong.

Whilst the majority of the walk to the café is downhill, there is a slight incline to begin with, and I do feel the exertion of this. I'm aware that I'm still visible from our doorstep and I don't want the PW to see me struggling after only a few metres, so I battle on. It does feel a bit like walking through treacle, but eventually I reach level ground, before the road goes downwards and my expedition becomes more manageable. Cookridge, the village where I live, ought to be called Mount Cookridge, because that's what it feels like walking down the hill towards the café. My knees hurt in a different way as the downhill walk is putting pressure on a different part of my joints. The walking stick in my left hand provides essential support. I am hindered along the journey by three things. Firstly I have a phobia of dogs, so when someone is walking towards me with a dog, I instinctively need to cross the road to be away from the dog. This is crazy behaviour to 99.9% of people, but to me it's normal avoidance tactics and something that I have done all of my life, though this does however, make my journey longer than it needs be in terms of the step-count. Secondly, selfish bastards who park their cars on the pavements, thereby forcing me to walk uncomfortably on grass verges or have to detour out into the road. One of the streets I walk along is notorious for this. I've often felt like putting fake parking tickets under the windscreen wipers of the culprits who all have driveways but are too selfish to use them, and would rather those with pushchairs or wide-load incapacitated buggers like me have to risk life and limb by walking in the road and playing chicken with the oncoming number 6 bus. Thirdly, sloping pavements, a long-time nemesis, where the incline of the pavement is intentional to aid water flow into the road and the drains, but to me feels like I'm walking along the side of a cone. My ankles and knees hate sloping pavements, the pain that walking on them causes me is depressing and that is no exception on this walk.

Two thirds of the way towards the café, I am overcome by tiredness and a thirst that is absolutely insane. This is a post-operative consequence, on the thirst chart I can go from zero to one hundred in seconds. My entire throat and mouth feels like dry and cracked riverbed in the desert. Thank God the PW made me bring a bottle of water. I lean on my walking stick and remove the water from my small man-bag, which I have slung satchel style over my shoulder. Holding the bottle between my left forearm and my body, I twist the bottle top off and it immediately falls out of my hand and onto the floor. I watch helplessly as it rolls away from me down the pavement, into the road and between the grilles of a roadside drain. "Bollocks," I say out loud to myself. Now I'm standing here with a bottle of water that I'm going to have to drink all of, or pour onto the floor. Despite my raging thirst and internal dryness, I only need a few sips to feel recovered. I walk the rest of the journey, holding the open bottle in my right hand, occasionally sipping.

35 minutes after leaving my home, I arrive at my destination, the café called 'The Yorkshire Crust'. I've never actually been in it before, but it has quite a trendy purple sign outside as well as a modest decked area on the pavement, I've always imagined that it must be quite posh inside. I look at the now half-full bottle of water in my hand and sip a little more to try and reduce the amount, which inevitably and surreptitiously I end up pouring onto the floor, before putting the empty bottle into my man-bag, where the remnants of water that didn't leave the bottle will likely give my bag a soggy bottom, *c'est la vie*. At least this has given me a minute to compose myself after the physical exertion of the walk.

I open the door to enter the Yorkshire Crust and am immediately hit by a wall of acrid smoke from either a frying pan or a grill. The Yorkshire Crust isn't what I had imagined at all, in fact it smells and looks inside like a bit of a typical British greasy spoon café rather than the refined continental type café that I had imagined it would be like. Prior to my operation, the smell of burning bacon fat would have sent my senses into overdrive resulting in me definitely ordering a full English breakfast or at the very least a bacon sandwich, but now all of that once-delicious food seems a bit alien to me. My body temperature rises quickly as the warm internal environment is in stark contrast to the cold and damp conditions outside. I approach the counter and order a large cappuccino, which I know will take me ages to drink, but that's good, as I need to sit down and rest.

My legs are aching quite badly and my knees are now more sore than they have been for a very long-time. The walk has been a huge challenge for me, but the opportunity to sit on a comfortable bench brings instant relief. The waiter brings over my cappuccino, which looks bath-sized. My immediate instinct upon entering was to go large and that is something that I need to address. In the hospital previously I hadn't gone large with my coffee, but now I have done without thinking about it. I am going to constantly need to keep reminding myself to be mindful. My coffee-drinking tactic is to sip slowly and even if the coffee is cold by the time that I've finished it doesn't really matter, plus I don't HAVE to drink all of it, although that does go against my upbringing and Barnsley ethos of drinking it because I've paid for it.

As I sit in the café four lads enter, all wearing what I call pyjamas, those fleecy grey tracksuits. I don't mind tracksuits for slobbing around at home or for sport/exercise but as casual wear I can't stand them, they're just chavvy to me. I'm then reminded of the fact that as I sit here on my mental high-horse, I'm actually wearing a pair of tracksuit pants myself as I'm afraid to put my jeans on (which require a belt), as the tight denim and belt may hurt my stomach. I really need to stop mentally judging others by their clothes, for all I know these lads might be top athletes who've just been training and not layabout stoners with the munchies. Even top athletes enjoy a full English breakfast now and again.

I immerse myself in my phone reading the news, but none of it fills me with joy and I put it down in the end remembering the promise that I made to myself to use my phone less. It's hard to fill the time mentally though. I mean, what do you do when you've got nothing to do? Maybe I should learn breathing exercises or to meditate, although sitting listening to the four chavs in front of me talk about *The Fast and the Furious* film franchise (which I consider moronic) isn't exactly relaxing.

I've been sitting in the café for 40 minutes by the time I've finished my bucket of cappuccino. It started off red-hot and painful, but it ended up cold and creamy. I enjoyed every mouthful if I'm completely honest. I pay my bill and leave. I text the PW and tell her that I'm going to get the bus home and not to worry about coming to get me. The PW replies that she has to go to a meeting in 30 minutes at her workplace, so if I want picking up to say now. I reply and reassure her that I'll be fine getting the bus. There is a bus stop a short walk uphill from The Yorkshire Crust. I arrive at the stop and just as I do so it begins to rain, and this bus stop doesn't have a shelter and now I'm going to get wet. *Bugger*, I think to myself. I don't have an umbrella, but I am wearing a hat, and my coat offers some protection. I look down the road and cannot see a bus approaching, so decide to chance it and walk to the next bus stop as I know that the next bus stop has a shelter.

Literally 30 seconds after beginning my painful limp towards the next bus stop, not one but two buses pass me, the second bus being right on the tail of the first one. I've often considered the number 6 bus service to be a bit crap, and today is no exception. The buses are supposed to be every 10 minutes, but experience has taught me otherwise. I arrive at the next bus stop and take shelter from the rain. My left knee is really hurting now and my right knee is joining in the pain for good measure. I know for a fact that my knee pain is aggravated by the weather, although when I've tried to convince doctors of this in the past, they've looked at me as though I'm telling them an old wives' tale. At the bus stop there is a number that can be texted to find out when the next bus is due. I text the number to find out that the next bus is due in 25 minutes. Every 10 minutes my arse.

I can be home in 25 minutes if I walk from here. Now I don't have any water, but I am energised following my cappuccino bath, and if the worst comes to the worst, I can raise my head to the falling rain and open my mouth, like you see people do in films, you know crap films, a bit like *The Fast and The Furious*. Although I can't actually put my hand on my heart and say that I know that there is definitely a scene in one of *The Fast and The Furious* films where that actually happened, but I bet that there is.

I set off walking up the hill. It is a mission, a real mission. After about 50 metres, I feel like I'm doing the three peaks, but not the Yorkshire three peaks, I'm talking about Mont Blanc, K2 and Everest. Did you know there is a ravine crossing on Mount Everest called 'blood and guts', named after the fact that so many have fallen there, with bodies in the ravine below frozen forever and irretrievable? It takes guts to cross the ravine where your blood could be spilled, and many people's has been, I've even seen on TV the red-tinged snow where injuries have happened there. The sloping uphill pavement of Green Lane with badly parked cars providing obstacles and dangerous detours into the road is my blood and guts. Thankfully the falling rain means that there aren't any dog walkers in sight, a small saving grace to be thankful for.

I have to stop approximately every 50 metres, and when I stop I catch my breath and pretend to be looking at my watch or phone so that passers-by don't become concerned about me. I'm going to do this, I am in pain, but I am determined. I push on in the face of adversity, imagining the driving rain to be the slew of icy inclement weather faced by climbers of Himalayan mountains as I painfully trek up Mount Cookridge. At this moment in time, this feels like the most painful physical challenge that I have ever attempted. My body is both hot and cold, my chest is tight, my throat is dry and my knees now feel like there are molten steel splinters embedded within them.

Bite-sized chunks is how I look at the journey ahead of me, I'll head to that lamppost, I'll head to that post box, I'll head to that street sign. Eventually after 40 minutes, I can see my house, and what a beautiful and welcoming sight it is. It represents sanctuary and a place for recovery. The last few steps that I take towards the front door even have a spring in them.

I get inside the house, strip off my outer layers of clothes, drink a glass of water and sit in my killer chair where I promptly fall asleep for over an hour. The exertion has been huge, and my body hurts everywhere, especially my knees.

When the PW arrives home, I tell her all about it. I am pleased with my achievement and the PW praises me as well as chastises me for not ringing her for a lift.

That night, after I make the very stiff and painful ascent to our bedroom on the second floor of our house, I know that I am going to sleep very well, and I take the last remaining dose of Oramorph to guarantee a quick send-off. The level of fatigue that I have feels like jet-lag after spending 30 hours on an aeroplane to Australia (which I've done three times).

Little do I know that when I close my eyes, that my banana journey is about to become more difficult, and when I say difficult, I actually mean excruciating. I close my eyes to sleep, as hell awaits me.

11 – Pain

I've had one of those incredibly deep sleeps where I haven't moved all night. I'm in exactly the same position as I was around 7 hours ago when I went to bed, lying on my back, knees slightly bent over my knee pillow, arms flat against the mattress by my side. I put my right hand instinctively towards the PW, but she isn't there. The space where I'd usually connect my hand to her bare smooth tummy is now empty but still warm, so she can't have been gone long. I peel the sticky CPAP mask from my face and press the 'off' button on my bedside breathing machine as I inhale the cold bedroom air into my lungs.

I sense in myself that something isn't right, then I have a flashback to waking in the night and feeling pain so severe that I passed out from it before I could react to it; or was it a dream, or more accurately a nightmare? I adjust my sleeping position by shifting my bottom and from nowhere, the most intense, sharp, piercing dagger to my both of my knees causes me to cry out. That wasn't normal. All of the above has happened in less than 10 seconds from waking, I was still groggy but now I wake with a start in the realisation that something is very badly wrong with me.

Yesterday's walk to the café and back had been too much, my joints were buggered, on top of this, the night had been damp and drizzly, the ibuprofen that is normally trickling around my system keeping pain and inflammation at bay has gone completely. The Oramorph sent me to sleep, but it has done nothing for my inflamed knees. I haven't had any ibuprofen for a couple of weeks now and the damp wet weather outside has let the arthritis into my already sore knees with a vengeance. What were stiff and painful legs are now impossible to move without agony striking (the likes of which I have never experienced in both legs at the same time before). This isn't normal pain, this is chronic, red hot lava, burning rusty corkscrews of pain stabbing into my knees from the outsides of the joints and from the back of them. It's easily ten out of ten if not higher on the pain scale. As I've written previously, I'm used to pain, it is a part of my life, but this more-than-extreme pain is something else completely. I feel paralysed, I cannot move at all, my legs are brittle and immovable. I cannot believe that after having major surgery and most of my stomach removed, that my old enemy of joint pain is now wreaking havoc within me. My stomach doesn't even hurt, but I need to pee and this is a waking nightmare.

My phone is next to the bed, so I ring the PW who is two storeys downstairs and explain my predicament. I hear movement, I hear cupboard doors opening and closing, I hear the familiar metallic click of my crutches being bashed together, and finally I hear the stairs creak as the PW ascends. She appears at the open bedroom door a few seconds later, crutches in one hand and plastic bucket in the other. "So you can't move at all then?" she enquires. "I'm in agony, love," I reply as I shake my head, "this is the worst pain ever." After peeling back the quilt gently the PW visually inspects my knees. "They are swollen" she says, "but not overly so." The cold bedroom air on my exposed knees seems to be making them hurt more, but not as much as when the PW gently put her hands on the sides of my knees which causes me to scream out in sheer pain. "Oh, love," she says sympathetically, "this isn't good, is it?" I shake my head. I'm actually holding back tears, caused by a combination of chronic pain and chronic frustration. I don't want to cry twice in two weeks, so I raise the dam wall to prevent tears appearing as my eyes glisten.

"I guess we'll be needing this then?" says the PW as she holds up a white plastic bucket. "I don't think I can even get out of bed to do that," I reply. "Well let's get some paracetamol in you," says the PW who drops two soluble paracetamol tablets into my bedside glass of water. "Drink that and I'll come back up in half an hour," she says as she gently puts the quilt back over my knees, though even the delicate weight of the quilt causes me discomfort. After the PW leaves, I try to distract myself with my mobile phone but the pain in my legs is constant, besides this, my bladder is stretching and aching. I'm just glad that I don't need to poo, the pain from my legs and overly stretched bladder is enough for me to deal with at present.

25 agonising minutes pass; it usually takes paracetamol 20-30 minutes to begin their job of relieving pain, and I'm not sure if they've made a difference or not but I really, really need to pee. The overriding urge to empty my bladder is now almost as pressing (literally) as the pain in my knees. I gently peel the duvet covers from my knees, as the shock of the cold bedroom air makes the hair on my legs stand on end and causes me to wince as I await a lightning bolt of pain to hit. The surge of pain does indeed follow but it's not quite as bad as I had feared. Maybe the painkillers are working, maybe I can pee all by myself like a big boy.

I decide to go it alone and attempt a solo pee. It's a risky business but mentally if I can do this then there is hope and that will make me feel slightly better about my current predicament. Every millimetre of movement hurts, removing my knee pillow from beneath my knee with my left hand – agonising pain, turning my body around to sit up – agonising pain, leaning forwards to hold on to the top of my bedside drawers to attempt to stand – agonising pain. I don't actually manage to stand at all unaided. My crutches are just out of reach, but as luck would have it, I have a telescopic back scratcher in my bedside drawer, which came in handy when I got so large that I couldn't actually reach places on my back to satisfy an itch. There is a chance of me reaching a crutch with the back scratcher and I'm going to take it. I'm briefly reminded of one of those films where somebody is faced with an impossible task, like sliding a bolt on the outside of a locked cell door with a bent coat hanger from inside the cell. I think that was from the movie *Split* starring James McAvoy, a definite recommendation from me the film is too. In the film, McAvoy's character kidnaps three teenage girls. One of them is faced with the impossible task of getting out of a locked cell, and eventually she does succeed in escaping, only to be eaten by McAvoy's psychotic character (so now you don't need to see it as much). The young soon-to-be-eaten lady shows that with sheer determination she can do it. During her escape scene, the clock is ticking and McAvoy's psychotic character is approaching, the suspense is unreal. Now as I extend my back-scratcher towards the crutch the suspense is rising, I need to do this before the PW approaches, not that she is going to eat me (she'd be going at it a long time if she were), but because I'd just like the dignity of being able to pee by myself. Lord knows I've suffered enough indignities over the past few weeks, it would do wonders for my self-esteem just to get a little pride back.

The back-scratcher connects with the crutch and I pull it towards me, catching it with my free hand. Now I have a second tool to help me stand along with my bedside drawers. Pushing on both the drawers and my crutch I manage to get myself into an extremely painful and crooked standing position. I'm using the word 'standing' loosely though, as I'm in more of a question mark shaped stoop. I manage to hold my balance with the crutch in my right hand so that I can let go of the drawers and pull down my shorts with my left hand. The bucket is on the floor, my aim needs to be true. With my shorts around my knees I unfurl my sleeping snake (or more truthfully snail) and take aim with my exposed walnut whip (the cold bedroom air isn't kind to him). I have to clear my mind, think of taps running, fountains, waterfalls until "ahhhhhh" the hot pee squirts out of me, and overall my aim is decent, but that first spurt definitely overshot and there is a small dark patch on the carpet. Another job for the PW unfortunately as I have no chance of reaching it. The momentary bliss of urination takes my mind off my pain, but as soon as the pee ends the pain returns.

I pull up my shorts and cannot see any easy way to get back on the bed and in the end, I just fall backwards onto it, giving myself an extra push with the crutch. I cry out as I make contact with the bed beneath me, and wave after wave of electro-shocking agony rocks me. As I lie there panting and sweating from the exertion, I hear the recognisable sound of the PW's stair ascent. I drag myself up the mattress fighting the urge to scream out as my knees feel like they are being burned by sulphuric acid. I momentarily think of the line "acid for blood" from the film *Aliens* (the second one in the Alien franchise, and the best one at that). Could this be a gout attack rather than arthritis? The pain is certainly up there with a gout attack, which is one of the most painful conditions a person can have, and I do suffer from gout. I've never had a gout attack in more than one place at once before and it's usually in a joint extremity such as a toe or my thumb. Maybe today is my lucky day and I'm having a dual gout attack in both knees, or both gout and an arthritic flare up together, which must surely be the Holy Grail of pain inducing punishment (gout and arthritis are intrinsically linked). I just don't know, but I do know that the pain that I am feeling is more severe than any pain that I've felt before.

The PW appears with a tray, upon which she has brought me a cup of tea, a smooth yoghurt and a plastic bag containing a flannel. "I've managed to pee by myself," I tell her, "but I missed the bucket a bit…sorry." She smiles. "It's a good job you married a nurse," she says jokingly. The PW removes the bucket before putting my tea and yoghurt on my bedside table. I'm lying too horizontally to be able to drink the tea without pouring it all over me, so again have to endure electrifying agony to raise my posture, the PW helping me by adjusting my pillows until I'm in a semi sitting position.

The tea tastes wonderful, everything still tastes wonderful and it brings welcoming moisture that soothes my cracked dry throat. I had completely been unaware of how dry my throat and mouth was due to the pain in my knees, but now I'm gulping back the tea greedily in order to satisfy an undeniable desire to moisten my insides.

Despite having the operation and having a shrunken banana-shaped stomach, I'm still able to gulp back my tea in a way that I hadn't anticipated before my operation. I had been expecting to be unable to gulp my drinks at all, instead only being able to manage a sip, but it turns out that I can still drink easily. I'm not sure if this is a good thing or not, but the pressing issue right now isn't my ability to quickly quench my thirst, it's the severe pain that I'm in.

"I think you need to ring your GP," says the PW as she removes a steaming flannel from the plastic bag that she has brought to the room. She gently peels back the quilt again and proceeds to give me a bed bath, which brings both skin tingling refreshment and tremors of discomfort as the wet, warm and slightly rough flannel cloth is gently rubbed over my knees and up my legs. The PW washes as much of my exposed skin as she can before the flannel loses its heat and starts to become cold. The wash is followed by a dabbing of a dry and fluffy towel, before the quilt is reapplied to keep me warm. The PW applies the flannel to the small dark patch on the carpet caused by my stray pee, before taking my toilet bucket down to the bathroom on the floor below. I'm literally being 'slopped out' as if I were in Wormwood Scrubs, although in prison, I'm pretty sure that beautiful six-foot blonde nurses don't actually slop out for you. I'm sure that part of the punishment of being there is having to carry your own bucket of pee and poo to be emptied in the toilet. My God, imagine the indignity of having to stand in line awaiting your turn to empty your bucket. I mean what would you actually talk about to your fellow slopper-outers? "Morning, Frank, looks like you had a good drink before bedtime, and I see that you had the vindaloo," and then there's the smell...let's leave this thought just there.

I ring my GP, and she isn't available, but I end up speaking to somebody whom I don't know, and ask her for the top-of-the-pyramid painkiller Oramorph, which I am of course denied. Even though I explain my predicament, my stomach operation, my inability to take non-steroid anti-inflammatory drugs (NSAIDs) and the agony that I'm in. No GP wants to jump straight in at the deep end by prescribing oral morphine, but instead placates me by offering me 4 days dosage of codeine, which I can crush up and take alongside the soluble paracetamol. In all honesty, I'd take anything if it touches the pain, so the PW goes to collect the drugs for me from the pharmacist and I begin my tag-team attack on the pain in my knees with both of these drugs every four hours.

The codeine makes me very sleepy, which is both a blessing and a curse. I take the codeine mostly through the day-time and then it sends me to sleep. In fact, I spend two whole days in bed, barely able to move. Through the day I'm taking the drugs and sleeping, but at night I'm not taking the drugs and I'm awake. The pain that I experience at night is severe, but through the day it's more bearable. The PW is a proper wonder throughout, regularly bringing me drinks, smooth yoghurts, custard, soups and anything that might nourish me and allow my body to strengthen in the hope that this will help to fight the pain. The bucket peeing and slopping out continues, drinks in means pee out. Thankfully I don't need a poo and a side effect of the codeine is to bung up or dry out my bowels, which is something that will come back to haunt me in a few days' time, for now I'm blissfully unaware of how my pain will evolve in other parts of my body. I have zero appetite, but I do get very thirsty very quickly, so the regular supply of liquid refreshment is much needed and appreciated.

48 hours after the agony in my knees began, I awaken with a new determination to get out of bed. I prepare myself by taking the paracetamol with codeine and waiting for 30 minutes until the drowsiness begins to waft over me. At the point I painfully sit up and lower my feet to the ground. The pain is real, it is severe, but I am determined not to spend a third day in bed. I need to move!

Using my crutches, I drag my flip-flops towards me until I can just about get my feet into them. That (despite hurting a lot) was the easy part. Next, I have to stand using the crutches. I've done this a few times now to pee, but only to pee and only to stand briefly. I stand for a few seconds before collapsing back onto the bed and crying out in pain. I don't want the PW to hear me, I want to show her that I can do something for myself, I want to show her that I'm not completely useless. I attempt to stand again. The pain is severe, but I have to do this. Using the crutches to take my weight and for support, I robotically move one leg then the other. I wobble and have to immediately balance myself, though the jolt of doing so sends sledgehammers into my knees causing me to inhale sharply, my eyes tightly close and my face contorts. I inch slowly, slowly to the bedroom door, finally gripping the door frame for comfort and support. The truly impossible and difficult task is what is next, the stairs and there are lots of them between our second-floor bedroom and the living room on the ground floor. There is no easy way to get down the stairs, I can't lower myself to slide down on my bottom and I can't easily use the crutches either. In the end, I abandon one crutch and brace my body between the wall to my left with the remaining crutch on my left arm, whilst I tightly grip the bannister with my right hand. I have to bend my knees or at least one of them. There is no other option, there is no other way. Bending my knees is the single most painful thing that I can do right now and there is no alternative. I'm just going to have to suck up that pain and do it, and I do do it and it nearly fucking kills me. I cannot even closely describe how agonising this is. Imagine your knee joints filled with razor blades, rusty potato peelers, corkscrews and red-hot gravel. That's how my knees feel. My mouth is beyond dry, sweat is pouring from my brow, I feel truly, truly awful. But step after step and jolt after jolt with fire burning deep into my joints and a feeling like I could pass out at any point I make it down the first flight of stairs to the landing. I feel victorious as I've escaped the confines of my bedroom, yet I'm only halfway there. After a momentary pause on the landing to compose myself and focus on the remaining flight of stairs I begin the final descent. Maybe it's the benefit of movement, maybe it's the codeine, maybe it's mind-over-matter, I don't know what it is, but I tackle the second flight of stairs more quickly than the first until finally my flip-flopped-feet are on cold, laminate terra firma, and I couldn't be happier. This miniscule mental and physical victory feels like I have won a major competition. I've literally just got a gold in the Paralympics for stair descent. I smile through the pain, I'm breathing rapidly with sweat from my dripping brow stinging my eyes, but I feel wonderful at what I have achieved. I look like a dripping fat shabby mess in my bed shorts, t-shirt and flip-flops, but I don't care. I've escaped my luxurious and comfortable prison cell. From this point onwards there'll be no slopping out for me, I'm going to pee into an actual toilet (so I think).

I edge my way to the living room door, using the crutch as a support in one hand and gripping anything I can on the wall with my other hand. I push open the door and make my grand entrance, 'ta da'! Mentally I'm already in there, but at my snail pace, dragging my useless burning legs means that there are several seconds between the door opening and my face appearing around the door architrave. I'm overjoyed to share my achievement with the PW, except she isn't there. I then see her through the conservatory to my right in the back garden pegging out some washing to dry. I limp and shuffle slowly to my killer chair before extremely painfully slumping into it with both of my legs flying out in front of me like the character Woody from *Toy Story*. I half sit/half lie in my killer chair, legs outstretched, feeling both happy at what I've achieved, but also extremely uncomfortable. Everything hurts, most of all my knees but my entire body is now aching with the exertion that I have put myself through.

After several minutes I hear the back door open and close and footsteps as the PW approaches the living room. "Oh my God," she cries out, "you're here!" I then proceed to tell the tale of my grim determination and escape to victory, of course embellishing the most dramatic "nearly fell down the stairs" moments. The PW brings one of our dining chairs from under the table, so that I can rest my legs on it whilst sitting in the chair, and this is momentarily comfortable, although it doesn't take long for the nagging pain to return.

When you have very little, the smallest things mean much more than they ordinarily would. On the LRD or the '3-day diet' any food intake was appreciated, and anything with an element of flavour was especially appreciated. After being in hospital, the first breath of outside air was precious, and now after two days' confinement in my bed, just being able to see my living room and sit with the PW means everything to me. I can't imagine what it must be like to come out of prison. I spend the rest of the day downstairs, the PW spoiling me with drinks, soups, smooth yoghurts and all manner of liquid items. I have no appetite, but I do have a continually raging thirst, so keeping lubricated is important.

I feel very cold whilst sitting in the room. I'm not sure if this is due to the lack of movement and blood flow or my depleting fat stores, so the PW keeps the living-room wood-burner going, whilst smothering me in soft blankets. The PW also makes me a hot-water bottle to go on my legs as heat might help the pain, although in the end it doesn't do anything other than make me warmer, which is still quite welcome. My hands don't seem to get warm, so I even wear gloves for a period. This is something that is new and weird to me. I'm never cold, I went several years not even wearing a coat in winter, instead just putting on a hoodie over my t-shirt. I remember Skip and Fruddy and I going up to the Lake District, Scotland and Northumberland for New Year in 1995, it was a bloody freezing winter too. Roads were closed, cars abandoned, our car broke down and there were snow drifts everywhere. But whilst everyone else was walking around wearing thick winter coats, gloves, scarfs, trapper style hats with ear flaps and winter boots. I was content to wear my Billabong hoodie, a baseball hat, jeans and trainers. I didn't own a winter coat, a pair of gloves or a scarf. We stayed the night in Melrose and it was -15 degrees Celsius, yes I did feel the cold on the walk from the youth hostel to the pub, but you can be assured that the beer blanket I was wearing from the pub back to the hostel certainly kept the cold at bay!

My first day in the living-room downstairs, whilst painful and uncomfortable, is much more pleasant than my previous two days were upstairs, and psychologically it feels more normal to be in the comfort of the PW and be in a more 'traditional' day-time space. I continue to take the painkillers, and the codeine still makes me drowsy, but at least in the chair I manage to stay awake through the day. I struggle to stand up from the chair, but when I need to pee then I have little choice. Unfortunately, with my crutches I just can't get into the downstairs toilet as the entrance isn't wide enough, so the bucket comes back into play again, and as I'm drinking more frequently now that I'm sitting with the PW, then the bucket seems to come out quite often. Every time that I need to stand it is a rigmarole, which involves me pushing with my right wrist on the chair arm, whilst the PW holds my left elbow and pulls. My knees hurt immensely, and whilst the pain doesn't in any way get any better, I do become more accustomed to dealing with it. By the end of the first day downstairs, I have probably stood and peed around seven times. I'm not used to peeing so frequently, but then again, I'm not used to drinking so regularly.

The PW switches off the TV and begins to prepare downstairs for bedtime with the usual routine of fireguard being put in place, lights being switched off and doors being locked. I push as the PW pulls to get me out of the chair. Using my crutches, I make my way to the bottom step of the two flights of stairs to our bedroom. To ascend the stairs requires knee bending and movement, and it is at that point that the wheels fall off my brilliant plan to go downstairs, as I realise that I don't have a prayer of making it back upstairs, my legs hurt too much and I just don't have the strength. I was worried that this might happen, however I would rather sleep in the chair downstairs and at least be downstairs in the daytime than be stuck upstairs. I tell the PW that I won't be joining her, and whilst she is upset for me, she knows that I am not making the decision to sleep downstairs lightly.

My chair is enhanced to bed status, with the addition of a quilt to pad it out and to wrap around me whilst sitting there with my legs rested on the dining chair. I take my last codeine of the day and it doesn't take long for me to fall asleep. Unfortunately, my sleep is short-lived, I wake up not long afterwards and stay awake for the entire night, I'm hot, I'm cold, I'm thirsty, I need a pee and did I mention that I'm in a lot of pain. By the time that the morning comes around I look and feel like death warmed up.

The next day is my last day of codeine, and I need to get this pain sorted out, I can't go on like this. I don't want to sit there depressed, feeling sorry for myself, I want to be proactive. So as soon as the doctor's surgery opens, I call. Again, my GP isn't in unfortunately, but I'm directed to another GP to whom I go through my long story with explaining my predicament, again making a plea for Oramorph, but this time really emphasising how much agony I am in and how disabled I've become. I choose my words wisely, I speak with conviction and emotion, but remain calm and focused. I feel like I'm Derren Brown doing mind control down the phone line. This time the GP understands and sympathises that the codeine isn't making any difference to my predicament, it's just sending me to sleep, and the GP agrees that there is nothing else immediately available to me that I can actually take that can help me. The fact that I have taken Oramorph previously and that the PW is a nurse definitely works in my favour, as I draw to a close and summarise my arguments. The culmination of which is the GP agreeing to prescribe me one small bottle of Oramorph, that should cover my pain relief for another 4 days after the codeine has ended.

Hearing that I'm once again being given access to this top of the pyramid pain relief brings me joy, as I believe that the Oramorph will lead to me being able to walk, climb stairs and use my legs properly again. I take the last of my codeine on this second day downstairs, deciding to see if it will help me in the end, but of course it doesn't, and I end up spending a second day supine in my killer chair. The second night downstairs I sleep slightly longer but I am still awake for half of the night. As soon as dawn breaks, I begin to take the Oramorph, following carefully the required dosage instructions. This isn't *Trainspotting* and I don't want to turn into a smack-head from the stuff, I'm very aware of Oramorph's addictive properties. What I don't take into account, or even consider is that like the morphine and codeine, Oramorph also acts as an antidiarrheal, it bungs my bowels up even further (at least it dries them out) and it's now been a few days since I had a poo. I do not want to think about needing to poo, I'm only focusing on the pain. How that will change in the next few days.

The Oramorph has a sweet chemical taste. It's neither pleasant nor unpleasant, but it's decidedly medicinal and very sticky medicine at that. My first day on the Oramorph isn't too dissimilar to my days on the codeine. I sit in my chair while the PW keeps me warm and brings me drink and liquids. I sleep a lot and painfully stand to pee in the now familiar white bucket when necessary. Psychologically though, the Oramorph gives me the belief that I can climb the stairs and that I will make it to bed tonight. By 19:00, I'm shattered and tell the PW that I'm going to attempt the stair ascent. I'm still in agony but I just can't face a third night in the chair. The PW can't do a lot for me to help me climb the stairs as they are too narrow, but she does stand reassuringly behind me so that I know that she is there as I begin my ascent. With my left hand I tightly grip the wooden bannister which creaks and groans as it takes my weight, and with my right hand I push hard with the crutch in order to uplift myself so that I can try and bend my knee slightly. I need to pull with my left and push with my right in a co-ordinated manner in order to get enough leverage to get one foot up onto the step. It hurts like hell, but I manage it. Then I need to pull with my left arm and brace myself with the crutch with my right arm as the PW pushes my bottom upwards so that I can lift my left foot onto the step. Getting both of my feet onto the first step takes a gargantuan effort, a lot of groaning on my part and very heavy breathing; it also takes about 2 minutes to climb this one step up. I'm completely knackered, my throat is dry and I need a drink of water, which the PW brings for me. The PW always has plentiful water. I still have another 27 steps to climb to our second floor-bedroom. This is going to take me an hour.

The effort, pain and stress is repeated time and again until 20 minutes later I have climbed the first set of stairs (something which in total should take 10 seconds if that) and reached the landing where there is a wooden rail that I can lean against. I am absolutely soaked with sweat, my legs are on fire, the pain has become so intense that it is making me dizzy. I feel sick, I can hardly get my breath and I feel as though I'm having an out-of-body experience. I'm almost hallucinating, my vision is certainly blurred and I feel like I might lose consciousness as happened to me in Tesco Express the other day. I can see myself leaning and crippled, a fat, sweaty, shabby mess. How has this happened to me? This is more than just a consequence of excess body weight, there is something else going on. Is it my body going into shock at the lack of NSAIDs in my system? Is this what cold turkey feels like? The biggest irony of this moment is that my newly created banana shaped stomach isn't bothering me at all. It is both of my legs, with the pain epicentres around my knees. Physically this is the worst that I have ever felt in my life. But I also need to remember that my body is physically weak after undergoing major surgery. The red-blood cells, which might otherwise have been directed towards my knees, are probably preoccupied inside my stomach.

I become aware of the PW's arm around my shoulders, holding me steady and in place against the wooden rail. She won't let me fall, the PW is a powerful woman, although if I did lose consciousness I don't think she would be able to hold my weight, she would at least be able to bring me down more gently than what gravity alone would. But then how would I get back up? That would be a nightmare. I breathe in sharply and focus. "I'm not going to make it up the second flight," I tell the PW. "You're going to have to sleep in the front bedroom," the PW replies. The front bedroom was originally our youngest daughter Becky's bedroom, but when eldest daughter Hannah went to university, Becky 'upgraded' into the back bedroom with Hannah being 'relegated' into the front bedroom when she returned home. Now both girls have long since moved out and we have two spare bedrooms on the first floor of our house. The back bedroom is the slightly larger of the two, but it has a lot of 'stuff' in it. I think all empty-nesters whose kids have moved out have a room like this, full of miscellaneous furniture items, bags of clothes, suitcases, old TVs etc. The upshot of this is that the back bedroom wouldn't be easy for me to negotiate with my crutches, whereas the front bedroom, which is comparatively empty, will be just fine.

The PW passes me my crutches, and I drag my burning legs to the front bedroom, a distance of about 2 metres, which feels more like 2 miles, so progress is slow. Even the carpet gripper, which holds down the carpets from the hallway and the front bedroom where they meet in the doorway is an impediment; despite it being only a 3cm border between carpets, its rough metal surface is harder to drag my feet across than the carpet is, and I wince as I lift firstly my right leg and then secondly my left leg over this most miniscule of obstacles. I can see the bed in front of me, it is a whole 3 metres from where I am stooping in the bedroom doorway. I'm going to do it, determination creeps in, the effort is Herculean, the pain is blinding, the light fades as I almost pass out, but at the last millisecond I snap out of it and back into consciousness as the PW pushes me upwards to take my weight. I am shaking as I drag myself across the bedroom floor. Not only do my legs feel like I'm dragging a pair of burning tree stumps, but my arms, which have been taking my weight via the crutches, are now shaking and I fear that they might give way. 1 metre to go, just one more metre. "You can do it, Stuart," I tell myself, while the PW is saying encouraging words in a very caring tone, but I can't register what the words are. I'm not with it, my cognisance is diminishing as I mentally begin to shut down. The pain has almost fully taken over and I know that if I don't make one final push now, I will end up on the bedroom floor. This isn't something that I want, falling down now is only going to make my situation and my pain much worse. I must do this. I scream out in pain as the side of my left knee finally brushes against the bed. I've made it, I've reached my destination, I hear an automated train announcement in my head; "the next stop is bed, change here for sleep and a good lie down, thank you for travelling on the Trans-Pain-ine-Express."

I turn my body around so that the back of my legs are pressed against the side of the bed, but now I have to lie down, and in order to do that I have to bend my knees, but I can't bend my knees, I don't know what to do, so I ask the PW for advice. She doesn't know what to do either. "Can you just fall backwards?" the PW suggests. I can't see any other way, whatever happens this is going to hurt. I start to slow my breathing and try to breathe more deeply, which makes me feel that I am concentrating and that I'm getting into the 'falling onto the bed zone'. I'm preparing myself for the PW to shout "Timbeeeerrrr" as I fall backwards, legs unbending flying out in front of me like scaffolding boards. It's going to hurt, there are no two ways about it, but I have no other choice. I release my arms from the grips of the crutches and take one final breath as I fall, fall, fall backwards. I'm a skydiver, I've just jumped out of an aeroplane, I can see the plane above me as my back is facing the earth towards which I am plummeting. I outstretch my left hand as if trying to grab the aircraft as it becomes smaller and smaller as it travels into the distance. Before I have time to pull the rip-chord of my parachute, I hit the ground, I'm going to die now, as nobody survives falling out of an aeroplane (actually a couple of people have). I scream out in agony, a long blood-curdling and intensely sharp scream that takes a layer of cells off my throat and vocal chords. I'm lying on the bed, my legs are half bent with my heels on the ground. I haven't died, but as the aeroplane that I jumped out of becomes just a dot in the sky, it suddenly becomes night and my world goes dark as the effort and pain finally win and I completely lose consciousness.

When I awake a few seconds later, the PW has already jumped straight to work, taking full advantage of the opportunity presented by my unconscious body and has somehow managed to turn my body by 90 degrees, so that my head is on the bed pillow and that my legs are on the bed. She has even put another pillow under my knees to slightly bend them, knowing that my legs will hurt even more if my knees are flat against the bed. I look up feeling confused, to see that the PW is standing above me looking concerned, but also smiling reassuringly, stroking the back of my right hand. "You did it," she says, and for a brief second I can't remember the pain. "Thank you," I reply. Then the pain returns in waves as my knees take their revenge, seemingly for the work that I have made them do. I breathe in sharply. "I'm going to get you some Oramorph," says the PW. I'm certainly ready for it, I'm ready for anything that might help alleviate the agony that I'm in.

The PW prepares the room for me as I gaze upon her through a pain- and morphine-induced haze. She sets my CPAP machine up on the bedside table, and my mobile phone is plugged in to charge. The PW also brings my iPad, a bottle of water, a milkshake, a yoghurt, a spoon and the white pee bucket. "If you wake up and you're hungry have some yoghurt," she says. I'm not hungry, I hope that I'll never be hungry again, but I can see me drinking the water soon enough as my throat is intensely dry. I take a sip from the bottle as the PW disappears and then reappears carrying the quilt from the bed in the back bedroom to cover me with. It hadn't occurred to me prior to falling on the bed that I would need to get under the quilt that I had fallen onto. That was going to be an impossible task now, so instead I have another quilt over me so that I'm sandwiched between two quilts. Despite the pain this does feel very comforting. "I'm leaving the heating on," says the PW, "but if you get too warm, just peel the quilt back a bit." I nod in reply. I can't find any words at the minute as the morphine is already kicking in and I feel very tired. "I've got my phone with me," the PW continues, "so if you need me just ring me." "I will," I reply. Finally, the PW bends over me and kisses me on the lips whilst cupping my cheeks in her hands. "You'll get through this," she says, and this time I manage a verbal response as I reply. "I will." I look sad and I feel sad as the PW leaves the room and ascends the stairs to our bedroom on the second floor. We have lived together for 13 years, and we have only once slept in separate beds before (when we're both at home), and that's because I was too drunk to get upstairs after a huge night out with a group of graduated students during which I drank most of a bottle of Southern Comfort (something which still shames me to this day). Yes, I have just slept downstairs in the chair for 2 nights, but that was different, a chair isn't a bed. This feels weird. "Night, night, I love you," I croakily call out of the room to the PW. "Goodnight, my darling, love you too," she calls back. I'm awake for only a few more seconds before the morphine adds an extra blanket of comforting, enveloping warmth to my body along with the quilts, then I fall deeply into an abyss of darkness in the hope that morphine plus rest will start to mend my tortured legs.

I awaken just over five and a half hours later at 01:37. The room is mostly dark and the house is silent apart from the blowing of my CPAP machine. I lie there with a dry mouth and my eyes open, looking straight above me at a metallic star-shaped ornament suspended above from the ceiling. The ornamental star is still, but reflects light from the street outside of the room that I'm in. It's not a relaxing thing to look at or focus upon, if the ornament fell it would land on my face and almost certainly injure me. I don't know which of my daughters put it there, and I can't understand why they put it specifically in that spot, but it looks and feels dangerous as it dangles like some sort of medieval torture device. If it fell while I was asleep and the long prong of the star (which was pointing downwards towards me), hit my throat, it would almost certainly puncture the skin and most probably kill me. The star is menacing and I adjust my head very slightly to the side, in the hope that if the star falls, it would just catch me causing a minor injury such as a cheek laceration, rather than taking me out altogether.

I remove the CPAP mask from my face, and the air blows noisily as I fumble to my right to find the off switch on top of the machine. When I press the switch, the blowing immediately ceases and the room is absolutely silent. This bed has a metal bedhead, so using one of the head straps on the CPAP mask I suspend it above me. I don't like letting the mask fall onto the floor, I always imagine that spiders will crawl inside it. Can you imagine the horror of me turning on the CPAP machine only for a spider to be blown into my mouth! The thought makes me shiver. I take a drink of water from the bottle. I have so far only moved my arm and my head, my legs are completely still, and for the moment, I can feel no pain from them, which is a complete blessing. I wonder if they are getting better, that would be miraculous. I gently adjust my lying position, but as I do so I can feel the heat in my knees rise to a simmer, I know that if I attempt to move any further the simmer will become a boil before eventually becoming red hot molten lava. I cease my movement.

I pick up my iPad, and the blue-white screen light causes me to squint my eyes to protect them from the glare as they adjust from darkness to light. I spend the next few hours writing, before eventually going back to sleep and reawakening when the sound of the PW coming downstairs stirs me. She puts her head around the door. "Are you awake?" "Yes, love," I croakily reply. "How do you feel?" she follows, and I respond, "my legs don't hurt in this position if I keep them still." I proceed to tell the PW about my night, waking early, doing some writing, and being glad about actually being in a bed rather than in the chair. The PW leaves with my CPAP mask in her hand. The silicone mask seal that presses against my face needs washing daily, otherwise the mask noisily leaks air and doesn't work effectively.

She returns some-time later with a cup of tea, which requires me to adjust my lying position into more of a sitting position, which hurts incredibly until I'm still, then the pain begins to subside again. The tea is very welcome and as the PW tidies my bedside area, I sip the warm liquid, which fills the cracks in my dried throat. "Are you going to come downstairs?" she asks, and I shake my head in reply. "No, I think I'll be staying up here for today."

In fact, I end up being stuck in the bed for 3 days. Only occasionally getting out and standing for a pee or a sponge bath. My Oramorph runs out in the interim, but my GP agrees that I can have one more bottle. My days and nights blur into one, I'm awake for 3-4 hours and then asleep for 3-4 hours. I write notes about my thoughts and experiences regularly, words which will eventually find their way into this book.

On the fourth day however something else happens, which causes me alarm and discomfort. I need to poo, it has been over a week since I opened my bowels and now they don't want to wait any longer. I decide to prepare myself with a spoonful of Oramorph, not realising that this painkiller was only making matters worse. I have to call the PW to escort me to the bathroom, as I support myself with my crutches. When I get to the bathroom I can't get onto the toilet, which is too low for me, my knees just won't bend that far. I explain to the PW that I need something to my left to support me

217

to allow me to more easily lower myself onto the toilet with minimum knee bend. The PW returns with a dining chair, which might work if I turn the chair and use the top of the padded seat to rest my flattened left palm on in order to lower and lever myself into position, whilst my right hand grips the window ledge, which is above the toilet to the right. The exertion is severe and once again I'm a sweaty mess, but I just can't get seated. The PW then brings a pile of large heavy textbooks to go onto the chair to raise the height of the seat. This might just work. I pull down my shorts forgetting what dignity ever was and with fire burning in my legs I attempt to lower myself onto the toilet seat. The pain is off the chart, but if I don't do this, then I'm going to end up going to the toilet in bed, and I'm not willing to let that happen. My backside lowers millimetre after millimetre. If you've ever seen the International Space Station dock with a visiting space craft, then my arse approaching the cold plastic seat is my shitter equivalent. I'm sweating, I'm straining, I'm gasping, I'm trying not to drop my cargo from the payload too early, although the jungle drums are beating hard in my stomach, and there is very soon going to be an expulsion. Finally, my bare arse cheeks touch the cold plastic of the toilet seat. The exertion of bending my knees so much combined with the shock of the cold seat on my arse skin causes me to cry out in pain. "It hurts so much," I pathetically whimper.

So now I'm there, what next? I muster all of my inner strength and push, and push, and strain and push until finally out comes the single longest and loudest fart that I've ever done in my entire life (at least it seemed that way, truthfully I may have beaten it after a night on the real ale and a full English breakfast the next morning). The tiled bathroom echoes my anal trombone and the PW and I both simultaneously burst out laughing. "Excuse me," I sob, before pushing again, and again, I raise my shoulders and push them down with the effort, my head held back and face contorted. The muscles in my neck are standing out like a dead-lifter's. Nothing, nothing at all, not a sausage (literally). There is a pain in the back of my lower stomach like there is something there, but it doesn't want to move. I'm dried out, the codeine and Oramorph are making me pay a terrible price for the pain relief, I can't poo.

After sitting there for around 10 minutes, I can't bear the pain any longer, and pushing on the pile of books on the chair next to me whilst pulling on the window ledge to my right, I manage to get myself almost standing, heavily leaning on the window ledge. My mouth and throat are dry, I'm soaking wet. I'm in agony. The PW pulls up my shorts helps me back to the bedroom. I'm exhausted and now to go with my leg pain, I have stomach pain, or "poo pain" as I refer to it to the PW.

The above process is repeated three more times on that same day, all with similar results, although my backlog of farts have now been spent, so on the subsequent visits, there isn't even a soundtrack to accompany the pain and entertain us. Nothing, no solids, no gasses, just pain. The trapped stool in my colon feels like a giant painful shitty hook.

At the end of a shitty yet shitless day, the PW brings me a drink. "It's got a soluble stool softener in it," she says, it's probably been in our medicine cupboard for 10 years, but I don't care. I need to get this beast out of me. I sip the oily drink and hope that in the morning things might move a little easier.

The next day, the stool softener does indeed have an impact, but not the expected one. The beast within me does indeed shift, perhaps dislodging its dry outer shell from my colon wall, but it stays buried deep inside. Instead, a disgusting putrid liquid, which was probably being held back by the butt plug inside me manages to escape and I poo nothing but liquid. It isn't even lumpy, it's a definite 'type 7' from the Bristol stool chart 'liquid consistency with no solid pieces' indicating 'severe diarrhoea'. I know that I definitely don't have diarrhoea, but my liquid shit was definitely a good imitator. After this ordeal, I decide to have a shower, I feel very unclean, despite my daily sponge bath. The PW is worried that I might slip on the wet tile floor, but if I wear my flip-flops that should give me enough traction.

The shower is a step-free wet-room and the hot water on my skin is blissful. It feels as though I'm washing off days of baked on sweat and grime. Washing my hair with shampoo is a pleasure. I brace myself in the shower using a crutch with a sock on the end to give the rubber stopper some traction in my right hand, and by holding an overhead bar that keeps the shower wall in place with my left hand. Psychologically this is a winner, I feel good for showering, and the distraction of the shower acts as an escape from the pain in my legs and bowels.

With the PW's assistance, I make my way back to the bedroom, where she towels me dry, and puts talc on my skin. As I stand there naked in front of the mirror in the bedroom, my legs look quite skinny, as do my arms. My stomach is still fat, but not as large as it used to be, there is definitely some shrinkage happening. I haven't weighed myself since the disappointment of my last weigh-in, which was frankly underwhelming. I don't want to become obsessed with weighing scales and getting on and off them in my current fragile predicament, which isn't worth the pain.

When I eventually get myself into a seated position on the bed, I can feel the dislodged and very hard turd in my colon, which feels like it is stabbing upwards into my banana-shaped stomach. I've never felt anything like this before, and I have to roll onto my side to relieve the discomfort. I visualise the turd as being like the top of a coat hanger, a shitty hard plastic coat hanger. I make a further two unsuccessful and very painful visits to the toilet that day, again the routine of lowering myself onto the toilet using the books on the chair and grasping the window ledge is repeated, and by this point, I'm getting out of bed unaided and making my own way to the toilet without the PW. I'm either getting used to the knee pain, or it is subsiding, either way it still hurts greatly.

This day marks two weeks since my operation, and I'm now onto the 'pureed food' stage of my post diet regime. This means that I can add to the smooth liquids, yoghurts and custards, other foodstuffs such as mashed potatoes and pureed meat and vegetables (a bit like baby food). I'm not too keen on the appearance of the pureed food, it looks horrible, although every single thing that I put in my mouth does taste amazing. On my first day of pureed food, the PW brings me some pureed chicken and potatoes in gravy, which tastes like heaven, although I can only eat a few spoonfuls before feeling full. My appetite is minimal and I'm also wary of eating much until I manage to clear the blockage in my colon. I take another stool softener drink before bed, and bravely decide not to take the remainder of the Oramorph (there are around two doses left), instead saving it for an emergency. I do continue to take the soluble paracetamol every 4 hours like clockwork.

The next day I awake early, it's 05:35, again I have severe pain in my knees, but certainly no worse for not taking the Oramorph, there is also a bubbling sensation in my stomach. I know that I need to try and go to the toilet again. I take my paracetamol and start writing on my iPad. I lose track of time and it is after 07:00 when I realise that I still haven't been to the toilet. The PW gets up for work, she mostly works from home, only going into the office for meetings, and today is a home-working day. I wait until she has showered before hobbling with my crutches to the bathroom. The chair and textbooks are already in place and I begin the now familiar and painful routine of lowering myself onto the toilet. As with every previous attempt I strain, I make grunting noises, I'm sweating and heavy breathing as I push, push, push until suddenly and without any warning, the blockage shoots out of me like a scud missile into the ocean, and the solid blockage is followed by a backlog of putrid liquid. "YES, YES, YEEEEEEEEESSSSS," I scream at the top of my lungs, it's the kind of scream I might have given if Barnsley had just scored a winning goal at a Wembley cup final in the dying seconds of the game. "Get in, you beauty." The PW shouts upstairs, "I take it you've been then?" I reply with one word, "splashdown!"

When I finally prise myself up from the toilet, I'm shocked at what I see. The blockage that has finally cannoned out of me isn't the shape of a coat hanger, maybe it was when it was inside me, but the beast staring back at me is the size and shape of a courgette and a good sized one at that. How that ever came out of me I'll never know. It is standing length ways in the water exactly as it landed, half exposed to the air propped against the back of the pan like a wonky obelisk or the Leaning Tower of Poosa. If I'd had my phone with me, I would have taken a selfie with it. I don't think

I've ever seen or done a bigger human poo. It is completely solid, flushing the toilet does nothing, this beast isn't going anywhere, so in the end I fill my pee bucket with hot water and attack it from above. This does the trick, a fracture appears in the structure and finally the beast breaks in two. After a further three flushes it is finally gone, what a beast, what a truly magnificent beast I have beaten, and next I'm going to defeat this bloody pain too.

The moral victory of quashing the beast gives me a new motivation, and a new strength to fight the pain in my knees. I have another shower, followed by a good clean shave, a spray of deodorant, a splash of aftershave and some fresh clean clothes. I have a spring in my limp and a new resolve. Today I'm going downstairs and tonight I'm sleeping in my normal bed with the PW. I am determined, and you know what, I do it. It isn't easy, it hurts like hell, but I do it.

Once I'm downstairs, on the advice of the PW I phone my GP and we discuss my knees. This time I actually get to speak to my own GP Dr Williams. I explain that I won't be taking any more Oramorph and I request cortisol injections in my knees. In case you didn't know, cortisol is your body's main stress hormone. It works with certain parts of your brain to control your mood and motivation, but it is also a very effective anti-inflammatory for arthritis sufferers. The GP agrees that it is worthwhile trying this as an option and makes me an appointment for 2 days' time. I have faith in the cortisol, I've read good things about it, and I need to be able to move, because in 10 days' time, I'm working at a conference in Edinburgh, which is something that I had agreed to do a year before. If I can't walk or stand, then I'll be unable to go to Edinburgh, and that for me is a red-line. I look forward to working this conference annually and for both the PW and myself, Edinburgh is something that we spend months looking forward to, in many respects it is how we begin our Christmas season.

My first day downstairs is wonderful. I write, I watch TV and I talk to the PW. I keep my mind focused away from the pain in my knees. I take a mind-over-matter approach. I'm in pain, a lot of pain, but I insist on standing up unaided and am managing to push myself out of my chair with my right hand as I lever myself up with the crutch in my left hand. I go to the downstairs toilet unaided, it's a painful struggle, but I manage it. I continue to take the paracetamol every 4 hours that I am awake. I eat a variety of pureed fruit, vegetables, meat and an extremely soft and runny poached egg, which honestly tastes incredible. I get the food down without struggling. I take my time and I leave a 30 minute gap in-between eating and drinking. I struggle getting up both flights of stairs to bed, but I do it. The pain doesn't go away, but I feel as though I am beginning to get on top of it.

The next day I have to get out of our house and into the car to get to the doctors' practice. I struggle hugely getting into and out of the car, but I do it. I cannot sit down in the surgery waiting room, as the chairs are too low and I'm afraid that I won't be able to get back up, so I painfully hobble back and forth on my crutches until it's my turn to enter Dr William's room. Once in, I'm required to get onto a trolley-bed, which isn't easy, but I manage it, albeit with plenty of gasps of breath as the pain needle jumps up and down. Dr Williams, like Mr Mehta and so many of the medical staff that I have encountered, is another superstar. She chats, asks questions and puts me at ease. Prior to giving me the injections, Dr Williams warns me that they might hurt, and I tell her that, "I'm more than used to pain now." The needles go in and I barely feel a thing. I have to wait a few minutes to make sure that I'm OK and then I'm sent on my way to hobble back to the car. I'm elated at getting the cortisol injections and am convinced that they will make a difference.

After a few more days my knees do seem to ease up more, but I cannot walk without the aid of my crutches or a walking stick. I continue to push myself up and out of the chair and I continue to go to bed in our second-floor bedroom every night, making my way fully downstairs every morning. The pureed food is enjoyable and I even push the boundaries with some very soft pasta, which I chew into nothingness before swallowing.

The pain in my stomach and colon dissipates and every poo that I do for the next few days is enormous, there must have been quite a backlog. My knees improve very, very slowly, but any improvement is good as far as I am concerned. In one last bitter ironic twist though, the continual pushing myself out of the chair causes me to sprain my wrist, which brings me as much pain as my knees, and I end up with my wrist strapped up in a support. Using crutches has now become even more difficult. I look like the walking wounded returning from the frontline, I am in considerable pain, but I am bloody determined that I'm going to make it to Edinburgh.

12 – Fear and learning in Edinburgh

I am a serial traveller and with travel like everything else that I binge on, I'm addicted. Typically, I travel for work or pleasure at least once per month (often internationally) and I love it. The surgery that I have undergone and recovery period following it have curtailed my international travel until the New Year. However, I like to think that I'm strong enough to fulfil a long-standing business trip obligation to Edinburgh, with the PW to keep a watchful eye on me of course. I generally have most aspects of packing and preparation down to a fine routine, but despite my preparedness, I always get some anxiety before embarking on a journey. This usually bubbles to the surface with some snappiness from me, often directed towards the PW, for which she immediately forgives me, as she knows me so well. I always apologise afterwards, knowing that I'm in the wrong.

Today on Sunday 24th November, 2019 we are heading to Edinburgh, which is something that we have done every single year on this weekend for the past 12 years. I work with a fantastic educational organisation called Businet on their annual student conference, the core theme of which is employability, which also happens to be one of my academic specialisms. My nerves and anxiety about this trip are usually concerned with: making sure that my presentation files are on my USB stick and safely backed up in 'the cloud; having my train tickets safely stored, and the trains being on time so that I make my connection in York. Today my anxieties are on overload, not only are they about all of the above, they are also concerned with how people will react when they see me, what and how much I will drink in the pub (an essential aspect to any conference), and what I will eat whilst in Edinburgh. I'm going to be with the PW so we will have to eat out and the difficulty of navigating a menu for something small and pureed, or at the best very soft, terrifies me. Whilst I am there mostly to work, socialisation is a significant aspect, and I want the PW to be able to relax and have a good time too, and not be constantly worrying about me. I don't want to share my fears with her, as I don't want her worrying about these things on my behalf too, although she probably already is.

I have had to pre-warn the conference organiser, David (who is a good friend) about my recent health issues including my bariatric surgery and recent terrible arthritis, and how this has left me physically weaker, prone to tiredness and less mobile. The hotel where the majority of conference guests, (including me) usually stay is The Old Waverley on Princes Street, which is conveniently close to the main Edinburgh Waverley railway station. However, The Old Waverley Hotel has a first-floor rather than a ground-floor reception, and there is no lift up to reception from street level. Combined with this, the majority of bedrooms do not have accessible showers, to get to the shower it is necessary to climb over quite a high bathtub, above which the shower is located. This is no good for me, as my legs are still in a poor and weakened state from the arthritis, and combined with this, I still can't use my right hand to grip and help me manoeuvre myself. Even when fully able bodied I hate climbing over baths to get a shower, we have a nice wet room walk-in shower at home, which replaced a previous shower over a bathtub. With climbing over baths there is a risk of slipping and it isn't the least bit accessible. I don't understand why so many hotels are designed this way instead of with a simple shower cubicle. I don't think many people in the 21st century really want to sit in their own dirt (and possibly other people's) in a hotel bathtub. In my opinion, a refreshing and cleaning shower is much healthier – or is this me looking solely through the eyes of a fat person who wouldn't be able to get in or out of a bath anyway without causing a tsunami and personal injury, as well as possible property damage.

I expect when I see David in Edinburgh that there will be plenty of joking. I can imagine his Sunderland accent now saying, "where've you gone?" and "they haven't made you any better looking." That's the kind of banter that genuine friends are allowed to do and I'm prepared for it, but actually David has been great, and has managed to secure me an accessible room at the nearby Ibis Styles Hotel. It will be a shame not to be with the other delegates and speakers, unfortunately needs must in my current unwieldly condition.

I have already made changes in my conference plans in order to avoid the dangers of calories and excess. The conference begins on Sunday and on the Sunday evening there is a European Aperitif, at which delegates bring food from their home countries to display and share out buffet style. There is usually a LOT of Belgian chocolate there, and I'm never shy at the buffet, there are typically also Dutch waffles, Belgian beer, smoked sausages, cheeses and a wide range of tasty and highly calorific treats. I reckon that in previous years I could easily do 1,500 calories at that event, after all I am a binge eater. I would move from table to table like a grazing buffet buffalo. This event is then followed by a visit to an Indian restaurant for all staff members, where poppadoms, deep fried Indian starters, curries, rice, naan breads, wine and beer are consumed. I would easily take on board another 2,500 calories there. The evening is typically rounded off with a breathless waddle to Rose Street and a few pints in one of the pubs along there, so probably another 1,000 calories or so, all in all making Sunday night a 5,000 calorie event. The prospect of this now terrifies me. This year, in order to avoid this red-flagged calorific danger zone, the PW and I are travelling up on the Sunday evening and are therefore missing out on these dangerously tasty events of temptation and consumption. Don't get me wrong, I love these events, but I can't put myself in such positions now. I do feel bad that the PW is missing out, but I know that she understands. Besides this, I'm still supposed to be on pureed food until Thursday, although that seems to be slowly going out of the window as 'soft foods' (albeit well-chewed) have already started creeping in. I'm glad that I have made these positively healthier changes to my conference itinerary, but I'm also sad to miss out on the fun stuff and socialisation. It doesn't take a genius to recognise that my over exuberance at the events described above are yet more jigsaw pieces that have sent me on my banana journey. Over the course of a 5-day conference such as this, I can easily gain 7 pounds in weight, which is pretty heart-breaking when I step on the scales afterwards, leaving me wracked with guilt and self-loathing. This would then be followed by me putting myself on an extreme 3-day detox diet. A constant yo-yoing of diet hasn't been healthy and it has taken me far too long to recognise and admit this to myself.

At the conference I present two sessions to a room of around 120 international delegates. I have a strong, clear and loud presenting voice, which is something that has developed nicely after 19 years of lecturing. I pride myself on my voice and my ability to project myself across a large and crowded room without a microphone in an animated and engaging monologue performance. Besides this, my presentations will require me to stand and move around the room for long periods, which is something that I haven't done for a while. This year I have some nerves about presenting, which isn't because of my fears of standing for long periods (I'm sure that my adrenalin will carry me a little), this is because I have noticed that my voice seems to have risen slightly in pitch, and some of the 'boom' seems to have softened to a David Attenborough style huskiness. When I speak now, I think that I sound like I have a sore throat, and I can only put this down to the sleeve gastrectomy narrowing my oesophagus at the stomach entrance, lessening the bass from my belly.

I am required to deliver a 30-minute presentation on Monday afternoon at The Royal College of Physicians. This is an introductory session, where I talk to the conference delegates about facing their fears at the conference (ironically); getting out of their comfort zones; a basic introduction to what employability skills they need to utilise at the conference, and I set them a group task, which is to write and perform a 60- to 90-second song, poem or rap about their experience of being at the conference. This terrifies them, but year after year I am delighted by the effort that they put in and what they perform back (at the end of the conference). Monday is usually an easy session for me, but with confidence issues in my voice, as well as a constant dry mouth, I am nervous about this.

Tuesday is typically a free day for me, so the PW and I usually go somewhere to explore. This year my weakened physical state will likely impact upon my ability to do as much as we have in previous years, but I am hopeful for the PW's sake that I manage to be able to do something worthwhile with her.

My biggest fear of the conference is for Wednesday, this is my headline day. I am the only speaker and have to deliver two sessions of 2 hours each on my keynote subject of employability skills. On a 'normal' year, in my animated and interactive presentation format, the Wednesday sessions tire me out, this year I'm facing this in an already tired state and I'm fearful that I'll either crash and burn or that I'll just be incapable of delivering, which would ruin the entire conference for a lot of people. I haven't confided this fear in David, I've told him that I'll be OK and he took me at my word. Now the pressure is on me and I need to make sure that I'm fully prepared with enough liquid energy and soft snacks to keep my throat lubricated and the fire in my banana-shaped belly fuelled, just to get me through it. Preparation will be of vital importance.

On the Wednesday evening, there is an end of conference celebration, which includes a buffet dinner. This typically involves the consumption of a lot of food and plenty of beer and wine to drink. After this I usually then compere the singing performances from the delegate groups, it is done in a mock *X-Factor* style, with a panel of judges and audience participation. It is great fun and it appeals to the entertainment management academic within me. This year, the buffet will be lost on me. I can see myself sitting there with a tiny bowl of couscous, and then having to wait 30 minutes for it to digest before I can sip a glass of wine (that is if I can tolerate wine). Meanwhile full bellies being patted alongside drunken laughter will be all around me. I really don't want to be the boring one at the party, sitting there quietly while all around me people are having a great time and wondering "what on earth is up with him?" At the same time, I don't want to be the topic of conversation about my bariatric surgery and, "that's what has made him so boring now." I want to be at the Wednesday evening social event, but at the same time I'm afraid of being at the Wednesday evening social event. I have to keep saying to myself, "face your fears, Stuart, just like those who will be performing their songs in front of an audience." One thing I have told David is that I don't think I'll have the energy to compere the singing competition this year, so I'm hoping that if I'm not capable, he will take on this role himself.

So today the day that we travel to Edinburgh, I weigh myself early in the morning and am delighted to see that my weight is 22 stone 9.5 pounds (144 kilos). This means that I have lost 37.75 pounds (17 kilos) since the beginning of the LRD, which was 36 days ago. This is an incredible achievement, the weight is literally flying off me at a rate of around 1 pound (0.45 kilos) per day. Despite the pain that I'm in, this is a real success and puts me in a great mood.

The bags are packed and we are both ready to depart on time, in fact we are both ready to depart early. In order to get to Edinburgh, we need to catch a taxi from our house to Horsforth station, and then two trains, one from Horsforth to York and one from York to Edinburgh. The time is 17:45, I open the Uber app on my phone, and there is a car 5 minutes away, so I order it. The PW then proceeds to take our bags outside while I set the burglar alarm and lock the doors. The car arrives quickly, and then I have the embarrassment of being useless at loading bags into the car, leaving it for the driver and the PW to do between them. As always, I ask the driver to slide the passenger seat all the way to the back so that I can squeeze my stiffened bulk into the vehicle. The journey to Horsforth railway station car park takes 5 minutes, and it is dark and rainy. At Horsforth station the driver and PW between them have removed all bags from the car boot by the time I've prised myself back out of the vehicle and onto wobbly standing feet. The PW helps me to secure a satchel around my neck and a backpack onto my back, whilst she wears a handbag and backpack, and also carries a shopping bag and pulls our very large and heavy wheeled suitcase, the PW is certainly porter material. I am no longer using crutches; in my left hand I have my walking-stick and on my right hand and wrist I am now wearing a heavy-duty support to suppress movement. The wrist has become extremely painful so I'm basically unable to carry or pull anything myself. It is disempowering and makes me feel much less of a man. With that said, this is 2019, so all hail the power of women and gender equality!

We are at Horsforth station 15 minutes early for our 18:19 train to York. There is nowhere for me to sit down, the outside seats are wet, and the inside benches are too low, I would struggle to get back up from them. I am again left wondering why designers of seating do not consider the more elevated needs of the less able bodied. I have to stand painfully, so I hobble around on the platform, as this is less painful than standing still. I glance at the LED sign board on the platform; my heart sinks and butterflies dance around in my banana-shaped tummy. The train to York is running 7 minutes late, this means that what should have been a 12-minute connection time between trains at York has been reduced to just 5 minutes. Now I am worrying about my slowness, will I be able to make the connection in such little time? The PW is on the phone to her sister, I hear her tell her sister that my legs are 90% better. I snap at her that the figure is no more than 60% as my anxiety about missing the connecting train comes to the fore and turns me into an arsehole. The PW corrects the figure to her sister, laughing about the accuracy of her assessment of my leg improvement percentage. I apologise for snapping.

The ramshackle old train eventually arrives, and I climb on board followed by the PW. There is a small performance for the other passengers of us de-bagging and stowing baggage in overhead racks, particularly when I get caught up in my straps. We then take our seats for the hour-long journey to York. This is my first train ride since I began the LRD and I immediately notice the difference in how much better I fit into the train seat, and how much less I encroach upon the PW's seat space. I ask her if she notices the difference and she tells me that she does. This makes me feel good about my progress so far on the banana journey.

As the train approaches York, it is action stations. Coat on, hat on, glove on (I'm only wearing one because of the support on my right wrist), satchel over shoulder, backpack on, walking stick in hand, go, go, go. As I stand at the train door waiting for the door unlocked light to turn amber so that I can press the button to freedom, I feel like a paratrooper awaiting the jump light to turn from red to green. The door unlocked light illuminates and my finger depresses the door open button in a nano-second. There is the screech of hydraulics and the door opens letting in the cold York air. Unlike a paratrooper I don't dive out of the train, I climb down gingerly using my walking stick for support. Once on the platform I turn to see the PW agilely stepping forward, baggage in tow, what a woman. I begin my fast hobble to platform 5 for the Edinburgh train, which hasn't arrived yet, but must only be seconds away. I have to guess where coach J will be on the long platform as I have reserved two seats in that coach (the platform signage isn't helpful), so thinking logically, it must be towards the back end of the train, I head in that direction. History repeats itself at York, as when I glance at the overhead LED signage, our train to Edinburgh is also delayed, this time by 14 minutes. I can breathe a sigh of relief, panic over, no need to rush now. I would sit down and relax, but at York just like Horsforth the seating is too low so I limp up and down the platform looking for the most likely location for coach J, whilst the PW sits down and bemusedly watches me.

The 19:37 train from York to Edinburgh arrives at 19:51. Coach J sails straight past me. "Bollocks," I exclaim loudly, before fast-hobbling down the train the length of two carriages (which feels more like ten) to get to coach J. The PW with our luggage is closely behind me. We board the train and there are two people sitting in the seats that I have reserved. I was expecting this, it always, always, always happens. "Excuse me, you're sat in seats that I've reserved," I say to a young couple in their 20s, one male, one female, both hipsters. The hipster couple look at me bewildered, before the hip young male says, "there aren't any reservations on this train," and points to the overhead reservation signs, all of which are black. The system is evidently broken, nice one, LNER with your expensive new Azuma trains that clearly don't work properly. Luckily, in front of the seats that I have reserved are two empty seats, and just to put a bit of icing on this stressful journey cake, they are accessible seats with double leg room, which will do nicely. Once again, the PW and I perform for the carriage as we put our bags into the racks. Before I take my seat, I remove a cushion from my backpack to sit on. Losing so much weight so far has meant a loss of cushioning fat from my backside. I have already experienced discomfort in an armchair after a couple of hours sitting, so this 3-hour journey on a hard seat, which isn't that comfortable is going to be problematic for my rump, hence the cushion.

The journey north in the dark is unremarkable. There is nothing to see apart from our own distorted reflections in the window. There is a small drama a few rows in front where a passenger is travelling without a ticket and gets caught out by the guard. It escalates quickly, every excuse under the sun, he's heard them all before mate. The guard stands his ground and the fare dodger is £62 lighter. I retrieve my laptop from my bag and start typing, in fact I skip forward from the chapter of this book that I had been writing and write the first 2,000 words of this very chapter that you are reading now. I don't know why, but I've always enjoyed writing on trains, the odd tubular confines of a train carriage somehow get the best out of me as the outside world whizzes by at 125 miles per hour (201 Km per hour).

En route the PW retrieves some soft pasta with tuna and a bag of Cheese Wotsits, as the PW is also a picnic wizard. I am supposed to be on pureed food, but it just isn't that practical. I try a small forkful of tuna pasta and chew it very well until there is only effectively a puree left to swallow. It seems to go down OK without a problem, so I have another, and another. I begin to register the sensation of fullness, so I leave the pasta for the PW to finish. Old me would easily have eaten all of the pasta along with sandwiches, crisps, fizzy pop and all manner of other highly calorific journey treats. Now I'm completely satisfied with just a few mouthfuls. A little later, the PW opens the bag of Wotsits, I try one and it dissolves on my tongue with very little need to chew before swallowing. That single Wotsit is a salty cheese taste sensation, I used to love crisps and salty snacks, I have certainly eaten too many in my lifetime. The nutritional value of them is minimal, they're just a tasty salty fatty mouth treat, they don't curb hunger. I have a second Wotsit and then a third before stopping. They go down easily, but I don't want to get back into old bad eating habits. Moderation is the key. I acknowledge that I can already tolerate this kind of food, but I must recognise that I need to avoid it. I really hope for my sake that I can remain self-disciplined.

In what seems like no time at all, we have passed Dunbar and are fast approaching Edinburgh. The stress rises as it's now time to pack away laptop and cushion, ensure phones and wallets are safely in pockets and begin the process of stretching creaky knee joints before pulling myself upwards into a standing position using the seat in front for leverage. I am sore from sitting in one position for so long and standing ignites a fire in my knees and ankles. I grab hold of my stick to steady myself, before retrieving my hat, glove and coat and getting dressed to face the outside world. The lights of the Edinburgh suburbs are suddenly all around us, raising the stress levels to get bags down from racks more quickly. I grab my satchel and put it over my shoulder, before the PW helps me to get my backpack on. She is already fully dressed and laden down with baggage, Sherpa style.

The train enters Edinburgh Waverley railway station, and suddenly the outside blackness and amber street lighting is replaced with bright white lights. Time to be fully alert, time for action. The train gracefully slows before stopping with a slight jolt. I was prepared for the jolt and was already holding on to a seat back to steady myself against the inertia. We disembark the train, and the PW once again strides down to the platform, bags in tow like an athletic baggage handler, this is no challenge for her. My egress is much more robotic, meticulous and awkward, but with the assistance of my stick and bracing myself in the train door, my feet touch the platform one slowly after the other with just a small amount of fire burning in my joints. I straighten my posture, stretch my back, and then I hobble along the platform towards the lift. We have to cross Edinburgh Waverley station by means of a pedestrian bridge, and then there is another lift to street level. We exit the final lift next to the iconic Balmoral Hotel on Princes Street. As the door opens the cold dampness of the Scottish night air penetrates my clothing and my flesh, and goes deep into my bones. Our breath creates clouds of vapour that barely move, there is no wind, just an overbearing cold dampness. This is perfect weather for an arthritic flare-up and I'm so glad that I've had my knees injected with cortisol. I hope that they will tolerate the weather whilst we are here, otherwise this will be a very difficult week.

We are staying at the Ibis Styles Hotel near St. Andrew's Square. To a 'normal' able-bodied person, this would be a 7-minute walk away from Edinburgh Waverley station. For me it is a 15-minute walk away and the PW walks loyally by my side without complaint, constantly reminding me not to rush and to take it steady. The PW is a very patient walker. The pains in my joints are temporarily eased and my spirits are lifted by the city of Edinburgh's Christmas theming and décor. It is still November, but the Scottish capital city is fully trimmed up for Christmas, with wreaths, fairy lights and light projections in abundance on the city streets. I get that Christmassy feeling, that lovely happy and warm glow inside that is a throwback to childhood. Despite the dank weather, Edinburgh always delivers a good feeling at this time of year.

We reach the Ibis Styles hotel and have to climb three old stone steps to get to reception. I manage this using both a handrail and my stick. Annoyingly there are bright white spotlights in the floor shining upwards; these are there for style and effect to showcase the building architecture at night, but to somebody with poor mobility who has to carefully look at the floor whilst negotiating steps in the dark they are blinding and a nuisance. This is certainly a case of style over practical substance and is not at all disability friendly. The hotel reception is open plan and nicely decorated, and is fairly new. The staff are friendly and welcoming, and there is not a Scottish accent amongst them; like the NHS this is the true face of global Britain.

We get to our room, number 110, and it is cavernous. The high ceiling, huge floor space, giant bed and very tasteful décor are most welcoming and immediately put us into a positive mood about staying here. The bathroom is a wet room and will be perfect for my mobility needs. One slight annoyance is that there are no electrical plug sockets next to the bed, they are at the other end of the very large room some 7 metres away. My CPAP machine needs to be next to my bed, and it needs to be plugged into mains electricity. I always carry a 3 metre extension cable with me when travelling, but even with this and the three metre CPAP electrical cable it isn't long enough. I am forced to call reception to ask for an extension lead, and fortunately they have a short 2 metre one, which the receptionist brings up for me. I am thankful for this but also slightly annoyed with Ibis Styles for once again putting style and décor before practical substance with regards to disability.

I'm sitting on the bed, aching, extremely tired and sweating. I am a mess, a hot sweaty mess. The PW is busying herself unpacking and putting things away, while I recover from the 15-minute walk. My body is telling me to go to bed, my head is telling me to go to bed, my heart is telling me that I should go and say hello to David and other members of the conference team, which means going to the pub. I haven't been in a pub since the day before I began the LRD, and I'm nervous about it. The PW tells me that I would be better off going to bed, but I feel bad about hiding away, so off to the pub we go.

What should be a 5-minute walk, once again takes me 15 minutes. The rain is pouring and we both arrive at the pub wet through. The conference team are all there, including David and his intern Franzi, along with the other conference speakers, and some tutors of the student delegates. I've known most of them for several years and they are good friends. They all look concerned at the poor physical shape that I'm in, wet, bedraggled and limping with a walking stick in my left hand and wrist support on my right hand. I smile through the pain and greet old friends with hugs and wrist-support inhibited handshakes. I do not know how much they know about my stomach operation and arthritis, but when asked, "how are you?" I feel that I need to volunteer some explanation for my poor physical state, so I explain about the terrible attack of arthritis that I have suffered. There is no ribbing, no micky-taking, no pub banter, just sympathetic looks and responses. They can see that I am physically hurting. I get told that I've lost weight and am "looking good" despite my obvious physical problems, which is a nice mental boost.

I go to the bar with the PW to get a drink and opt for a half-pint of ale. This would certainly have been a pint in days gone by, but now a half-pint is sufficient. The PW carries the drinks back over to the others, who are sitting on tall stools at a tall table. They have pulled two extra stools over for us, but I am incapable of climbing onto them. I struggle on tall bar stools at the best of time, having 'little legs' as the PW puts it. My legs are only 27 inches (69 cm) long, even for somebody who is 6 foot (180 cm) tall, I have a long body but short legs. With the added complication of completely stiff arthritic knees, for me climbing onto a bar stool at this point would be akin to me trying to mount a high horse. There is some ensuing fuss about me being comfortable, which I am embarrassed about. I don't want everyone else to be worrying about me, when they should be having a good time in the pub. I insist that I am OK standing at the tall table. The PW knows that I'm lying, but goes along with it in the interim, while my knees and ankle joints feel like they have been injected with hot lava. I begin to do the fat man standing dance, which is to sway and constantly shift my weight from one foot to the other in an attempt to move the pain around whilst giving micro-seconds of relief to non-weight-bearing joints. It doesn't take long for the others to see my obvious discomfort and on their insistence, we decamp from the tall table to a more accessible booth where I can sit on a bench. I am embarrassed to have to make everyone do this on my behalf, and I apologise profusely. In return I get ribbed about it "always being about Stuart." I needed that, it breaks the ice and melts my awkwardness. They are good people, and I shouldn't be embarrassed about accepting help.

The rest of the evening is just like old times, there are jokes aplenty as well as stories about past conferences, as the Businet team is like a family, and despite my pain and tiredness, I am happy with my decision to go to the pub. The ale tastes good, but I can only sip it, it lasts me around 45 minutes. After this I have a gin and tonic. I am not supposed to drink fizzy drinks, so I have plenty of ice in it and stir it vigorously with a straw to dissolve the bubbles. This drink is refreshing and goes down slightly quicker, but after two drinks I am satisfied and do not want to consume anymore. This is definitely a new me.

Once back at the hotel, I reflect upon the evening, telling the PW that I am glad that we went to the pub, as this was something of a challenge for me, I can see that she is happy at my relief. I lie in bed with my CPAP mask affixed and machine turned on, air blowing into my lungs. The small amount of alcohol consumed combined with my already tired body quickly sends me off into a deep but happy sleep.

Breakfast in a hotel is my next-morning challenge. The pureed option is yoghurt, and it is natural unsweetened yoghurt, which to me tastes like gone-off milk. I contort my face at the first taste of it. "I can't eat that," I tell the PW, but she likes natural yoghurt so eats it for me, which I'm pleased about because I don't like wasting food. In previous years at The Old Waverley Hotel, breakfast was a highly calorific highlight of the day. The breakfast at The Old Waverley is a hot buffet, and hand on heart it is one of the finest cooked breakfasts that I have ever had anywhere. We would stay there for four nights, which meant four delicious breakfasts would be consumed. My breakfast plate would be loaded up with the following: three rashers of thick salty bacon, two pork sausages, three hash browns, two fried eggs, two thick pieces of black pudding, and; a mountain of haggis in the centre of the plate (it's a Scottish breakfast don't forget). But hold on, the beastly breakfast doesn't end there, the giant mountain on my plate would then be turned into an erupting volcano with the addition of several large spoonfuls of baked beans, which would coat and drench the entire plate like lava. To the uninitiated it might have looked pretty disgusting, to me it was bloody lovely! This mountainous plate would often be followed by a second round of haggis and a few more baked beans. To end on a sweet note, I would have toast coated with butter and Scottish marmalade. This breakfast would easily be in the region of 2,500 – 3,000 calories, and following it, I would usually go back to bed for a snooze while my body worked overtime to digest the fatty food that it had been assaulted with.

For just a second, I think wistfully about The Old Waverley breakfast. There would be no such breakfast at The Ibis Styles Hotel, where the options are only continental. In the end I settle for a slice of cheese and a hard-boiled egg, both of which get cut into small pieces and chewed to a pulp before swallowing. That very small amount of food completely fills me up. Gone are the days of giant Scottish breakfasts, gone but not forgotten. I enjoyed every one of them, but like all other tasty things that I went overboard with, they are yet more pieces in the path of my banana journey that I will need to avoid in future.

After breakfast, the PW and I go for a slow stroll around wet Edinburgh. Princes Street is one of the city's main arterial routes, the pavement of which is completely clogged with shoppers, tourists, workers and local residents. Everyone is in a hurry in the wet weather, everyone that is apart from me. I even get overtaken by an old dear with a walking frame, go girl! I seem to be hobbling against the main flow of people, although maybe that's my imagination. I'm amazed at how ignorant a lot of the pedestrians walking towards me are, as if they are trying to play chicken with the fat man with a walking stick. I get several tuts from disgruntled people who at the last minute have to alter their dead straight line to walk around me. Every "tut" served at me is volleyed back with a vicious "piss off, twat" or "get lost, dickhead." I might be a fat man with a bad limp and a walking stick, but I don't suffer fools, and I will stand up for myself. None of the pedestrians on the receiving end of my verbal wrath retaliate, probably because I look like a nutter with a big stick, or possibly because they think that I have Tourette's on top of all of my other problems.

At lunchtime we go to The Kenilworth Tavern, a lovely traditional old pub on Rose Street. There are benches against the walls, which makes sitting down easier for me. I order an Americano coffee with a splash of cold milk and a glass of still water, and the PW orders a pint of cider. We meet Businet friends Flo, Julia and Matthias, who are having lunch at the pub. When they see that I have a coffee rather than a beer and when they realise that the PW and I are not eating, the inevitable question is asked by Flo. "So what exactly is your medical situation?" I'm glad that he asked, I feel like I need to properly explain, and it's easier doing that to a small audience than a larger one. Flo and I have known each other for quite a few years now, and my change in behaviour is obviously noticeable to them all, he knows exactly what a boozer I used to be. It's time for me to be upfront and honest, so while they sit there eating fish and chips and drinking pints of Guinness, I tell them the whole story from start to finish. They all sit silently nodding whilst eating as I explain about my surgery, processing

239

the enormity of what I have gone through and why. They are all supportive and give positive remarks back to me. I had been worried about explaining myself, but the process was actually therapeutic, it is a relief and a burden off my mind.

My next fear to face on this wet afternoon in the Scottish capital is my short 30-minute presentation, which I am giving to all 120 international conference delegates. I approach the venue, which is the wonderfully preserved event hall in the historic Royal College of Physicians. I have presented here before on many occasions and have even performed book signing sessions here in years past, when my book *Employability Skills* was the conference gift to delegates. Unfortunately, that particular book is now out of print, so I can't do that anymore, maybe next year I'll be signing this very text there! It is always a privilege to present in this venue with such high ornate ceilings, decorated with statues of historic figures and supported by gigantic marble columns. I arrive as the delegates are having a coffee break, allowing me easy access to get myself set up away from staring eyes who may wonder why a fat man with a stick and a wrist support is addressing them. David is in the room, as are other presenters including Dale, who will be following my session. I cannot afford to run over time as we need to be out of the venue by 17:00, and Dale needs 30 minutes from 16:30 for his session, so on top of all my other worries, no pressure, Stuart!

The clock strikes 16:00, the delegates are seated and before I've had time to worry about the strength of my voice, David is introducing me to an enthusiastic audience. I cannot let David down, and I cannot fail in front of this audience of international students and academics. As soon as the first of my slides appear on the big screen, the adrenalin kicks in and I go into my flow. My vocal chords find their strength, my husky voice firms up and the no-need-for-a-microphone boom in my voice box returns. I have the attention of the whole room as I go through my slides. I am facing one of my biggest fears head-on, that I might not be able to project myself and give a good presentation anymore. I am proving to myself that I can do this, and my voice, body language and showmanship grow in strength as I talk to the audience about facing their fears of participating in an international conference in a language that isn't their own and working with strangers from other countries. The distraction of presenting makes me forget about the pain in my legs, adrenalin is a great analgesic, and I present for most of the 30 minutes without using my stick for support. Towards the end of my presentation, I set the students their singing/rapping/poetry task to a mixture of frightened murmurs from the introverts and enthusiastic exclamations from the more outgoing personalities. At the end of my session, I receive a round of applause that really lifts my spirits and makes me realise that I've done something good, the audience is happy, and their claps are my positive feedback.

Dale follows my employability session with an introduction to experiential learning for the delegates, setting them a complex political group task. Feeling very positive, but also very tired, I grab my stick and hobble to the very back of the room where I collapse not very gracefully into an empty chair. I find a bottle of water and drink thirstily, my mouth, throat and oesophagus feeling like a desert. I rehydrate myself with a sense of relief in my heart. I think that I've still got what it takes to perform, although my long Wednesday sessions will be the real test. The PW comes to meet me at the conference venue, and we slowly walk back from there to our hotel. Once in the room, I get undressed, get in bed, put my CPAP mask on and sleep solidly for two hours. Whilst I haven't had a highly energetic day, my body in its weakened state is left shattered by the little that I have done.

On Monday evening we meet the other speakers, tutors and Businet team in the Abbotsford Arms on Rose Street, another lovely old traditional pub, with the all-important benches around the side of the room for my comfort. The team have saved me a bench space in the corner, which is perfect for me and allows me to stretch out my legs. Tonight I decide to have a pint of ale, which again I sip, and it lasts me an hour, I don't feel overly full by drinking it, but I do not want another pint afterwards, so have a glass of dry white wine, which lasts me for the rest of the evening. Everyone is ordering food apart from me, and the PW orders a cheeseboard platter, knowing that I can nibble on a little cheese. Once again, I feel the need to explain to those sitting closest to me why I'm not ordering food, so I discuss the operation with them, and once again there are nods of understanding and supportive words in return. I don't know why I was so afraid of telling people in the first place.

Tuesday is a free day, so after a meagre breakfast of a boiled egg and part of a cheese slice, the PW and I head out into Edinburgh. It is throwing it down with rain, and as I can only hobble at a snail's pace, we take a taxi from the hotel to the Surgeons' Hall Museums, which the PW as a healthcare professional is interested in visiting. I am happy to go along, it is a museum that I have never visited and I want to see how the 'new' lighter me copes walking around visitor attractions. After taking a lift to the reception, we pay our way in and begin to walk around looking at the exhibits, where everything is going fine to begin with, and it is certainly very interesting and informative. But then very slowly I can feel my temperature rising, I begin to perspire, I catch a glimpse of my forehead glistening in one of the glass cases. My throat goes completely dry and I feel dizzy and a little sick. I need to sit down, but the only bench that I can see is far too low for me to get onto and back up from. I go to the reception and ask if there are any slightly higher chairs or benches, extending my wrist support as I speak as evidence of my ill health. I am advised to go to the second floor of the museum, where there are some other benches. I tell the PW that I need to sit down but not to worry about me, but she evidently does.

I take the lift to the second floor and find a wood and leather bench, which is lower than I had hoped but I manage to collapse onto it. I retrieve a bottle of water from my bag and sip thirstily. I am a hot, sweaty and very unfit mess. I must look a sorry state to those walking around the museum who see me. In the end I stay sitting down for over an hour, while the PW explores the museum. She comes to check up on me every 15 minutes. I am physically shattered and just want to sleep, but I try and put a brave face on it by saying that I am fine, though I know that she knows that I am lying. I feel deep guilt for spoiling our Tuesday together so early on in the day, and I continually apologise to the PW, who keeps telling me that I have nothing to apologise for. It doesn't make me feel any better about myself for what must be a disappointment for the PW.

242

We leave the museum and slowly trudge along the wet Edinburgh streets. Umbrellas and waterproofs are all around. I cannot hold an umbrella with my right hand because of my aching wrist and I need to use my left hand for my walking stick, so I just accept the fact that I'm going to get wet to add to my misery. The PW suggests that we go into a pub for some shelter, rest and a drink, and I agree. We go into The Advocate, which is near the Royal Mile. We decide to order some food, so the PW orders sausages and mashed potatoes, knowing that I can eat a little bit of the mash, and I order a starter, which is two haggis fritters. I order a glass of water to drink, not particularly fancying anything alcoholic, while the PW has a gin and tonic. The food arrives and even my starter looks enormous to me. Deep fried haggis is not particularly healthy, but I know it will be soft, and I'm in Scotland and I want to try some haggis! There are two haggis fritters and some salad. I eat the salad first and it goes down well, I have a spoonful of the PW's mashed potatoes and I eat one of the haggis fritters. It all tastes wonderful, but then I am full and can eat no more. The PW eats a little of my second haggis fritter but doesn't really enjoy it.

We leave the pub and I limp painfully back to the hotel, so we arrive like two drowned rats. I undress and climb into bed affixing my CPAP mask and turning the machine on. The PW decides to go for a walk around the shops, I close my eyes and sleep heavily for the next three hours. Later that evening when we go to bed for the night, I cannot sleep, possibly because I slept so heavily during the day, but also because I am nervous about my capability to deliver the lengthy presentations that I am due to give, which could make or break the conference. Today I couldn't even stand in a museum for an hour, and tomorrow I have 4 hours standing in front of an audience. The pressure is on and it keeps me awake.

Wednesday's breakfast is small, just a yoghurt as I'm too preoccupied to eat anything else and I'm not hungry anyway. At breakfast I see a friend whom I haven't seen for a number of years, called Petra, also a Businet member of staff. I first met Petra at a Businet conference in Berlin in 2006, I was sitting next to her at the conference's last night gala dinner. I remember the night well as the meal was steak and vegetables and I wolfed mine down hungrily. Petra asked me if I would like to have her steak. I remember asking her if she was a vegetarian, and she told me that she'd had a gastric band fitted. I'd heard of a gastric band, but never met anyone who'd had one before. The offer of an extra steak was obviously something that I wasn't going to refuse. Petra told me that the band largely prevented her from eating meat as it would get stuck. This is something that had stayed in my mind ever since and through that chance encounter, 13 years later when I was discussing which of the three procedures I could opt for, this was one of the key reasons why I chose not to go for the band. The Berlin Businet conference opened many doors for me and through that event I made a number of professional academic contacts and friends. Another person whom I had sat at a table with for a meal at the top of the Berlin TV Tower was a very nice gentleman called Geert Timmers. We kept in contact via email for a short while after the conference, but as is typically the way with the busy connected world, we went from exchanging family photographs and friendly greetings, to more infrequent communications and eventually nothing. 8 years later, Geert was on board Malaysian Airlines flight MH17, which was shot down by Russian-backed separatists with a Buk missile over Ukraine killing all passengers and crew on board the aircraft. I guess you never know what is around the corner. RIP Geert.

It was good to catch up with Petra at breakfast, and we spoke at length about the trials and tribulations of bariatric surgery, as well as arthritis and the debilitating pain that it causes. Like myself, Petra is an arthritis sufferer, and she knew the pain that I was experiencing only too well, so we arranged to meet for lunch later between my presentation sessions.

At 08:45 I leave the hotel accompanied by the PW, who wants to make sure I will be OK walking to the venue. The PW is my perambulation warden. I'm wearing a pair of trousers that I have not fitted into for 4 years, so this is quite a nice mental boost. The venue, the Royal Society Edinburgh, is another beautiful historic building, which it is a pleasure to present in. The event space only has capacity for 70 people, so I need to perform my employability keynote twice, once from 09:30 – 11:45 and again from 13:15 to 15:30. Today will be a real test of my energy, voice and ability to stand for a prolonged period of time.

My session is divided into two halves. I begin by telling the story of my life: from childhood; through school; to employment in a Barnsley hotel; to backpacking to Australia; finding employment with a fledgling Vodafone in Sydney; climbing the ranks and working managerially for a Vodafone subsidiary in Melbourne; travelling around the world through New Zealand, Fiji, Hawaii and across the USA; returning to my hometown of Barnsley and unemployment; moving to London but not settling; becoming disillusioned with London and applying for university; becoming a student at Leeds Metropolitan University; becoming a Lecturer, then Senior Lecturer and Teacher Fellow at Leeds Metropolitan University (now Leeds Beckett University; working with educational institutions across Europe with the EU backed Erasmus program; becoming an author and having four academic text books published (to date); how one of those text books (Employability Skills) kick-started my relationship with Businet in 2006, and; how this relationship has led to me making great friends across Europe and working with colleges, business schools and universities in Germany, Belgium, the Netherlands, Spain and beyond. I discuss how opportunities and sometimes good fortune have shaped and influenced my life and career, and how we all 'climb a ladder of life', where we do not necessarily know where the ladder is taking us, as the future is never set. The story of my life and career is contextualised through life-long learning and employability theory.

My story takes me an hour to tell, and I do so with the use of photographs from throughout my life. There is absolute silence in the room as the audience sit transfixed (apart from giggling at my various hairstyles in the photos) as I tell my story, from very humble beginnings to the person that they see before them, who has done quite well for himself, but still firmly has his feet on the ground and is always searching for future opportunities. I don't discuss my health during this story as the focus is on employability, but maybe in future my banana journey will become integrated into this story for a wider 'life' context; now there's a thought. I like to think that I am a good storyteller and do get told this in feedback from delegates.

The second hour of this session is more of an interactive seminar. The delegates are put into small groups of four or five and have to listen to me speak for short periods before being directed into undertaking four tasks of 5 minutes each, which require teamwork, communication, discussion, confidence, leadership and public speaking. The second hour covers the following areas: defining employability; when skills are developed in education and beyond; the needs of the labour market; the challenges for students in identifying the skills that they have; applying for jobs; being reactive to feedback; self-reflection; strategic planning; and life-long learning.

As soon as I reach the first task for the delegates to undertake, which requires them to discuss and write a definition of employability, I hobble out of eyesight around a corner and collapse into a waiting chair, which I had already strategically placed there. I am absolutely exhausted, my knees and ankles feel as though they have rusty knives embedded in them. My pain levels are easily at nine out of ten after I have been standing for just over an hour. This is the longest straight period that I have stood for several weeks, and in my weakened state it has really taken it out of me. My mouth is bone dry and I am sweating. Luckily David and the other tutors in the room know that I need support here, and step in to walk amongst the delegates to ensure that they are focused on the activity. During this couple of minutes of respite, I drink several mouthfuls of water and take pain medication. Then I'm back on my feet and carrying on with the next part of my talk, before giving the delegates their second activity and again finding a valuable couple of minutes of respite. This process is repeated over the next hour, until my session is completed.

At the end of the session, I receive enthusiastic applause; the audience can see that I have battled through pain to deliver a successful keynote and are appreciative of my effort. I thank them all for their attentiveness and participation and then hobble off around the corner to once again collapse into my chair. I am sweating and in severe pain but I am happy. I have done it, despite my weakened state, my voice projected, I managed to deliver the session standing (apart from my short respite sits) and I have faced and conquered my fears around whether or not I would still be capable of performing for a long session. I sit for 10 minutes, just to get my breath back, to cool down and to take on more water. The PW arrives and sees that I am hurting, so she helps me to my feet and we walk a very short distance to a tapas restaurant a couple of doors away where we meet Petra and David for lunch.

When I arrive at the restaurant, I have an hour until my next session begins, which means an hour to take on board more water, more painkillers and some food for energy. The discussion at the table is about the shared memories of the old times that we have spent together. We all have fond memories and this is a very pleasant distraction from the pain that I am feeling. I manage to eat around three quarters of a single salmon tapas for my lunch before I feel too full to eat anymore. I am supposed to have a 30-minute gap between eating and drinking in order to get the most from the nutrients in my stomach without washing them through my system. On this occasion I do not have time for this, it is difficult to stick to this rule when eating out, as it is so customary to have a drink with a meal. I decide for now to relax this rule when in restaurants rather than stress about it but will stick to it rigidly when eating at home (and I do). Despite the fact that this is supposed to be my last day of pureed food, my stomach has tolerated everything (which has been either soft or very well chewed) that I have eaten so far, and I am thankful for that small mercy.

It is soon time to return to the Royal Society Edinburgh for my second 2-hour session (which is an identical repeat of the first session). This second time around, my confidence is greater, but so is my physical pain and exhaustion. At the end of the second session, I have to sit down for 20 minutes to recover enough to be able to walk the short distance back to my hotel. The PW accompanies me to make sure that I am OK, and she lifts my spirits by telling me that as she was entering the building one of the exiting delegates was telling his friend that my session was "amaaaaazing." I am satisfied that this was a job well done, despite the toll it has taken upon me.

Once back at the hotel I sleep solidly for 3 hours, whilst the PW goes shopping and sightseeing around Edinburgh. My alarm awakens me from a very deep sleep and I am confused as to whether it is 19:00 or 07:00 when I look at my wrist-watch. I sit up in bed gathering my thoughts slowly, whilst recognising that my right knee is now hurting as much as it did before I had the cortisol injection. Standing for over 4 hours today has damaged me physically, and in terms of recovery from my arthritis has possibly put me back a week or more.

That evening we go to the final conference dinner, where the students are performing their songs/raps/poems, from the group task that I had set them on Monday. My pain levels are through the roof and my legs are stiff like the tin man from *The Wizard of Oz*. I realise once seated, that I am incapable of standing to compere the competition as I have done in previous years, so David very kindly steps in and does this on my behalf. The evening is great fun for the students, and that lifts my spirits too. I eat a very small amount of food before feeling full, and a little later I drink a few glasses of red wine, which actually helps numb the pain in my legs before I limp alongside the PW back to our hotel and an extremely welcome night's sleep.

Thursday is the day that we return home from the conference. Ironically it is the only day of blue sky and good weather that we have seen in the 5 days that we have been in Edinburgh. That in itself is a small spirit-lifter. After checking out of the hotel, I settle myself down onto a bench in the lobby to do some writing, whilst the PW goes for a final walk and shop. David calls in to express his gratitude to me for coming, and I appreciate that very much. He has become a good friend over the years, and I'm glad that I didn't let him down, as much as I am glad of his support during the conference, when I was flagging.

The journey home is long and painful, but eventually we make it back home for 18:30, where I collapse into my armchair in pained exhaustion. The PW makes a keema curry for dinner, which tastes delicious, but I only manage a few spoonfuls before feeling full. We eventually go to bed for 22:30, which is later than I had anticipated. The exertion of the past 5 days catches up with me as I sleep solidly for 12 hours. When I do awake the next morning after my usual ablutions and shower, I delicately climb onto the weighing scales and am amazed to see that my weight is 22 stones and 0.75 pounds (308.75 pounds/140.05 kilos). I have lost weight in Edinburgh at the Businet conference, and this has never, ever happened to me before. I am in agony, but also slightly delighted as my total weight loss since beginning the LRD is now 46.5 pounds (21 kilos), which equates to just over 1 pound (0.454 kilos) per day.

Despite this being an already very long chapter, I think it is worthwhile me reflecting upon and summarising the lessons that I have learned from Edinburgh, so here they are:

- Ask for help instead of struggling. I wouldn't have coped in The Old Waverley Hotel with its stairs and shower baths, and this would have made me miserable;

- Be strategic, make plans to avoid red-flagged calorific events that may either make you ill if you do participate, or make you miserable if you are there but cannot participate in them;

- Talking about your bariatric surgery can be therapeutic. If you are explaining this to genuine friends, they will understand why you have had surgery and they will be positive and supportive of you. Everyone I spoke to at the conference about my surgery was most understanding and very positive to me with their comments in return;

- Don't worry about what hasn't happened and what might not be. I had worried unnecessarily about my ability to be able to speak and present to a large audience, thinking that my voice had changed post-surgery, but in the end this was unfounded and my voice was as strong as ever. I had worried about how I would be in social situations involving food and drink, but in the end I still had a great time, I just consumed less;

- Know your limits in terms of energy and exhaustion, I worked at this conference only 3½ weeks post-surgery. It was exhausting, and I should have factored into my plans how much energy it would take out of me and how much extra sleep I would need, also my free day between speaking days should probably have been a rest day;

- Pureed foods aren't very practical out of the home, I have experimented with well chewed soft foods during the pureed stage of my post-operative diet and have tolerated these just fine, I found by cutting my food into small pieces and chewing it very finely that it all went down well;

- Moderation is key, particularly with foods that are not so healthy (such as when I had a haggis fritter), and of course with alcohol, which should be drunk slowly. In pubs I was quite satisfied with the small amount that I did drink, and I didn't feel like I was missing out;

- Don't be a martyr, if somebody offers you help and you need it, then accept it. I would have been in debilitating agony in the pub if I had stood instead of accepting the offer of the group moving from tall bar stools to a booth;

- Drink plenty of water and carry water with you at all times, the sudden mouth and throat dryness that can strike post-surgery is quite unpleasant;

- If you overdo it, you might suffer for it. I know that I did overdo it in terms of standing at the conference, and I believe that I have put the recovery in my arthritic joints back by at least a week, and;

- Finally, it is possible to partake in events and still have fun and enjoy yourself without going to excess in terms of food and alcohol. Up to this year, every Edinburgh conference that I have attended has been about eating and drinking as much as it has been about working. The balance has shifted for me this year, I have still really enjoyed my time in Edinburgh without eating and drinking to excess, and I've actually come home with a weight loss, which is certainly something for me to be very happy about.

13 – Disappointment

The Wonder Stuff are one of my most favourite bands of all time, in fact I'll be bold and say that they are my sixth favourite band of all time, my top ten favourite bands being (in order): Public Enemy; The Prodigy; Pop Will Eat Itself; The Beastie Boys; The Levellers; The Wonder Stuff; N.W.A.; Run DMC; Ice-T, and Grandmaster Flash & The Furious Five. There's a definite 1980s/early 1990s hip-hop/indie vibe going on here. I think it's safe to say that the music that you love in your late teens and early twenties, will be music that you will love for the rest of your life. One of the best gigs that I have ever seen was The Wonder Stuff headlining the main stage on the Friday night of The Reading Festival in 1992. I remember the event well, although possibly I shouldn't as I was completely off my head. In those days, The Reading Festival attracted a smaller audience than today, maybe around 50,000 attendees. The Wonder Stuff were due on stage for their headline slot and I was somewhere near the back of the arena, I was wearing a balaclava to keep my face warm, as the late August night air had a definite chill, so only my eye holes and mouth were visible. With my accompanying wardrobe of army camouflage trousers, and tie-dye T-shirt, I was quite a sight. It took me about 4 minutes to claw my way from the back of the arena to virtually front row centre shouting "intifada" (at the time I didn't know what this meant) as I pushed my way forward. Yes, I was a bit of a gig nutter in those days when alcohol was concerned. Reading 1992 was glorious and by far the best and most varied three headliners ever to grace the main stage: The Wonder Stuff; Public Enemy, and Nirvana. Yes, I've seen Nirvana, in fact I was virtually front row centre for all three headliners, as I loved them all. This also happened to be Nirvana's last ever UK gig before Kurt Cobain took his own life. RIP Kurt. The event was also compered by the legendary DJ John Peel, an iconic and cult figure of my youth who sadly died in 2004, RIP Peely. Nothing and nobody lasts forever, so I live by the mantra of seizing opportunities while I can. In terms of festivals, it would be very difficult to beat the variety and quality of those headliners nowadays, particularly with today's overproduced beige and plastic off-the-shelf headliners who travel on a merry-go-round circuit of overly commercialised sponsored festivals that are ready-made for them to headline. The festival experience went downhill from the mid-1990s onwards in my opinion, although maybe the toilets have got a bit better.

Tonight, the night after I have returned from Edinburgh, The Wonder Stuff are playing at Leeds O2 Academy, and I have tickets for the PW and me to go. We are supposed to be meeting my good friend Col, whom I have known since high school and who came and lived with Skip, Fruddy, Paul and me in Sydney 25 years ago. Thinking of Col makes me think of Australia and my travel diary from 1994-1995. I used to play a game with Col where I would read out an entry and he would have to guess the date, he was unnervingly good at it too. I grab my old diary and find the entry for the 29th November, 1994, which happened to be a Tuesday, it simply reads:

"First day back at work, boring day. Fish finger sandwiches for tea with a couple of beers, read some of 'Natural Born Killers' before bed."

That was pretty much a nothing day. It was just after Skip and I had been north to Queensland for a long weekend to meet a mate of Skip's called Wes, and we stopped at his huge and impressive open plan house on the Sunshine Coast. We got absolutely smashed all weekend in Mooloolaba and then had to endure a 14-hour bus ride back to Sydney, knackered, hungover and feeling like shit. Monday was a write-off and I threw a sickie at work, Tuesday being my first day back at work still feeling the worse for wear and with very little energy. I dread to think how many days in my life I have written off because I was too hungover to function properly. Coincidentally I had a fish finger for my dinner today, just the one with a spoonful of baked beans, lovingly prepared by the PW, which is all I can manage at the minute.

In terms of meeting Col at The Wonder Stuff gig tonight, I am struggling to stand up unaided, walking is extremely painful and I need my stick to get about. I know that if I do go to the gig there will be nowhere to sit as my ticket is standing, I'll get bashed around by the crowd and this will further put me back in terms of recovery from the arthritic flare-up that is still very much entrenched in my aching legs. With a heavy heart, I let Col know that I won't make it, which I'm extremely disappointed about, as I know how much I would have enjoyed myself there (under normal circumstances), and how great it would have been to catch up with Col. This is now the second event that I have missed post-surgery due to my health (the other one being Jonathan Pie the day after my operation).

The PW is also disappointed not to go, but cannot find anyone else to go with. I feel bad about this, but know that I am making the correct decision, it's a bit of a case of short-term pain for longer-term gain. In the end we have a quiet Friday night in without alcohol. After the exhaustion of Edinburgh, this is actually very welcome.

Saturday is a day of rest for me while the PW, inspired by Edinburgh, sets about decorating the house for Christmas. I sit in my chair with my right leg up offering comments and direction, but largely am quite useless at doing anything else. We watch terrible Christmas romance films to make us feel seasonal. I resist the temptation to provide a mocking commentary, knowing that it would spoil it for the PW who is in her Christmas element. My left leg is fairly well recovered at this stage, but my right leg is still incredibly painful.

Sunday is a big day, as we are going to my parents for Sunday dinner and they have not seen me since I was on the LRD. I don't want to get into the habit of weighing myself too often, I think it can become problematic and obsessive to fixate on the numbers on the screen of our bariatric digital scales. I weighed myself only 2 days ago, however as today is a special day I want to weigh myself again. We are visiting my parents, and I want to be able to give them the most up-to-date figure for my weight loss. This is the first time that I have seen my parents in a month, a couple of days before I had the operation. I step on the scales and see that I have broken the psychological barrier of another stone boundary, I am 1 pound less than I was on Friday, which means that I'm now into the 21 stones rather than the 22 stones. My weight is 21 stone, 13.75 pounds (307.75 pounds/139.59 kilos), I'm only just into the

21 stones, but I'm ecstatic. It's literally been 8 or 9 years since I saw that my weight was 21 stone something. My total weight loss to date from the beginning of the LRD is now 47.5 pounds (21.55 kilos). This is around the same amount of weight as a heavy suitcase that would be taken on holiday, imagine shedding that amount of bulk from your frame, and I've still got quite a long way to go.

The drive to my parents' house in Barnsley is busy but uneventful. I didn't struggle too much getting into the PW's car but getting out is more of a challenge. My stiff arthritic right leg is unwieldly, and it takes some effort to get both of my feet out of the car and onto the ground. I hobble stiffly and painfully to their back door to enter the house. There is one step up and on a normal day this step is a little too high for me to be able use comfortably, and today it is feels like I'm straddling Uluru. Painfully gripping the door frame I prise myself up the step, over the weather bar and into the house. To an able-bodied person, such small things would be insignificant trivialities, to me they feel like an assault course.

It is great to see my parents, it always is. None of us are getting any younger, and I want to appreciate the time that I have left with them as much as possible. I was once offered a teaching job at a university in Florida; it would have been quite a dream ticket in terms of working conditions and salary compared to what I'm used to in the UK, but it would have meant leaving my parents behind and only seeing them a couple of times per year, I just couldn't face doing that. This year, all three of us have had varying health issues which have prevented us from going away on holiday together, which is something that we usually try and do during the late summer. They both comment that my face looks thinner, but when I remove my thick fleece hoodie and jacket and they see me in just a pair of shorts and a T-shirt I can see that they are surprised and impressed by how much my body shape has already changed. I proudly lift my T-shirt to show them how my belly doesn't overhang my shorts and how neat a job the surgical team have done on me. The scarring is minimal, and the bruising has all but gone, I sense their relief at seeing this, as I think that they were fearful that I would be left with a huge disfiguring Frankenstein scar across my belly.

I had spoken to my mum in the week and pre-warned her that I could only eat a tiny amount of food, so she would be best cooking for three people instead of four. I'm not quite sure that she fully understood as she has seemingly cooked for five people, with the full buffet style selection of roast beef, Yorkshire puddings and vegetables on display. Struggling to stand and carry things whilst using my stick, I ask the PW to put me some items on a small side plate. I end up with a little taste of each item, and every mouthful is heaven. I have to eat slowly and meticulously, chewing everything down to a pulp. I register the sensation of fullness around a third of my way through the plate, so I stop. My intention is to warm it up in the microwave later and try again, however as I'm sitting there chatting with the plate in front of me, I pick at it gradually. Over the next 40 minutes, the stone-cold food is picked at until it is gone. Whilst the meal size overall would be considered less than a young child's portion, it is easily the largest meal that I have eaten since I had the operation. I probably shouldn't have picked at it like that, but my mum's food is simply the best food.

An hour later, pudding is served. Mum has made 'Apple Snow', which is stewed apples mixed with sugar, cream and custard. A sweet and fatty calorific taste extravaganza! In the olden days I would have wolfed down a full bowl and gone looking for more. Today I just try a few spoonfuls, and whilst it is lovely, my body tells me that I've done enough for today food-wise. Mum's Sunday dinner (with Dad's Yorkshire caviar mushy peas) is another culinary success. Whilst I have eaten a very small amount, I do not feel as though I have missed out in any way, I have got to try everything that was there, and it tasted as good as ever. More importantly, I got to see my parents, and they got to see the emerging new me, I hope that they are proud of me, in fact I know that they are.

Whilst Sunday was a big day for me in terms of seeing my parents, Monday is an even bigger day in terms of what I have to do next and the new challenges that face me. Monday is my first post-operation appointment with dietician Mary at Leeds General Infirmary (LGI). Following this, I have to make my own way to Stoke-on-Trent for another long-standing engagement at Staffordshire University, where I have been appointed to the position of External Examiner, which requires me to visit the university once or twice per year. My appointment in Stoke is early on Tuesday morning, so I am travelling over on Monday and staying overnight. This requires me to pack an overnight backpack containing my extremely heavy CPAP machine and accessories, a change of underwear, flip-flops, phone charger, power-bank, iPad, a packed lunch and dinner, half a litre of water and my medication, including the remainder of my Oramorph, in case of painful leg emergency. My backpack weighs 8 kilos but it feels more like 8 tons on my back. It is ironic that the weight that I have already lost is more than double the backpack weight. You might think that I ought to feel lighter on my feet after losing so much weight already, but the truth is the arthritic flare-up in my legs has completely taken the shine off the benefits that I should be feeling when it comes to walking and movement, which is disappointing, but never mind. I have to keep telling myself that things will get better.

The PW isn't working today as she gets every alternative Monday off in exchange for working longer days, so she accompanies me to LGI. We take a taxi to the hospital, which is located in the city centre of Leeds. Ordinarily we might have taken a bus, but I cannot face this with my right leg being so stiff and painful. The roads are busy, and despite ordering a taxi for 09:00, we are slightly late for my 09:40 appointment, which causes me stress, I hobble as quickly as I can with my walking stick in my left hand, while the PW carries my heavy backpack.

It is good to see Mary and she tells me that she can see that I have lost weight just by looking at me. We go through the usual procedure of going for the weigh-in first. I remove my coat as per usual, but unlike other weigh-ins, I am not wearing removable flip-flops, shorts and a lightweight T-shirt. I am wearing my knee brace beneath heavy denim jeans, a heavy cotton T-shirt and a pair of trainers on my feet. Today is my first weigh-in where I have no concerns whatsoever about what the scales will say, because I know how much weight that I have lost. For the first time ever, I don't even look at the scales or ask Mary what they say, because I know that my naked weight loss only yesterday was 47.5 pounds.

We move from the weigh-in room to Mary's office. Mary asks me about what I am eating, so I tell her that I'm trying to eat a normal diet as much as possible now, albeit with tiny portions. At first, she seems happy enough with this, but then when I mention some of the foodstuffs that I have been eating, such as noodles and soups, Mary seems disappointed and makes it clear that I am not getting enough vitamins, minerals, proteins and fibre from some of my food choices. It also becomes apparent through our conversation that I am not taking on nearly enough dairy, and that after years of avoiding fatty milky coffees, now I should be drinking these between meals to boost my protein intake as well as other essential vitamins and minerals. I feel like a bit of a fool, this guidance is in the documentation that was given to me, but for some reason I have become fixated with the numbers on the weighing scales more than my overall bodily health. Could this lack of protein even be prolonging my arthritis? Am I losing weight too quickly in a way that is unsustainable and potentially damaging to me? I do tell Mary that I have seemingly developed a bit of a liking for cheese, which before the operation I was not fussed bout. This then turns the conversation to Edinburgh, and me talking about having some cheese for breakfast most mornings, which Mary approves of. I then mention the challenges of being away from home working at a conference and the problems with socialising around food and drink. I mention that one evening I drank a pint of beer, which took me an hour, and then followed this with a glass of wine, which took me the rest of the evening. Mary is not particularly approving of this, she again seems disappointed and I immediately feel quite guilty. She tells me that I should not be consuming that level of alcohol until 6 to 8 months after the operation, not 3 weeks. I'm annoyed at myself in case she thinks that I'm a waste of time and a lost cause, who is going to lose weight and then just revert back to bad habits putting it all back on again and wasting everybody's time as well as my own life. I try and explain that my alcohol intake was a fraction of what it would have been, and I also tell her about how I avoided dangerous calorific intake situations, such as the European Aperitif and following Indian meal to try and bring some balance and positivity to what I'm telling her. Like Janine before her, Mary is very supportive, and I feel bad if she might feel let down by me so soon after the operation. I take her advice on board, there will be no beer for me in Stoke tonight. I was hoping to leave LGI today feeling uplifted and motivated, but instead I'm a little disappointed in myself.

The PW and I leave LGI, and now I'm wearing my heavy backpack, which I have to get used to wearing whilst painfully hobbling with my stick. We walk in the general direction of Leeds train station and call into a Wetherspoon pub for breakfast. We choose this particular venue as there are wall mounted benches that I can sit on more easily than chairs. Wetherspoon's do a brilliant large breakfast, which consists of two fried eggs, two rashers of bacon, two pork sausages, baked beans, three hash browns, mushrooms, tomato and two slices of toast, and according to the pub menu it is 1,420 calories. It is a delicious breakfast, and one that I have greedily consumed on more occasions than I care to remember, all washed down with bottomless coffees. Now I sit there in the pub at 10:30 in the morning, surrounded by a combination of: fellow breakfast eaters; early-morning barflies taking advantage of cut-priced drinks, workman in high visibility clothing and white hard hats who are on breaks and drinking pints of lager (worryingly), and Christmas shoppers having a pre-shop brunch.

I look at the menu and feel overwhelmed by what I see. Now with my shrunken banana shaped stomach I cannot even begin to imagine getting through an ordinary sized breakfast, let alone a large one. I settle for something called Eggs Royale, which is two poached eggs with salmon and rocket, covered in Hollandaise sauce and served on an English muffin, according to the menu it is 497 calories, and whilst I won't be able to eat the muffin due to its bulkage, the rest of the meal sounds delicious and should go down easily. This breakfast is something that I would never have contemplated ordering before the operation, my default would always, always, always have been the large breakfast. My breakfast arrives and is delicious. The eggs are cooked to perfection with runny (but not overly runny) yolks. I eat too quickly at first and pay the price with a little stomach pain. Slow down, Stuart. As I cannot drink within 30 minutes of eating, I have to consume the breakfast without the usual pleasure of a bottomless coffee. In solidarity with me, the PW orders Eggs Benedict which is almost identical to my breakfast, but with ham instead of salmon and 11 more calories, and she also enjoys a bottomless latte, which I have to confess to sucking the froth off.

From the pub I hobble to Leeds station, stick in hand and pack on back. Whilst it is only a short distance it is a slow and difficult journey for me, and the PW patiently walks by my side. Tickets are purchased and the PW accompanies me to the platform barriers. Here we say our goodbyes, hug, kiss tell each other that we love each other, and then do it all over again. The PW tells me to be brave and that I can do it. Unlike Edinburgh, the PW isn't accompanying me to Stoke, I have to do this all by myself and I am genuinely daunted by the prospect of this journey and the potential difficulty of the task ahead of me. I put my ticket into the barriers, they open and I pass through. I turn and wave to the PW who smiles and waves back. I feel incredibly sad at leaving her behind, I wish so much that she was coming with me. I walk a few more steps and turn again and wave, then I'm on the escalator, I turn again and as the steps rise the PW disappears out of sight. Now I feel lonely, incredibly lonely. I remember her words, I need to be brave, I can do this.

I'm going a long way around to get to Stoke from Leeds. The sensible journey would be Leeds to Manchester Piccadilly and then Manchester Piccadilly to Stoke. Instead I am going from Leeds to Sheffield, Sheffield to Derby and then Derby to Stoke. The total journey time including waiting times between trains is around 90 minutes longer, but there is method in my madness. If I went for the fastest journey, I run the risk of not getting a seat between Leeds and Huddersfield, or even worse, Leeds and Manchester. The TransPennine Express trains are notoriously overcrowded from Leeds westwards, and even with the addition of some new rolling stock, there are still too many trains with insufficient seating, and too many selfish travellers who won't give up their seat to someone who needs it more than them. I have stood all the way between Leeds and Manchester for an hour on several occasions, and it is a painful experience without an arthritic flare-up. It is something that in my present state that I cannot contemplate.

The train from Leeds to Sheffield is a Northern Rail two-carriage unit, which is not overly busy and has extra legroom seats for people with mobility problems. I secure one of these seats and ride comfortably to Sheffield. At Sheffield I painfully climb down to the platform where I have a 5-minute hobble including two lifts and a footbridge to the East Midlands Railway (EMR) train to London, which calls at Derby. My transit between platforms is slow but without incident, and as I arrive at the platform the train pulls in. This train does not have extra leg room seats for people with mobility issues, but the spacing between seats is adequate for my journey to be comfortable. On the ride to Derby I eat my small lunch of a quarter of a crust-less quiche, with three cherry tomatoes and some salad cream. It tastes wonderful, and I eat it slowly savouring the flavour of every bite. I follow this with a codeine tablet and two paracetamols, which currently I'm taking every 4 hours, I have to wash these down with a mouthful of water, so I'm bending rather than breaking the 30-minute rule, albeit for medical reasons. The journey is without incident and I again climb down painfully from the train onto the platform at Derby, which is in bright winter sunshine. The weather certainly lifts my spirits and after so many dark, wet cloudy days it is a welcome relief, particularly as the high-pressure weather system behind the sunshine is arthritis-friendly.

I have 30 minutes between trains at Derby, which is quite some time when I cannot sit on the platform benches as they are too low for me to be able to get back up from. I make the most of the sunshine by hobbling up and down the platform with the sun on my face. Eventually the EMR train arrives on the platform, and this is when things start to go wrong. The train is a class 153, which won't mean a lot to most readers, but: these trains were built 22 years ago; it is a single carriage train; the seats are extremely close together with no extra legroom for those who need it; it is very much accessibility unfriendly, and it is completely packed with passengers travelling between Derby and Crewe, which is the train's final destination. Everyone boarding the train is anxious to get a valuable seat, people push in front of me to board until finally one person takes pity on me and allows me to struggle onto the train. Once on board, I immediately realise that I cannot fit into the seat as my leg won't bend enough. In the end I have to sit next to another passenger on a left-side aisle seat, with my arthritic right leg sticking out into the aisle. My journey time is advertised as being around 45 minutes, in the end it is 55 minutes of pure pain. Even with my leg stuck out it hurts, and I am continually having to pull it to the left to prevent other embarking and disembarking passengers knocking it as they pass. Despite this, I get several knocks on my foot, each of which sends a shockwave up my leg that feels like a red-hot poker being jabbed into my knee cap. Getting off the train at Stoke is agonising, but I have never been so happy to get off a train before. This 55-minute journey has probably worsened my pain by 80% and set my recovery back even further. I vow never ever to set foot on a class 153 train again.

I take a taxi to my hotel, which is The Premier Inn. The journey is thankfully quick and the taxi more comfortable than the train that I've just got off, and the sky has darkened as the sun has set. Check-in at the hotel is quick and easy, and my room (which has been booked by Staffordshire University) is an accessible one with a walk-in shower. I'm thankful to Staffordshire University for making this adjustment for me, from what was originally a standard room with a shower-bath. The room has one slight problem for me in that the bed is too low. Whilst I'll be able to fall onto it without a problem, I'll not be able to get up from it. I limp to reception apologetically to explain the situation, and they have a solution – elephant's feet! I've never heard of elephant's feet before, but essentially, they look like grey upside-down plant pots, which the legs of the bed can stand in, raising the bed by around 20 centimetres. They work perfectly and the bed is completely accessible to me. I painfully undress into my sleeping attire of shorts and a vest. I can't bend my right leg enough to remove my sock so leave both of my socks on. I set up my CPAP machine, take painkillers and awkwardly fall into bed, where I sleep for 1 hour and 20 minutes in complete exhaustion.

I barely get out of bed all evening, apart from to use the bathroom. I feel like I need nothing but rest and comfort. At some point I remember that I have my dinner to eat (which is a repeat of my lunch), a quarter of a crust-less quiche, cherry tomatoes and salad cream. Whilst I'm not hungry it goes down very well and once again tastes delicious. I decide to look at my Leeds Beckett email for an hour. I don't have to, but the email building up is causing me stress again, and there are currently 81 unread messages. After an hour, all have been read and the majority that needed answering have been responded to. I know that the PW is having a meal out tonight with friends (and a deserved break from me), so I simply send her a Facebook message to tell her that I've arrived fine at the hotel, I'm in pain, but I've eaten and am now in bed ready for an early night's sleep, I finish by telling her that I love her. At 21:15 my CPAP mask is affixed, the machine is turned on, the lights are switched off and I fall into a deep sleep. It is a strange sleep, I seem to wake up like clockwork every 4 hours, which is the duration between my pain medication, so I take my pain meds twice during the night and go straight back to sleep again afterwards.

I awaken early the next morning at 06:30 with my alarm on a gentle tone, I feel well rested having been horizontal for the best part of 12 hours. I want to give myself plenty of time to get ready so that I don't stress any more than I need to. My first decision is to shower or not to shower? At present I am wearing yesterday's black and white striped socks, I'll need to remove these in order to shower, I don't have the PW here to help me now, but there is insufficient bend in my right leg for me to take off my right sock. If I do manage to get it off, I'll not be able to get another one on, and I haven't even thought about how I'm going to get my trainers back on. The realisation dawns upon me that I might have to go to my meeting at Staffordshire University wearing flip-flops and socks on my feet. What a way to make a first impression with new colleagues. Maybe they'll think I'm trendy? After all flip-flops have been rebranded for Generation Z as 'sliders', which is a marketing term that incidentally repulses me. They are not sliders, they are flip-flops, they flip and flop when you walk, end of. As far as I'm concerned, a slider is a dial or lever that controls sound on a musical instrument or music player. I realise that there are also mini burgers that are called sliders, but I find that to be a pretty stupid marketing term too. What makes Generation Z sliders even worse is that it has become a popular fashion to wear them with socks. My generation have worked so hard over the past 40 years to eradicate the memories of our parents wearing flip-flops with socks in the 1970s, yet now it has become a repulsive high-street trend for fashion conscious sheep to follow. The children of Generation Z will no doubt look shamefully at the fashion crimes of their parents as did my generation and will hopefully work hard once again to eradicate the memory of flip-flops with socks. Either that or they'll do something even worse, such as wear Crocs with socks. I can just imagine the advert for this, with rapped lyrics as follows:

"I'm rockin' my Crocs with socks,
I'm rockin' my Crocs with socks,
I've got a slick top-knot with fresh hip-hop,
I'm rockin' my Crocs with socks,
I'm rockin' my Crocs with socks"

This song is a nightmare waiting to happen and it is embedded within my cranium thanks to all those flip-flop and sock wearing fools. I've even seen students in Leeds wearing flip-flops with socks on winter days when it's been throwing it down with rain, the bloody idiots. Today I am going to have to join their ranks thanks to my inability to bend my right knee and put a pair of trainers on. I suppose that I could go with a trainer on my left foot and a flip-flop on my right foot, but I'm not quite sure that I'm edgy enough to get away with that particular look. I resign myself to that fact that I'm wearing flip-flops with socks today. I suppose it could be worse, my socks could have holes in, thankfully they don't, although close inspection of the material over my right big toenail shows that they're not far from fraying. I hope that they hold on, just for one more day.

Unable to shower, I have a vigorous flannel wash all over my body, which in all fairness feels very refreshing. I dry off and painfully pull on new boxer-shorts, and very trickily the knee brace for my right leg, which I set tightly. My jeans are dragged on next, which is more of a struggle than I would have liked, but I manage to do it inch by inch very slowly, even though the exertion leaves me sitting on the bed out of breath and sweating. I lie back for a minute to recover, bringing my legs onto the bed. I close my eyes momentarily and awaken 25 minutes later; now I'm really stressing. I still have to pack my rucksack, finish getting dressed, have breakfast and get to the university. In the end after getting dressed I decide to take breakfast as quickly as I possibly can do, however an inspection of the restaurant reveals that the seating is too low for me get up from anyway, so I skip breakfast in order to concentrate on packing my backpack, which takes me longer than it ought to. By the time I've checked out of the hotel and ordered a taxi, I am sweating and dishevelled, and do not look like a professional academic.

I arrive at Staffordshire University an unkempt sweaty limping mess complete with flip-flops and socks. I get to the meeting room and am relieved to see that there are some height adjustable chairs. I get myself a coffee and a chocolate biscuit (the breakfast of sweaty flip-flop-wearing champions), then take a raised height seat. I am set to be in this room for 2 hours, before moving to another campus for lunch and to meet other new colleagues.

The morning session is informative, and I learn about the university and its vision of connectivity. It is presented well, but like all English universities in a fee-paying competitive HE system, the ideology seems driven by marketing; sadly in our present HE system it has to be. This is something that I'm ashamed to say a Labour government with Tony Blair as Prime Minister and Gordon Brown as Chancellor of the Exchequer began in 1998 with the introduction of tuition fees. Successive Tory governments have worsened this position still by strangling universities further financially and raising tuition fees to unsustainable levels, paid for through loans, which a significant proportion of graduates will never pay back. I wonder who will end up paying for that particular magic money tree?

During my time sitting there, I have to keep moving my leg around as I seem to be unable to get it in a comfortable position for more than a few minutes. The pain becomes distracting to the point that I begin to lose track of what is being said, I take an extra codeine tablet. I need to focus and try and ignore the pain. I mentally do what I can, but I realise that after the morning session is over, my pain levels are such that I am going to be unable to participate in the afternoon session. I meet a representative of my school and profoundly apologise to her for not being able to participate in the afternoon. I am very disappointed in myself for making such a poor first impression and feel as though I have wasted the university's time. I pride myself in my professionalism in the workplace, and dread to think what an impression I have left. I promise to return in January, once my leg is better and at my own expense. I consider my options in terms of my return journey to Leeds. I simply cannot face the horrendously cramped and painful conditions of an EMR class 153 train from Stoke to Derby, so I order a taxi from Stoke to Derby instead. One lucky Stoke driver is about to become £50 better off and I'll have to take this financial hit myself.

As I'm standing on the university campus waiting for my taxi, I become a witness to an extremely uncomfortable, unnecessary and aggressive verbal altercation between a male university employee and a man who owns a business next to the university. There are road works taking place outside of the university, which meant that the business owner could not park his car outside of his premises and has instead parked his car on campus in a no parking area (and also without a permit); the business owner is wrong to have done this.

The altercation takes place literally three metres from where I am standing and I am shocked and disappointed by the aggressive attitude of the university employee towards the business owner who comes to investigate why the attendant is looking at his car. The business owner tries to explain himself, but the attendant escalates the situation through a raised voice. He is verbally aggressive and repeats the phrase, "Not my problem, I don't care, shut up," several times. Then the employee uses foul language, which the business owner matches like for like. The university employee has no idea who I am at all, for all he knows I might be a senior member of university staff, although my flip-flops and socks probably suggest otherwise. Maybe there is a history between these two, maybe the business owner is a regular offender and the employee has reached the end of his tether, I honestly don't know, but this situation should not have unfolded the way that it did. I can definitely see the need for some retraining here in terms of negotiation, communication and conflict resolution. Thankfully the two men separate and leave before physical blows are traded, both swearing at each other before going in opposite directions and I am left alone in shock at what I have just seen unfold in front of me. Whilst it cannot be denied that the business owner is in the wrong parking his car where he has, I have to judge the university employee at fault for escalating the situation through his overly aggressive manner and language.

As I stand there awaiting my taxi, digesting what I have just witnessed, the business owner returns to move his car. His body is square and angular, his face contorted, his movements mechanical. I can see anger and adrenalin coursing through him. I feel as if I need to say something to him to calm him down before he gets into his car to drive, so I tell him that the university employee should not have spoken to him like that. He expresses his frustration about being unable to park by his business and at being spoken to like he was by the employee. I remember a piece of advice, which somebody once gave me to calm me down when somebody had made me very angry. I decide to pass this advice on to the business owner. "Can I give you a piece of advice, which somebody once gave to me when I had been wound up like you have been?" I say. The business owner pauses, surprised at my question. "Go on," he replies. I tell him, "there are seven billion people on this planet, so don't let one arsehole spoil your day." He digests what I have said for half a second, then his square shoulders drop, becoming round, his arms loosen, and his scowl turns to a smile that spreads across his face releasing endorphins, which hopefully restore a happy balance to his troubled mind. He pats me on my shoulder, looks into my eyes and smiles, and says, "thank you, you are a good man." I think we both needed that. The business owner then gets in his car and leaves with a wave. We are both less troubled souls for that exchange. I feel as though I have done a good deed for the day.

My taxi arrives 5 minutes later, and I'm soon on my way to Derby. I explain to the driver that I will need to call at a cash machine, so he pulls into a garage on the outskirts of Stoke. I climb out of the taxi with considerable discomfort and hobble with my stick to the cash machine. After withdrawing the money, I hobble back towards the car, I'm feeling sorry for myself in my painful and expensive situation, when a man crosses my path in front of me. He looks at me questioningly as if to say, "cheer up, it might not happen." I then notice that he is wearing three-quarter-length shorts, and underneath them are a pair of false legs and feet. He is walking unaided without a stick and for all intents and purposes, exactly like any man with a pair of flesh and bone legs and feet would walk. I feel disappointed at my own self-pity, I need to think more positively. I stiffly get back into the taxi for the hour long journey to Derby station.

At Derby I am pleased to see that there is an EMR train to Sheffield due in 15 minutes. I stand on the platform waiting for the train to arrive. I know that it will be a long train with good space between the seats as it is coming from London, I also assume that as the end destination is Sheffield, which is only two stops away, it won't be too busy. The train pulls in and I hobble towards the door. Plenty of passengers get off the train, and there are quite a few people on the platform huddled around the door awaiting to board it. I am towards the back of this scrum who probably all want a double seat to themselves. Thankfully, a very fierce grey-haired old lady physically extends her arms and holds half of the scrum back to allow me to board the train. I thank her for doing this and find a comfortable seat with sufficient leg room for the 35-minute journey.

Once at Sheffield, my pain worsens as I have to stand on the very busy platform waiting for the delayed 'fast train' to Leeds via Barnsley for almost 30 minutes. It is beginning to get dark and before long rush-hour will be here, along with thousands of commuters and standing room only. I can't afford to wait for that to happen. Eventually the train arrives 10 minutes late due to a signalling failure outside of

Sheffield station. The train is a Northern Rail class 153, the same class of train that yesterday I vowed never to ride again, and the same class of train that I've just paid a taxi driver £50 to avoid between Stoke and Derby. To say that I'm disappointed is an understatement, very pissed off is a more accurate interpretation of how I'm currently feeling. I board the train with the horde of other awaiting passengers; there are two seats that are marked as being extra-legroom for passengers with mobility issues, but upon close inspection there is no more leg room than with any of the other seats. The class 153 has made it to the top of my most hated train list, overtaking the dreaded class 142 'pacers'. It's amazing how these dreadful cattle trucks are endemic in the north of England, you certainly wouldn't see rubbish like this in London, and that's because Tory transport ministers look after their own. I hope so much that Corbyn wins the general election and renationalises the railways, which should put passengers before the profits of greedy corporations. Thankfully I find a fold-down seat, which is too low, but by grabbing onto the back of the chair in front of it I can lower myself down and pull myself back up. The position of the seat means that my bad leg is partially stuck out into the aisle. The 1-hour journey to Leeds is once again a very painful ride on a class 153, as I try and keep my leg out of the way of other passengers, and when I don't manage to do this, I receive a painful jolt for straying into their paths.

I pull myself to my feet as we approach Leeds. My face is contorted from the exertion and my forehead dripping with sweat. I struggle to pull on my backpack without knocking other passengers off their feet, and give out a few chants of "sorry." I need to get off this train amongst the herd of other passengers and not be left to the back, otherwise the scrum of passengers at Leeds waiting to board this train for the return journey will prevent my egress. My climb down to the platform is stiff and robotic, I am in severe pain. Leeds railway station is now in the grip of rush hour and everyone is impatient, pushing and jostling. Leeds is the second busiest railway station in the UK outside of London, yet the city has only one railway station, which is another sign of the underinvestment of successive governments in public transport. Leeds should additionally have an interchange station where the railway line passes Leeds bus station. Maybe one day it will happen but it's currently a pipedream. I need to get out of the way of the commuter horde, who like a Roman legion are trudging unstoppably, so I stand against a wall and let everyone pass until I begin to see patches of floor space. I limp to the lift, over the footbridge and down the lift to platform 8. From here I hobble towards and out of the ticket barriers. I could try and get a train to Horsforth, but I know how busy the rush hour train will be and knowing my luck it will be a class 153.

It is dark in Leeds and feels damp but it isn't raining. There is a huge queue for taxis outside of the station but not a taxi in sight. I hobble around the back of the station and open my Uber app, which tells me there is a 20-minute wait and that my journey will cost me between £29 and £40. I am not willing to pay this, when the fare should be half of that, so I very painfully hobble away from the station. The streets of Leeds are packed with commuters and Christmas shoppers and drinkers. I've had enough, any positivity that I was growing seems to have now died off, any amount of Christmas spirit within me has reduced so much that it is now a negative number. Misery consumes me as I hobble on for another 5 minutes until I find a quiet backstreet. I try the Uber app again; this time the fare is between £15 and £20 and there is a car 4 minutes away. I order it, and it arrives exactly on time, which is a small mercy that I am thankful for. I painfully climb aboard for a journey home that should take 20 minutes, but in this rush hour takes double that time.

The PW meets me as I awkwardly get out of the car, grabs my heavy bag and gives me a supporting arm, before guiding me indoors. She helps me out of my stiff cold clothes and into warm comfortable ones, and her energy and spirit soothe me as I tell her about my painfully disappointing day. She says all the right things, the PW uses positive words. She gives me a small plate of leftovers from my mum's Sunday dinner, which tastes fantastic, but goes down with some difficulty due to me being so dry inside, and due also to it being the only food that I've eaten today since my breakfast biscuit. We have an early night in bed and through sheer exhaustion I sleep solidly for 12 hours.

I pushed myself going to Stoke in such a poor physical condition, I shouldn't have gone at all, but I felt an obligation to go as I didn't want to disappoint my new colleagues, and now I have no idea what they must think of me. I'm disappointed in myself for a whole lot of things.

14 – Tis the season

December marches on relentlessly. The television adverts have become fixated on buying unnecessary presents for other people, many of which will spend years in cupboards unused, or will be passed on to somebody else who doesn't want or need them either. The type 2 diabetes lorry is all over our TV screens, as is the repugnant word 'holidays', which is an awful Americanism that has entered the British vocabulary. What is so wrong with using the word 'Christmas'? While I'm on this subject, 'Xmas' is not an acceptable abbreviation of Christmas either. I'm not religious or even a particularly huge fan of Christmas, but to me some things are sacrosanct. I'm also revolted by the emergence of the term 'gifting', we don't 'gift' in the UK, we give Christmas presents, why must we bow down and let the cultural imperialism of the USA spoil our traditions? Don't even get me started on Black Friday either, that most repulsive of American traditions crossing the Atlantic which serves only to exploit weak-minded fools into spending money that they don't have, on things that they don't need, which often haven't been financially reduced in the first place.

We don't have Thanksgiving in the UK (yet). Black Friday is an American tradition that is about people being paid at the end of the month after Thanksgiving and being financially 'in the black', meaning that Americans have money in their bank accounts, which invariably greedy corporations want in their bank accounts. I grew up with the understanding that black Friday was a bad day, a day of tragedy, particularly when it fell on the 13th of the month. There are numerous black Fridays from throughout history, here is a small selection of them. 14th October 1881, 189 Scottish fisherman mostly from Eyemouth were drowned in stormy seas, this event became known as 'The Eyemouth Tragedy'. 18th November, 1910, 300 women suffragettes marched on the British Parliament in London to demand equal rights. Many of them were subjected to horrific beatings and sexual violence by the Metropolitan Police and male onlookers. 13th January, 1939, 71 people were killed in Victoria, Australia by out of control bushfires, this event became known as 'The Black Friday Bushfires'. 13th June,

1975, 5 men were killed at Little Houghton Colliery in Barnsley after an explosion ripped through the coal face. 12th March, 1993, 317 people were killed and 1,400 injured from co-ordinated bomb attacks in Mumbai, India. At the time Mumbai was called 'Bombay', and the event became known as 'The Bombay Bombings'. All of those examples are actual black Fridays. Now the corporate marketers have ruined the true tragic meaning of black Friday and turned it into something positive for themselves, but certainly not for the gullible fools who fall for it and are then left in financial difficulties afterwards. To the reckless consumer who cannot control their impulsive spending, black Friday is still a tragedy, they just don't realise it until the bills arrive, or worse still the bailiffs. Seeing Black Friday promoted as an event in the UK, or even 'Black Tag' events, just makes me sad for humanity.

I'm sitting here writing this on what has now been branded by the marketers as 'cyber week'. Those marketers can all fuck off, although I have just bought myself a brand new 5th generation iPad Mini online, not because television or sneaky social media adverts have told me that I should, but because after travelling to Stoke, I've realised that I need something even more lightweight than an iPad to work on while on the move. My iPhone is good for this purpose, but just not big enough for typing comfortably, so I've gone for the in-between option of the iPad Mini, or should it be called the iPhone Maxi? I've bought the version that you can put a SIM card in, so I can be even more connected to the news and social media that I don't want to look at. The real reason I've gone for the SIM card version of the iPad Mini is that I want to be able to work more freely than at just the locations that have Wi-Fi (when it works), as all of my work and personal documentation, photographs and music are 'up' in the cloud. Working in academia is fortuitous in that I have free access to 2 terabytes of cloud space, and I do make the most of that, believe me. One final thing that I would like to say about this fairly expensive purchase is that I 'found' the money to pay for my iPad Mini in my bank account. Not going out drinking every weekend, I seem to have accumulated wealth that would otherwise have gone down my neck and then been pissed against a urinal wall. Cheers to a life with a lot less beer and a bit more money for nice things!

The British general election takes place next week, I have tried so hard to avoid news and social media, but it really isn't easy. A couple of nights ago just before bedtime I went on a bit of a Twitter and Facebook political binge, where I shared as many anti-Tory memes and news posts as I could do, before being asked by the PW, "will you put your phone down now, I'm trying to sleep?" Incidentally the PW is also my phone warden. The net result of that political binge, was me having a million thoughts rampaging through my fully-alert brain, and lying there in the dark, awake for over 3 hours thinking about how awful life would be for at least another 5 years when the Tories win the general election, and what a shit Christmas 2019 would be, when the only JC being celebrated will be the Middle Eastern refugee born in a barn in Bethlehem and not Jeremy Corbyn. Do you want to know what the real sting in the tale of this general election is though? The day and date that the votes are counted and the Tories officially get put back into government to ruin the lives of ordinary working-class Britons (who will moronically vote for them), is Friday the fucking 13th of fucking December, 2019. Never has the term black Friday been more appropriate. Tis the season to be angry.

In terms of eating, I still don't feel hunger but through being at home I have got myself into the good habit of usually eating three main meals per day, breakfast, lunch and dinner. My breakfast is usually yoghurt or porridge. I can eat a standard sized pot of yoghurt (if it is smooth), or just a few tablespoonfuls of porridge (with a blob of jam on top), before feeling full. My lunches vary, I'm still officially on the soft-foods stage, although I'm eating pretty much anything that I want to if I chew it well enough. Yesterday I had some grilled ham with baked beans, today I had about one fifth of a standard ready meal lasagne, with a few bits of chopped salad. Dinners also vary, yesterday I had a boil-in-the-bag cod in butter sauce with a spoonful of mushy peas, today I made a minced beef, spinach and onion curry. The total size of the pan of curry that I made would have only just been enough for the PW and me previously, now I just eat a few tablespoonfuls and there is enough left for me to have some more for lunch tomorrow. I love my spicy food and my curries, and whilst I am only eating a few mouthfuls, I never feel as though I am missing out. I eat with a teaspoon and chew everything at length. I stop when the sensation of fullness hits and despite me eating less than a child's portion, it feels as though I have eaten a full meal, which is great psychologically. In-between meals I may eat a few grapes or have a couple of crackers with a small amount of cheese. I am conscious of the need to up my protein and dairy intake, so am being mindful of this with my food choices. Tomorrow's special Saturday breakfast (which always used to be a full English breakfast) will be a poached egg with half of a sausage and a spoonful of baked beans. I'm sure it will be delicious, but I'll have to chew it to a pulp. I have also found that the 30-minute gap between eating and drinking is easily achievable at home, certainly more achievable than it is when eating out in restaurants.

Now that I'm eating small amounts of normal foods again, I have noticed that one of my eating habits has changed. Ever since I was a child, I have always saved 'the best' until last. This means that when I'm faced with a plate of food, I'll mentally grade the content from best to worst. The worst always goes first, so for example if I have salad or vegetables (apart from potatoes) on my plate, they will be the first to go. Second to go will then be either potatoes, in whatever form they take, boiled/roast/mashed/chips, or if I'm not having potatoes, then pasta or rice, depending on what I'm having. The headliner is saved until last, this is either the meat (or vegetarian equivalent), pie, quiche, burger, pizza slice or whatever it is that I'm having. The PW calls this my 'war mentality', in that people used to do this in the war when food was rationed, so they would savour the flavour for longer of the most favourite food that they were eating. I am the only person in my family that saves the best until last, and I have no idea why I do it. Anyhow, this has now had to change, because now that I can only eat a small amount of food, my war mentality of save the best until last runs the risk of me filling up on the less desirable items on my plate, and then missing out on the headliner. I'm now taking a less judgemental approach to the order in which I consume the food on my plate, concentrating instead on getting a bit of all of the different flavours and textures. Of course, if faced with my favourite 'wet foods' of curry and rice, chilli and rice, or a stew, saving the best until last doesn't really work, as it is all the best.

I haven't mentioned poos for a while, and thankfully after my last painful instalment about them, I am pleased to report that my poos are mostly regular and in good order. Even better, my body has now shrunk so much that I now can sit comfortably on our downstairs loo (I outgrew this toilet around 8 years ago), which is a small personal victory for me. Prior to me having the operation I would usually poo once per day, usually in the morning after getting out of bed. This routine mostly hasn't changed at all, the only spanner in the sewerage works has been the codeine/co-proxamol pain medication that I'm taking for my arthritis. This can have a slightly 'drying' effect inside, and I have gone a couple of mornings without pooing if I have had to take a full dosage of painkillers the day before. I try and combat this with a little Lactulose, which is a stool 'softener'. Less food in, obviously means less poo out, and my stools have shrunken in both size and quantity. They are generally a solid and healthy type 4 on the 'Bristol Stool Chart' (like a sausage or snake, smooth and soft). They actually look like the same shape as baby carrots with a rounded end and a tapered end. Anyway, that's enough of me writing shit for now, let's get on with December.

Sunday 8th December soon comes around. I have decided to weigh myself at weekends, and the news is good, my weight has dropped to 21 stone, 9 and ¾ pounds (303.75 pounds/138 kilos). This means that my total weight loss after 39 days is 51.5 pounds (23.4 kilos), which equates to 1.3 pounds per day since the operation. My weight loss this week has slowed down a little from last week, but it is still satisfactory.

The PW and I are heading into Leeds city centre to meet our long-time good friends Rob, Julia and Linda. This will be the first time that they have seen me since the operation, and this will be the first time that I shall drink alcohol since Edinburgh. I'd like to think that I could go and meet our friends and remain teetotal for the afternoon, but I'm a realist, it's our Christmas meet-up and I'm having a Christmas drink, just not too many of them. We meet in The Head of Steam, which is a newish pub on Park Row in Leeds city centre at 14:00. I chose this pub specifically as it is large and has a lot of benches, which are easier for me to sit on than stools. I'm wearing the knee brace on my right knee and using a crutch in my left hand, though my right knee is still very painful, as is my right wrist. The Head of Steam is a great pub for having a varied and often quite potent beer selection. I really do love my real ale, I particularly like strong flavours, whether they be pale ales or dark stouts. Stronger flavours often correlate to the beer being stronger in terms of alcohol by volume (ABV), so for me, the stronger the better is a principle that I go with when selecting which beer to drink. As a general rule of thumb, I won't usually consider ale that is under 5% ABV. I remember what Mary told me last week that I shouldn't be drinking alcohol yet, and I know that the guidance in my post-surgery booklet says to avoid strong ales as they are more calorific and likely to increase appetite. I'm just going to have to be naughty today and break the rules. This is a one-off occasion, so I decide to just go with the flow and see how I get on. I make the conscientious decision to drink half-pints rather than pints though, so at least I will be taking 50% less calorific and carbohydrate heavy liquid on board.

We spend 2 hours in The Head of Steam and during that period I drink three half-pints, all of which are in the region of 5% to 6% ABV. Pre-operation, this would almost certainly have been three pints. The conversation about my health is quick to arise and at first the discussion is about my visible physical difficulties with my arthritis. This soon turns to my bariatric surgery, so I tell the story about the operation that I have had and why. Rob, Julia and Linda are all aware that I have had the surgery, as the PW (with my permission) told them about it some weeks ago. They all comment how much thinner I look already and are taken aback at how much weight I have already lost in such a short space of time. I can see that their words are genuine and that they are all pleased for me. I explain to them about my changed eating habits in terms of portion size and how this has not bothered me at all, as I don't feel hunger, I also explain to them how drinking for me is still quite easy, and that I don't really feel a great deal of restriction, but I am choosing to drink less, as I'm not really supposed to be drinking at this early stage.

We move to another bar called Tapped, which is a specialist craft beer and real ale bar. Here I have a half pint of a strong 9% beer, which is a thick, dark and very potent drink. The PW always has a sip of my ales, even though she hates beer, and she likens this one to engine oil. There are no benches available in Tapped, so the others sit on bar stools around a table while I perch adjacent to them on a high-chair. The conversation turns to the forthcoming general election, and there are all sides represented among us, but because we are grown-ups and not morons we can debate and agree to disagree, although Rob does enjoy winding up Linda.

We move over the road to The Griffin Hotel, where again we find a bench. Even though I have only drunk two pints, I feel as though I have had enough beer, so I opt for a gin and tonic (with plenty of ice and stirred well to get rid of the bubbles). The politics talk has ended and we all end up breaking off into smaller conversations about a range of things, including stories from days gone by, what the kids are doing, and preparations for Christmas. I'm getting tired, as a combination of codeine, alcohol and physical exertion begins to take its toll, but I can see that the PW is really enjoying herself socialising and being out of the house. I have been something of a ball and chain to her for the past few weeks and I want her to have a good time. When her glass empties, I suggest one more gin and tonic, which she is happy to oblige with. The PW can see that I'm getting tired, she reads me extraordinarily well, so after the next drink is consumed, she is happy for me to order a taxi, and we finish the night early at 19:00. I actually feel physically shattered at this point and am ready to go home and go to bed. On previous meets for Christmas drinks, we would have stayed in the pub until around 20:30, before going for a curry, getting home after 23:00, and having consumed several thousand calories more. I would easily have drunk at least 8 pints of beer before, so I've definitely cut my alcohol intake down dramatically, and I've still had a great time with good friends and plenty of laughs.

The alternative medicine knowledge and wisdom of taxi drivers knows no bounds. Over the past few years when I've had an arthritic flare-up and have had difficulty getting in and out of taxis, I've had several drivers propose a variety of solutions to me, which in their opinion will improve the pain and functionality of my inflamed joints. These have included rubbing something called 'dog oil' into my knee twice a day (it's what they use on racing greyhounds apparently); taking magnesium tablets to reduce pain; wrapping freshly shorn lambswool around my knee to insulate it from the damp and cold; drinking cranberry juice as an all-round health booster, and eating more cruciferous vegetables such as broccoli and sprouts to fight inflammation. I found dog oil online, and ordered some, but it was heavy, greasy and didn't smell good, it did nothing for me. I'm now taking magnesium tablets regularly, but they don't seem to make a difference to my pain levels. I haven't yet found myself a lamb to shear, so I've put that one on the backburner. I drink cranberry juice every now and again, but it doesn't seem to make any noticeable difference when I do drink it. I do eat cruciferous vegetables regularly, again I haven't noticed them making a lot of difference. I think you need to have a certain amount of blind faith for some of these 'cures' to actually make any real difference.

This evening's taxi driver home has a new and innovative solution to fight inflammation and reduce joint swelling and pain, this is to drink turmeric lattes. He explains to me that he (like myself) cannot tolerate non-steroid anti-inflammatory drugs (NSAIDs), such as ibuprofen and naproxen, as he has severe stomach and bowel problems. Like myself he is also an arthritis sufferer in his knees, as well as in his back. The driver told me that a traditional cure for arthritis in Pakistan was to take turmeric mixed with a little vegetable oil, he had done some research online and adapted the traditional approach to taking turmeric into making turmeric lattes. He ordered turmeric online that contained an ingredient called curcumin, and then mixed this with a few drops of olive oil, some honey and a splash of coconut milk, before topping up with hot milk, stirring well. He told me that at first, the taste takes some getting used to, but that he has one every day, and after a few weeks of drinking these, his arthritic pain reduced and has never returned to being as bad as what it was. I'm so desperate to get rid of the pain and stiffness in my legs and wrist that I'm willing to give it a go.

When we do get home that evening, our Sunday dinner consists of cheese and biscuits with pickles, and it is a taste sensation, and this is then followed 30 minutes later by my first turmeric latte, lovingly prepared by the PW. This is not a taste sensation, in fact it is quite disgusting, but I persevere with a twisted face and just a couple of gags, after which we go to bed, me with a bad taste in my mouth that not even Listerine can shift. I continue with one turmeric latte per day after this, the taste does get a little easier to get used to but overall, they are still fairly unpleasant.

A couple of days later, I am back at my doctor's surgery for a check-up, this time into my left knee. I am definitely hobbling better on this occasion, than I was on my previous visit, when I had to have my right arm around the PW for support, along with a crutch in my left hand. The doctor immediately notes how much better my 'walking' is, along with how it is easily noticeable that I have lost weight. This is a good mental boost for me. We have a discussion about my wrist, and the doctor, after examining it, believes that my problem with it may be tendonitis, rather than arthritis, caused by overuse of the joint to push myself out of chairs when both of my legs were really bad. The only realistic solutions to help fix this are anti-inflammatory tablets (which I cannot take), or anti-inflammatory gel rubbed into the wrist (which I am doing), along with resting and not using this joint as much as possible. There isn't going to be a quick fix solution to my right wrist, so unfortunately, I'm just going to have to ride it out. The codeine that I'm taking for my knee definitely helps to reduce the pain in my wrist, but it is a pain masker, rather than a wrist mender. I leave the doctor's in good spirits (Dr Williams has a very positive manner) and also with a newly prescribed bag of medication. After weeks of being in pain, I have to tell myself, tis the season to get better.

It is general election week, and as much as I am trying to avoid the news and social media, I am like a heroin addict who thinks they can cure themselves with just an occasional small 'fix'. Unfortunately, as the week marches on, these fixes increase in size until I'm mainlining heavy doses of political news and internet memes over several hours per day. This impacts upon my functionality. I'm beginning to procrastinate from doing jobs that I have set myself by spending too much time online and sharing political anti-Tory news stories and memes.

This week Alexander Boris de Pfeffel Johnson has snatched a phone from a journalist's hand rather than answer a question about why a child was left on the floor at Leeds General Infirmary (LGI), because there were no beds, and hidden inside a refrigerated milk truck instead of answering another journalist's questions. The Tories have also been up to dirty tricks, claiming that one of Matt Hancock's (Secretary of State for Social Care & Health) aides was assaulted outside LGI by a protestor, which was a complete and utter lie that was then spread by BBC (Backing Britain's Conservatives) journalists on social media. The Tories also got their friends who work in private healthcare to try and discredit the story about the boy on the floor at LGI, but it didn't take long for internet detectives to expose the links between those making discrediting claims and the Tory party. The lying Tories are in complete denial that the NHS is collapsing under their lack of funding and austerity. Unfortunately, too many gullible and foolhardy Britons think 'getting Brexit done' (whatever that means) is more important. The polls are eroding the projected Tory lead, but I'm still not hopeful for at best a Labour win, or in second place a hung parliament. I can't stop myself from having my say online about this, if I can change the mind of one potential Tory voter, it will all be worth it. The impact that this has had on me is that two nights before the election, I could not sleep after reading news articles on my phone at bedtime (a bad habit that I'm supposed to be getting out of). I ended up getting out of bed at 02:00 and not going back to bed until 06:00, which is not in the least bit healthy.

The day after seeing Dr Williams, the pain in both of my knees and wrist has reduced to the extent that I do not take any painkillers; this isn't intentional, but as I haven't felt pain, I haven't felt the urge to take them. Whether it is a coincidence or not I cannot say, but I am wondering if the anti-inflammatory properties of turmeric really have made a difference. I've only been taking turmeric lattes for 4 days; could this really be the miracle cure that I've been looking for? I don't know, but the newfound freedom of movement that I'm feeling makes me more agile and improves my mood and functionality in terms of jobs to do, as my long list of planned jobs has hardly been touched due to my pain and limited movement. Despite their pretty grim taste, I'm going to persevere with the turmeric for now at least.

One of the little jobs that I want to do is to update and increase the number of photos on our digital photo frame, which stands in our living room. I take thousands of photographs each year, which end up in 'the cloud' and never get looked at. The photo frame is barely ever turned on as the pictures are old and haven't been updated for years. The frame also doesn't have a random function so they appear in the same order. At present the frame has 1,500 photos on it, most of which are over 8 years old. I spend around 10 hours over 2 days going through my photo collection, correcting the orientation of some photos from landscape to portrait and adding them to a SD Card to go into the frame. The memories of looking through the photos are wonderful and it is a labour of pure love.

Previously when adding photos to the frame, I would shy away from including any pictures of myself that contained full body shots. I couldn't stand looking at the shape of my fat self and certainly didn't want these images to be on display. Now I no longer care and eagerly add any photos I can find with myself on. This is definitely a point of reflection, as prior to the operation I would have thought that I might want to erase all memories of the old fat me, but this is not the case at all. It's almost like I'm getting some kind of twisted pleasure from looking back at photos of my former fatter self and thinking that, "at least I'm not that big anymore." The memories evoked by the photos are blissful; the PW and I lead a very busy, fun and varied leisure life outside of work, we are regular travellers, we go to many gigs and events, we participate in the arts, and by not displaying these photos, I have been denying myself the joy of remembrance. It seems so silly and vain now when I think about it. My efforts result in over 6,000 more photographs being added to the frame, giving it a total running time of just over 10 hours of very happy memories. I will say though, that there are an alarming proportion of photographs where I am holding a drink in my hand, maybe we just take more photos in pubs, cheers anyway! Tis the season to be reflective.

Election day is upon us. I awake early at 05:17, and I know immediately upon sensing consciousness that I won't go back to sleep. After a couple of minutes, I open my eyes, peel the silicon seal of the CPAP mask off my face and switch the machine off. The PW stirs and asks me what time it is, and when I tell her she reacts in a positive way with the words, "would you like a cup of tea?" the answer of course being a resounding "yes." What a perfect wife I really have. The PW makes a lovely cup of tea and then goes back to bed to read for an hour. After a less painful hobble downstairs than I've experienced for about 5 weeks, I switch on my laptop and have a good hour of political social media activism. I need to get the political thoughts out of my head in order to declutter my brain, so this helps my mind a great deal. My most 'liked' post on Facebook that I write is below.

"Remember if you're going to the polling station today and you really want to 'get Brexit done', that it's probably best to put a X in both The Conservative Party and The Brexit Party boxes. Better to be safe than sorry."

It makes me giggle as I write it, but can you imagine if anyone was gullible enough to believe this? Hopefully if people are gullible enough to believe the newspapers, then maybe they might just be. I'm not holding out any hope whatsoever for this general election, I'd love a Labour win, I'd love to see a truly left-leaning Prime Minister, but I'm a realist, the largest demographic age-wise in the UK are those around 50 years old. They are more likely to be right-wing than left-wing, and they are more likely to vote than the under 30s, who are more left-wing, and less in number. I'm from Barnsley, and I'm a fan of Barnsley FC, so I'm used to disappointment. Election defeats like getting thrashed at the footie are a realistic part and parcel of my banana life, usually commiserated over with several pints of beer. After a solid hour of activism on social media, I decide to call it a day. I don't want my day taken over by this, and I don't want to build up my hopes anymore, I'm prepared for the true meaning of black Friday tomorrow. I then decide to do another little job, which the limited movement in my painful wrist has been preventing, and that is wrapping up some Christmas presents, just to feel all seasonal. After all the Amazon parcels, which have been arriving on an almost daily basis, aren't going to open and unwrap themselves.

In the afternoon I have a look at my Australia diary from the 12th November, 1994, which happened to be a Saturday. I won't write out a copy of everything I wrote on that day as my entry is quite long, but I can tell you that I began the day with a hangover after a heavy session on Friday night. I went music and CD shopping in the afternoon, spending around AU$80 on four CDs, I had a pizza for my dinner, and then went out on the beer for the second consecutive night of the weekend, getting home after hitting a club until 04:00 on Sunday. After this I called in our local bakery on the way home at around 05:00 and bought some freshly made pizza dough and a ready-to-eat garlic bread. Once home, I drunkenly bashed the pizza dough into a circle, before covering it in cheese, onion and tuna and putting it in the oven. While it was cooking I ate the garlic bread and drank more beer. Then I ate the not properly cooked pizza with yet more beer before going to bed around 06:30. Is it really any wonder at all that I got fat?

As predicted, Friday 13th is indeed black Friday, despite Jeremy Corbyn getting more votes than Tony Blair did when he won the 1997 general election; the Tories have won a landslide victory, Labour heartlands that have been decimated by Tory austerity (but who blame the EU for their troubles) have propped up and strengthened their true enemies and slave masters. I hope all those working-class Northerners that have voted Tory can afford private health insurance, because they're probably going to need it. The SNP have had a resurgence in Scotland, and will now almost certainly hold a second independence referendum, which they will win. There will be a hard border in the Irish Sea between Northern Ireland and the rest of the UK. There are going to be significant changes to the political map of the Un-united Kingdom over the next few years. Corbyn, you reignited passion amongst young voters, but there just weren't enough of them. The middle-aged onwards had their minds poisoned against you by the Tory-supporting media. Thank you, Jezza, for everything that you have done for the Labour Party, but it's time to admit defeat in the face of a 'democracy' that is deeply bent by media control, and step aside to give either Jess Phillips or Keir Starmer (I can't contemplate anyone else right now) a shot at leading the reds into victory in 2024. At least the Brexit Party didn't get a single MP, not that it makes any difference to the overall outcome. Disappointed? Yes. Despondent? Yes. Surprised? No. To top it all off, my right knee is killing me this morning, maybe those turmeric lattes aren't really working after all. Tis the season to shut myself in a darkened room with a properly enforced news and social media blackout and a good supply of codeine. Black fucking Friday indeed. Oh, and it's my first official day back at work too, bugger.

My first official day back at work is a short day, as I also have my first post-op appointment with Mr Mehta on the same day in the afternoon. I go to work on crutches and with my wrist support on. It feels weird and slightly alien being back on campus. I notice the changes since I was last there. The leaves have fallen off the trees, and the new sports building that was still under construction when I last saw it, is looking much nearer completion now. There are also notably fewer students around, as many will have already decided to go home early for Christmas, missing the last teaching week (next week) altogether. The PW drives me in, and then I hobble to the classroom, where Jess (one of my cover tutors) is delivering an exam preparation session to my final year consultancy students. I enter the room to a mixture of welcomes and what seems like an air of cynicism amongst a couple of them. Do they know the true nature of my absence? Are they holding it against me? Is it just the end of a long semester and they're all knackered? Am I being paranoid? I just try and be myself, but I feel like an outsider in my own class and on my own course. I make my excuses after 45 minutes and leave, hobbling to my office to attempt to make some inroads into the mountain of email in my inbox. En route I bump into a couple of colleagues who knew about my op, and they say positive and encouraging words to me, which is good to hear and helps put my slightly troubled mind at a little more ease.

After work, the PW collects me by car and we drive over to St. James's Hospital, where I have a post-op appointment with Mr Mehta. We arrive on time and park without stress across the main road from the hospital. It is a short 5-minute walk to Bexley Wing, where I check in at 'surgical outpatients'. I recognise it as the same location where I met Mr Mehta for the first time. We have only been in the waiting room for a couple of minutes when I'm called forwards to be weighed, which takes just a few seconds. A couple of minutes later, I'm called forward by a female doctor, who introduces herself as a member of Mr Mehta's team. The doctor has a very good manner, but I must admit I'm a little disappointed, as I'd wanted to see Mr Mehta personally. We go into a side room, where the doctor asks me about my progress, my eating habits and if I've had any problems. I tell her that I'm recovering well from the operation, am probably a week ahead of where I should be in terms of what I can eat and am tolerating just about everything that I am eating. I explain that my main issue has been a lack of exercise due to my arthritis, which the doctor completely understands. The doctor presses against my wounds and tells me to cough each time; she is inspecting the wound sites to see if there are hernias behind them, and thankfully there aren't. I have plenty of questions to ask, but as usual struggle to remember them. Why on earth didn't I just write them down?

The appointment only lasts 10 minutes, and we leave the room to head back to reception. I'm glad the appointment went well, but I am sad that I didn't get to see Mr Mehta as I have brought a small thank you present to give to him. Just as we get to reception, Mr Mehta appears from a side room and I cannot contain my excitement. I poke the PW and say to her "it's Mr Mehta," although she can plainly see him with her own eyes as he is directly in front of us. The PW retrieves the present for Mr Mehta (which actually only arrived today while I was at work) from her bag. The PW has wrapped the present up like a Christmas present, complete with a gold bow. The PW is also a great present wrapper. "Mr Mehta," I say aloud, and he turns and says "hello." He must see dozens of patients each week, and I'm not 100% sure that he remembers me, but I thrust the present in his direction and say, "I just wanted to give you this as a token of my appreciation for everything that you have done for me and to say thank you." Mr Mehta seems taken aback, though he smiles and takes the gift. "Thank you so much," he replies, "that's really very kind of you, but you really didn't need to do that." I say to him, "it's just something small and silly, but I came up with the idea with my marketing head on, and I thought it might make you laugh." Mr Mehta then asks how I've been since the operation, so I give him the highlights of weight loss and arthritis, but I can see he is a busy man with other people to see in the waiting room, so after a very satisfying Mr Mehta handshake, we leave. I say to everyone there, "thank you and merry Christmas" before leaving in a really positive mood. I hope Mr Mehta likes his present, it's literally a silly £7 gift ordered online. I don't know if anyone else has come up with this idea before, but I hope not. I'd love to see his face when he opens it, hopefully he won't own another coffee mug that says "Mr Mehta Makes You Behta" across the front.

That evening we get to our first post-operation gig, which is to see a Beastie Boys tribute band called the Beat-Sie Boys at the legendary Brudenell Social Club (BSC) in Leeds, which is my most favourite music venue. The Beastie Boys are my fourth favourite band of all time, but due to the sad early death of band member Adam Yauch (MCA) in 2012 from cancer, they are no more. Adam was the same age as I am now (47) when he died, which makes me consider how important it is to live life to the full and make the most of the time that we have on earth. RIP MCA. After already missing both Jonathan Pie and The Wonder Stuff gigs, I'm determined not to waste tickets to this event too, even if it is for a tribute band.

We take a taxi to the BSC. I have my wrist support on and a crutch in my left hand. There are hundreds of people standing outside of the extremely busy venue and billowing clouds of cigarette smoke and e-cigarette vapour enveloping them. The air smells of tobacco and beer breath, as we make our way through the heavy and quite inebriated crowd into the venue. It is extremely busy at the BSC tonight, as there are three gigs on, one in each of the event rooms. I'm not used to being in a crowd and am worried about getting knocked or jolted, which could prove to be very painful for me. My crutch also slips on the wet floor, but thankfully I manage to stay upright and don't take a tumble. The gig is fantastic, the Beat-Sie Boys in character as the Beastie Boys do a fantastic job. It is testament to the lingering popularity of the Beastie Boys and the quality of the act on stage that 300 people have each paid £8 for a ticket to attend this gig, which lasts for 90 minutes. I stand for the entire gig, supported by my crutch and do so with very little pain. My weight loss means that my ability to stand for long periods has improved. I would have been in severe foot and ankle pain standing for 90 minutes at a gig prior to the operation, but now I stand there largely pain free, apart from a few twinges in my arthritic right knee. During the 90 minutes that we are there, I drink two half pints of ale, though in days of old I would easily have drunk at least five pints of ale at a gig such as that (including before and after gig drinks). I now know that I can enjoy a gig without being half-cut, this is a whole new world to me.

The next morning I weigh myself on the scales and the PW measures me. I have lost a further 3.25 pounds (1.47 kilos) this week, but the headline is that I have now lost 30 cm (12 inches) off my waist. This is significant, 30 cm or 12 inches is in imperial measurements a foot, the size of a school ruler! A foot of my waist has gone in 2 months, now that to me is pretty amazing.

We head to Chester for the weekend, and I'm wearing a coat that I haven't worn for 8 years as I outgrew it, but now it fits me perfectly, in fact it is quite loose. We haven't been to Chester since mid-October, and we liked it so much on that visit that we decided to return and try and see all of the things that we didn't get to see. It rained a lot during our first visit to Chester, so we spent a lot of time in the many excellent pubs that the city has to offer and I drank a very large amount of beer, I estimate between 12 and 15 pints over the weekend. The weather forecast for our visit this time is good, so I intend to behave differently this weekend, knee permitting.

This time we stay at the Mercure Abbots Well hotel, where I have booked an accessible room knowing that I won't be able to climb over a bath to take a shower. The hotel also has a swimming pool, and after checking in we decide to go for a swim before going into the city. I like swimming, and don't shy away from the swimming pool when we are in a hotel that has one, but I am always self-conscious about my fat body, which is usually the most rotund one there. Today is different, although I'm still fat, I'm not as fat as I was before, and I feel more confident in myself. The wounds from my operation are visible (although not drastically), but they don't bother me and I'm not ashamed of them in any way. In actual fact, the minor wound scars and bruises combined with my wrist support and crutch make me look like I've had a tumble or been in an accident of some sort. People can think what they want to about what might have happened to me, I really don't care, and if anyone asks me about my injuries I'm going to say that I was in a biker gang fight. After getting out of the pool I shower and then dry off, and as I'm drying I tie the towel around my waist and it fits. The towel doesn't untie and fall to the floor, it stays firmly around my waist, and this is something that I'm really not used to and it feels good. Tis the season to be a little bit proud of myself.

Chester has a lovely old city centre, with ancient walls, a Roman amphitheatre, cathedral and Tudor buildings aplenty. There is a blue sky, and I'm feeling very positive about the day, and a chance to do some filming, something that I haven't done for a good long while. I've had to forfeit my crutch today for my camera/walking pole, which isn't as supportive, but I can't use both the crutch and the pole at the same time, so I'm opting to put my filming over supporting my arthritic knee, which is a decision that I hope that I don't regret. We head into the city centre and predictably the sky darkens and the heavens open. I've only been to this city twice, but I feel like I can now say with some authority that it always rains in Chester. Soon the rain becomes oppressive and we seek solace in a pub. The PW is hungry, so she orders a salad to eat and a pint of cider to drink, she doesn't take half-measures, the PW is a pint woman. I scan the pub menu for something small, and there is a 'small plates' section, so I order small fish and chips with mushy peas and nothing to drink. In fatter days I would have scanned the menu looking for the largest meal on it and would definitely have washed it down with a pint. When our food arrives, the waiter looks confused, I can tell that he can't see a big bloke like me eating either a salad or a small fish and chips. The PW points towards the salad and we are given our correct meals. I manage to eat nearly all of the small fish, the mushy peas and four chips, but then I am stuffed, I feel as though I've eaten 'Jaws', not something that wasn't much larger than a fish finger. The PW happily finishes off my chips, she knew that I would leave them.

We go back out into the rain and wander the streets before exploring Chester's Roman Amphitheatre, the very lovely St. John the Baptist Church and the ruins next door and the Queens Park Bridge before walking in very heavy rain on the Handbridge side of the River Dee to a pub called The Grosvenor Arms. We decide to call it a day here, as it is pouring with rain, it is getting dark and by this point I've managed to hobble an impressive 9,794 steps. The pub is noisy, loud voices are competing with both music and TVs blaring out commentary of the football. The volume in the pub is oppressive and I would normally only stay somewhere as cacophonous as this for one drink, but the gin tastes good and the rain is heavy, so we stay for two drinks before getting a taxi back to the hotel, where we intend to eat in the restaurant tonight.

That was the plan anyway, it turns out that the hotel restaurant no longer opens on Sunday nights, so we resign ourselves to the fact that we're ordering a takeaway. We have a bottle of wine in the room, so our big night in Chester is spent in bed under the duvet drinking some very fine New Zealand Sauvignon Blanc (I just have a single glass), eating a delivery pizza and watching the *Family Guy* Christmas special. The pizza is thin crust and I chew it very slowly until it is a complete mulch before swallowing, I manage two slices before feeling full so stop eating at that point. We just get one pizza between us, and it feels wrong eating pizza as it is definitely on the red flagged naughty list of foods to avoid, but two slices won't break the bank considering my calorific intake for the day overall. I would have definitely eaten an entire 12-inch pizza to myself in days of old and probably some of what the PW ordered too. Despite the weather, Chester has been good, and again I've demonstrated to myself that I can still enjoy a range of different things to eat and drink, just in moderation. I'm sure that we will return to this city in the summer when the weather is better, as we still haven't climbed and walked around the city walls, which is something that we would both like to do. Last time we came to Chester I was too fat and unfit to be able to climb the steps and walk the walls, and on this visit my knee is too sore to be physically able, so fingers crossed for the next time. Tis the season to be hopeful.

A few days later I decide to test the waters with social media again, but it is a mistake; the toxicity of postings both political and otherwise is stressful and unpleasant to read, and my brain currently needs nice input, not venom, anger, stress or hatred. The fallout from the general election is that a combination of Labour anti-Corbyn v Labour pro-Corbyn battles are taking place in cyberspace, alongside a swathe of anti-Tory posts that are highlighting a backtracking of promises made about the NHS already. Besides the political posts are the usual angry rants about somebody's bad day that they are having, or those viral Facebook posts that end with a call to 'see if anyone is listening' and share, share, share, I can't stand looking at any of it. Social media when used for creativity and good can be a wonderful thing, but right now, reading it worsens my mood and gets my mind and blood pressure racing. I realise that I might have to knock both Facebook and Twitter on the head for a good long while. I can tolerate a bit of Instagram and in fact make a few photo posts on that platform, but I have become disinterested in scrolling through everybody else's photos, which all seem to highlight the same things that they did the last time I looked, albeit with a bit more tinsel and Christmas spirit.

Reflux is something that thankfully I haven't really ever suffered from, unless of course I've decided after a night on the ale to eat a curry at midnight, which to be fair, I've probably done at least monthly for the past 25 years. Under those circumstances it is only right to expect a burning rude awakening. I've taken an Omeprazole tablet every night for the past few years, not for reflux prevention (although it does serve that purpose), but to give my stomach a lining in case I need to take an anti-inflammatory painkiller during the night. Post-operation I'm taking Lansoprazole daily; these are similar to Omeprazole in that they reduce stomach acid so prevent reflux, as well as preventing me from getting strictures (narrowing of the oesophagus). I'm supposed to take these tablets morning and night for 6 weeks following the operation, and then just take one at night from then onwards.

Reflux is something that is associated with the sleeve gastrectomy surgery, and a lot of people seem to suffer from it post-operation. I've read in the Obesity UK Facebook group a number of posts from people who have had such bad reflux, that they have had their sleeve revised into a gastric bypass. The only occasion where I've had reflux badly was in hospital, after I drank a lot of liquid for my CT scan. It is now the early hours of the morning. I'm sound asleep, I came to bed early at 20:00 as the PW had been out to the ballet with her friend and I was home alone bored. I had my dinner, took my painkillers and went to sleep quickly, waking briefly when the PW got in bed. Now I have been awoken by an intense choking burning pain. I am coughing uncontrollably, and my throat is on fire. I can hardly breathe, even though the CPAP mask is blowing air into my very sore lungs. I don't know what is happening. Am I asleep? Am I awake? I hear the PW groan, "are you alright, love?" but I can't answer as I'm coughing so uncontrollably. Sitting up is difficult as it requires use of the muscles in my aching right knee, but somehow I manage to push myself to the edge of the bed and tear off my CPAP mask, coughing and spluttering as I do so. I think that I might vomit and in point of fact, have basically done so right up to the back of my throat, but thankfully not into my mouth and CPAP mask. The acid bile that has risen from my stomach has severely burnt my throat and oesophagus and the pain is searing. I've never experienced such an intensely burning and painful reflux before and it has shaken me up. I sit their trying not to cough anymore as every expulsion of air hurts my very sore throat. The acid reflux feels like burning lava, and I'm shocked by how traumatic the experience has been. I take another Lansoprazole tablet in an attempt to neutralise the acid in my gut. I wash it down with half a pint of water, which I sip. Every swallow hurts as does every movement of my throat muscles. The PW is sound asleep again. I sit on the edge of the bed for 35 minutes completely exhausted. I fall asleep sat there a couple of times before jolting myself back to being awake. Eventually I lie back down and put the CPAP mask back on. I really hope that this is a one-off and won't become a regular occurrence. I try to think what I did that may have caused this to happen, and the only thing that I can think of is that I went to bed quite early and not too long after my dinner. Maybe I should have waited longer between eating and sleeping? From this point onwards I will most certainly be doing that.

I have another hospital visit this week, this time to Wharfedale Hospital in Otley. I like this hospital, it has a friendly, relaxed and chilled ambience, and feels very local. I'm glad that it has so far survived the constant financial cuts to the NHS, although it has seen departmental closures as some Leeds NHS services become more centralised. This time the hospital visit is to collect my specially made corrective insoles from the orthotics department. Unfortunately, I cannot try the insoles on inside my trainers whilst at the hospital, as my arthritic right knee is so stiff that I cannot bend my leg enough to put the trainer on myself and the PW isn't here today to help me. So I just collect the insoles and go back home with them, spending £25 on taxis doing so. It seems like a bit of a waste of my time and money, but if they work it will be worth it. I don't feel convinced in them being the answer to correcting my walking problems if I'm completely honest, but only time and footsteps will tell.

The weekend before Christmas is upon us and that means another session on the weighing scales. The headline is that I have lost more weight, but I'm disappointed that the amount has again fallen, this week I have only lost 1.75 pounds. I fear that the weight loss plateau is definitely approaching. I did drink at the weekend, and I have eaten more food and not all of it was healthy, so maybe I shouldn't be surprised. One other point to note is that 2 days ago marked the 'official' date from which I am allowed to eat 'normal' food, not that this makes a lot of difference, as I've pretty much being doing that (albeit in small amounts) for most of the past 2 weeks anyway.

This will be a busy weekend for the PW and me as we are going to yet another hospital (my fourth different hospital this month) and then on to visit our daughter Becky in Hertfordshire. This time we are both going to the hospital as visitors and thankfully not with me as a patient. This isn't just to any hospital either, this is a visit to a hospital with a name that is infamous and often misunderstood due to the hospital's association with some patients who have committed terrible crimes; today we are visiting

Rampton Secure Hospital in Nottinghamshire. This hospital has housed patients including 'Angel of Death' Beverley Allitt, a serial killer who killed four children and attacked nine others whilst working as a nurse in 1991; Ian Huntley, responsible for the Soham murders of Jessica Chapman and Holly Wells in August 2002; and Charles Arthur Salvador, formerly known as Charles Bronson, who has been referred to as 'the most violent prisoner in Britain' in the media. Rampton is one of three high security psychiatric hospitals in England, alongside Ashworth Hospital in Merseyside and Broadmoor Hospital in Berkshire. It is a hospital and not a prison, although with its huge razor-wire topped multiple fencing you could easily be forgiven for thinking that it is a prison. The hospital is run by the NHS and not the Ministry of Justice (who are responsible for prisons in the UK). The people who are resident in Rampton are referred to as patients and not prisoners or inmates, they wear their own clothes and not uniforms. Their rooms whilst secure and often locked, are called rooms and not cells and are on named wards and not wings as in a prison. Rampton currently holds 350 patients; around 300 are male and 50 female, all of whom have mental illnesses including patients with dangerous and severe personality disorders.

The PW and I are visiting Rampton this weekend to see our nephew Jacob and give him his Christmas presents, this is something that we do each Christmas, and we also usually visit him in the summer. Jacob like anyone has a back story, he had a difficult childhood, which led to troubled teenage years that were punctuated with drugs and alcohol. This led to him spending time in and out of young offenders' institutions. Jacob felt like he had underlying mental health problems and he needed help but putting him in prison wasn't the answer. He went to a police station in Leeds and asked to be detained under the Mental Health Act as he felt violence inside of himself that he feared he couldn't control. He was told to go away and take himself to hospital, so Jacob threatened to smash up a police car, at which point he was arrested.

Jacob was assessed and sent to a privately run medium secure psychiatric hospital, which he had little faith in. Jacob self-harmed whilst in the medium secure hospital swallowing 22 batteries. He was put in seclusion (isolation), from which he broke out of, resulting in riot police being called to the hospital. At this point it was decided that Jacob needed high rather than medium security, so he was sent to Rampton Secure Hospital on the 10th of August, 2006 (Jacob remembers dates perfectly well). At the time of our visit, Jacob has been in Rampton for 13 years and 4 months. By February 2020, Jacob will have been in secure hospitals for 15 years continuously. He is 32 years old and has spent nearly half of his life in either a young offender institution or a secure hospital. When you consider the gravity of his 'crime' of threatening to smash up a police car, this just does not seem right. The other side to this is that Jacob does need treatment and monitoring, Jacob's ward is classified as a high dependency unit (HDU) and he has been diagnosed with having an enhanced personality disorder (EPD) and post-traumatic stress disorder (PTSD). This can lead to sudden flare-ups and bouts of violence, for which he is put in seclusion until he is in a fit state to go back onto the ward. Flare-ups are often triggered by the behaviour of other patients, or by Jacob's own frustrations at the situation that he is in. As Jacob has got older, his flare-ups have lessened. People can and do grow out of the behaviours associated with EPD, and that is a hope that we have for Jacob and a hope that he has for himself. There is certainly some evidence to suggest that Jacob's condition is improving, as he sometimes voluntarily asks to go into seclusion if he feels that a violent flare-up might be approaching.

It is Jacob's long-term plan to eventually get out of Rampton, to go to medium and then low security hospitals before being released. He wants to go to college, learn skills and get a job like many other people do. Jacob has been aiming to do this for some time now. On what seems like a cyclical basis, Jacob makes progress to being allowed to go into a medium secure hospital, but near the point of transfer, anxiety gets the better of him, he flares up and is then sent to seclusion, thus nullifying his chances of transfer and then the whole process begins again. Jacob has been in hospital for so long now that he is likely institutionalised.

Because he is in hospital and not prison, Jacob is entitled to Employment & Support Allowance (ESA) and receives £111 per week from the government. His spending options are limited to the hospital's own retailers or the Argos catalogue (goods are purchased through a third party). Jacob is not allowed any internet access, he can buy telephone credits (for monitored calls) and is allowed to subscribe to Sky Television services including movies and sports. He has a TV in his room and is allowed a Gameboy handheld console when in HDU. When Jacob is in a treatment ward he is allowed an additional games console to connect to his TV, although nothing with communicative ability is allowed. He is allowed a maximum of four electrical items in his room (in addition to his TV), a maximum of 24 CDs or game cartridges (DVDs are not allowed), and no more than 5 metres of cable in total across all of the devices he has in his room at any one time. This often means that he has to get consoles and controllers modified in order to reduce their cable length.

Games and gaming are a major passion for Jacob and other patients, as a repetitive routine and boredom are real issues when patients can spend up to 23 hours per day locked in their rooms (this is when in segregation). Jacob will periodically ask me to get him a particular game or console, which I usually purchase second-hand from eBay. He can reimburse me from his benefits via a cheque prepared by the hospital. Besides games, Jacob can buy food from the hospital shop, which includes sweets, crisps, cakes and other 'naughty' but nice treats. A fairly sedentary lifestyle and a diet rich in salty, fatty and sweet treats combined with the effects of medication, has led to Jacob becoming a big lad. He is not quite as big as I was, but it is fair to say that just like me he is overweight.

Luckily for Jacob, my weight loss and size reduction means that I now have a good number of T-shirts, hoodies, shirts, shorts and jeans that are now too big for me, but are a pretty good fit for him. It is more than a likelihood that I will be providing Jacob with clothing certainly for the next few visits. In terms of my T-shirts, hoodies and shorts sizing, I've gone from being somewhere between a 4XL and a 5XL to somewhere between a 3XL and a 4XL. Prior to our visit, the PW had got me to try on a number of my old clothes, and for every item of clothing that I had previously outgrew that now fits me comfortably, I gave an item that is now a bit too big for me to Jacob. This has resulted in Jacob receiving eight T-shirts, a shirt, a hoodie and a pair of shorts on this visit, all of which he is happy to receive.

The visit goes very well. Jacob is pleased to see us and is in good spirits. As well as giving Jacob my old clothes and exchanging Christmas presents, we drink coffee that Jacob prepares, I eat a couple of fancy Christmas chocolates and a cake bar, which Jacob has purchased for the visit (I feel slightly guilty about eating these, but it is a special occasion), we chat about life in general, family, my operation and we discuss Jacob's background and life in Rampton.

The visit is conducted on Jacob's ward in a small but comfortable private visiting room that has two members of staff present throughout the visit. We have 2 hours with Jacob, before the visiting time is over, and we are escorted back to the reception through a total of 12 locked doors and gates. I can't ever imagine anyone getting out of here by means of escape, in the case of Rampton, secure means secure. The site is huge but extremely quiet, and Jacob is the only patient that we see during the entire time that we spend there. Saying goodbye and leaving is sad for all three of us, it will be some months until our next visit, but we do speak to Jacob several times per week on the phone. Tis the season to realise just how lucky we are.

After leaving Rampton we head south down the A1 to Hertfordshire, to visit daughter Becky, her partner Brendon and puppy Hera in a small rural village on the outskirts of Stevenage. They moved here on the day that I had my operation, and we have not seen them since, which has been especially hard for the PW who used to see Becky regularly when she lived in Leeds.

We stay in a nearby Days Inn Hotel, which is right on the A1 road. I had requested an accessible room. I'm not sure what the Days Inn definition of accessible is, but there is a significant step up into the shower cubicle, which has a narrow door to enter it. At least this is better than having a shower over a bath-tub. The pain in my right knee is slowly but surely easing, and I'm still hobbling with a very obvious limp. Some days I need my crutches to help support my body weight when walking, but some days I can manage with my walking stick or a walking pole just for balance and a bit of support. I am lucky this weekend that I can manage with just my walking pole, but am hobbling very slowly, and I also get out of breath quite easily. Despite my weight loss I am unfit due to a lack of physical movement and activity caused by my arthritis.

We are both really looking forward to seeing Becky, but my feelings are also mixed with anxiety over meeting her dog Hera, which is a 9 month old puppy that is a bull-mastiff/Staffordshire bull terrier cross. My cynophobia (fear of dogs) is a realistic aspect of my everyday life and is something that I just have to deal with. Due to this, we meet Becky, Brendon and Hera in their local pub rather than at their home, which is Hera's territory. I felt that in a neutral setting that I might feel a bit more at ease and indeed I do, I even stroke the dog and let it sniff me. What I didn't know prior to the visit though, is that this particular dog isn't keen on men who are dressed in dark colours, so it is sod's law that I am dressed head to toe in black. Hera doesn't seem to mind my fashion faux pas in the pub at least anyway, although some other men dressed in black do get barked at.

We stay out for a couple of hours. There are lots of drinks, photos and conversation. I manage to drink two pints of ale before stopping drinking through a feeling of being bloated, as I now know that my beer limit is low and that my days of big boozing sessions are over. Prior to my operation I had been worried about this lifestyle change, but now that I am living this way it doesn't bother me in the slightest. I'm still socialising and I'm still enjoying myself.

Later that evening we head to Becky and Brendon's house. Unfortunately for me, my cynophobia kicks straight in when Hera barks and growls at me in the house, something that she hadn't done all of the time that we were in the pub, I'm on her patch now and she is letting me know it. I'm nervous and anxious and this prevents me from relaxing and enjoying myself. We are having cheese and biscuits for our supper, but soon I lose my appetite with fear and hyper alertness. I close my eyes and try to sleep a little, which is a little antisocial but at least it stops me constantly watching the dog. I think that I do a good job of masking my fear, but later that evening back in the safety of our hotel room I confide my feelings to the PW. I am taken aback at her response, which uncharacteristically is not at all sympathetic, and is very critical of me. I just wish that other people could see dogs through my eyes the way that I do. My fear of dogs stems from me being attacked and savaged by a dog as a child that was in somebody's home, so it is in people's houses that I am most nervous of dogs. That night I have a troubled and anxious sleep about returning to Becky's house in the morning.

The next day, my cynophobia and anxiety is at its peak, but I try my best not to show it as I don't want Becky to be upset by it. The visit to Becky's house by day actually goes much better than I expected, the dog barks at our arrival (as all dogs do) but it seems less bothered by my presence during the daytime and doesn't bark or growl at me after this. We have a lunch of cheese and broccoli soup, although I can only manage a very small amount before feeling full.

After lunch Becky, the PW and Hera go for a long dog walk. I go for a hobble around the village to take some photographs and do some filming of what is a quintessential English village with thatched roof cottages, Tudor buildings, a war memorial, a stream with stepping stones, some lovely churches and of course the village pub, in fact there are three of them. On my walk I go into one of the pubs, but just have a coffee to warm me up; how indeed I have changed. Later we have Sunday lunch in the pub, and while Becky and the PW enjoy a roast beef dinner with Yorkshire puddings and all the trimmings, I manage to eat only half of a goat's cheese tart starter. I do feel a tad of food envy looking at their beautifully presented meals, but I know that it would be absolutely wasted on me. It was really lovely to see Becky after so long, she might not be my genetic daughter, but I love her as though she were, and as far as I am concerned she is my daughter. She mostly refers to me as Stuart, but sometimes she calls me Dad, and when she does it gives me a very warm and satisfying feeling inside that she officially recognises the role that I have played in her upbringing.

On the drive home that evening, I again talk to the PW about my cynophobia and how it affects me. This time she listens more sympathetically having had time to digest what I had said to her previously. I will return to Becky's house, of course I want to see my little girl again, but I'll probably not go at night and I certainly won't be wearing black. I make it clear to the PW that the dog can never, ever come to our house, which is my only dog-free safe place; to me that would absolutely be a red line being crossed, in fact it would be a red line being decimated. The PW doesn't say anything in response to this and I'm fearful that at some point in the future she might try and go against this. I don't push the issue any further, I don't want an argument in the car, there are not many things that I will not discuss with a view to negotiation, but this is absolutely one of them. I'll never ever accept a dog in my home and the PW will just have to accept that, just like I as an intelligent man have to accept that my fear of dogs is irrational but real and is something that is a part of who I am.

It is now 3 days to Christmas and whilst I consume little, I eat some things that I shouldn't. My first taste of pork pie is not a disappointment, neither are some Christmas chocolates and fancy crisps that the PW has bought. In point of fact, almost everything that I put in my mouth tastes much better than it used to. I think that my taste buds have become really sensitive with a reduced food intake. I have to tell myself that this is Christmas, so I'm allowed to be a little less strict on my diet, but I'm also fearful of the next time I step on the weighing scales.

On Christmas Eve we go for a drink on Town Street in Horsforth, though we don't have a long and boozy session like we might have had in previous years. I manage 3 pints of beer over 4 hours and we are home by 23:00. It is nice to revisit this place where we have spent so many Saturday nights out drinking, socialising and watching live music, but I now know that my limits are reduced.

Christmas Day is action stations for me. My parents, sister Carla and nephew Aiden are coming for lunch (it is Christmas lunch and not Christmas dinner as it is served in the afternoon and not the evening, you begrudgingly know that I'm right). The Christmas lunch is my domain, the PW is on light duties today (I think that she has earned it) and I'm up early preparing the turkey, stuffing it with fruit and putting bacon lardons, chopped onions and butter under its skin before putting the bird in the oven by 09:00. The turkey needs 3 hours to cook and then 2 hours to stand before carving, which guarantees that the meat won't be too dry. It's a strange meat, turkey, it is a healthy meat, but it is only really eaten as a roast by most people at Christmas. I do wonder why it isn't eaten more year-round like chicken, pork, lamb and beef. I must confess that I personally am not overly keen on it, and I think truthfully a lot of people aren't that bothered about it either, we just punish ourselves to eat it on Christmas Day because it has become traditional to do so. I think if a Christmas lunch survey was carried out in the UK, that the most popular item on the Christmas Day lunch plate would be pigs in blankets, which is just plain old sausage and bacon, something that is eaten all year round.

This year the Christmas lunch that I cook includes the following items (in addition to the turkey): home-made pigs in blankets made from streaky smoked bacon wrapped around Bramley apple sausages; stuffing muffins, my own stuffing recipe consisting of sausage meat, chopped onion, chopped tomatoes, Italian herbs, bacon lardons, honey and a packet of sage and onion stuffing mix, which is all mixed together with a little stock and then cooked in a muffin tray (hence the name stuffing muffins); a steamed gammon joint, which is left to stand for 2 hours before slicing and then being laid in a roasting tin, drenched in honey and put in the oven for 20 minutes; steamed broccoli; steamed sprouts and bacon; honey roasted carrots and parsnips; roast potatoes; mega-mash, which is my own mashed potato/mashed carrot combo mixed together with butter and milk before mashing, and then with a fried onion stirred into the mash mix after mashing, the mash being then spread in a shallow dish and grilled to brown on top, and; my own special gravy mix which along with juice from the meat, includes tomato puree, half a bottle of amber ale, fried onions, bacon lardons and some blended potato. I'm cooking for six people (five in reality due to my small portion size), but when the food is presented buffet style, it looks like I'm cooking for ten people.

I don't eat breakfast today, instead I spend the entire morning grazing (a terrible Christmas habit), and worse still, besides me grazing on the food that I'm cooking, the PW has put on display a variety of chocolates, nuts, flavoured pretzels and crisps (this is a Christmas day thing in our house). These are all snack foods that are on the naughty list, but it doesn't stop me hoovering them up every time I walk past them. They are highly tasty, highly calorific, highly fatty, low in nutrition and they don't fill me up, so I just continue to eat, eat, eat them. They are there in front of me and I mindlessly and without any self-control pick at them all day long.

My family arrives around 14:00, which coincides with the Christmas lunch project crescendo, the final hour of pulling everything together, manoeuvring items in and out of hot ovens and finally presenting the food to a hungry audience. I'm shattered by the time that lunch is served, I've been on my feet for most of the past 6 hours, my ankles are swollen, my right knee is sore, but worst of all I'm not in the slightest bit hungry due to my perpetual grazing. So while everyone else fills their plates, I put a small piece of gammon, half a pig in blanket, a bit of stuffing, a bit of mash and some gravy on my plate and I can't even finish that. The food sits at the bottom of my oesophagus slowly squeezing its way into my banana-shaped stomach amongst the digesting items that I've been grazing on, leaving me feeling a bit queasy. My Christmas lunch 2019 is officially my smallest Christmas lunch since childhood, and my least enjoyed Christmas lunch ever, which is completely my own fault.

Despite my unenjoyable lunch, Christmas Day spent with family is lovely, my parents continue to be pleased with my weight loss progress and my sister and nephew are both amazed at how different I look, as the last time that they both saw me was back in October. The exchange of presents is always nice. I receive noticeably fewer food items this year and the PW has bought me a smart watch with an activity tracker in the hope that it will encourage me to be more active. I hope that it does this for me too. It's especially nice having my nephew here, seeing him opening presents and the looks of delight on his face. Children really are what Christmas is about, and when your own children have fled the nest it does leave something of a void. The whole day is lovely, but sadly all too soon it is over and my family are heading home, I'm not sure when I'll see them all again and what I'll weigh when I do. Tis the season to be thankful for having a wonderful family.

Boxing Day (26th December if you're not British, it's actually St. Stephen's Day) comes with a nasty surprise for me; the time that I spent standing up on Christmas Day has damaged my right knee and put my recovery back, and I'm in a lot of pain and hobbling around on crutches again. This is something that I really didn't want or expect to happen, particularly as in 2 days' time the PW and I will be flying to Poznań in Poland for New Year and then from there to Eindhoven in the Netherlands. All I can do is rest it and take painkillers, so I spend the next couple of days in my chair with not a lot of activity for my new smart watch to track. Periodically it does vibrate and the word 'move' appears on the screen. I do as I'm told and have a pained shuffle around the living room when instructed to do so.

The day after Boxing Day I get back on the weighing scales, and it isn't good news, in fact Friday the 27th December is officially another black Friday for me. My fears over a weight plateau are confirmed, my Christmas eating excess is evident, my weight loss is zero, I weigh exactly the same today as I did last week. December has thrown up a lot of special occasions; the visit to Chester, Christmas drinks with friends, visiting Jacob in Rampton, visiting Becky in Hertfordshire and then Christmas. I have a lot of special occasions in my busy life, perhaps too many and I need to remain mindful of the fact that just because it is a special occasion it doesn't mean that I should eat or drink the things that made me fat in the first place and actively undo the hard work that I've done since October. This is something of a wake-up call to me and something that I'm going to have to keep in mind over our New Year holiday.

Since beginning the LRD in October, my total weight loss to date is 3 stone, 12.75 pounds (54.75 pounds/24.84 Kilos). The overall weight-loss picture is still positive, however going from losing 7 pounds per week to losing nothing, clearly shows me that

I need to take back control of my special occasion eating and drinking habits. Tis the season to be more mindful.

15 – New Year, new journey

It has become something of a tradition for the PW and me to go away on holiday for New Year, as we don't particularly want to spend this occasion in a local pub, many of which charge entry just to be in there. I fail to see the attraction of paying an entry charge to drink in a pub that I drink in anyway, what's special about that for New Year? I also remember a time before the disastrous Millennium when pubs never did this, so why should they now? The greed of pub owners and pub chains in charging entry has only served to make having parties at home more popular than going out to pubs and clubs. In essence, the licensed trade's greed has been a nail in its own coffin. As a kid, I loved New Year parties on the cul-de-sac that we lived on. We used to go around 'Aunty Mary' and 'Uncle Walter' Joyce's house. They weren't really our aunty and uncle, but in those days it was respectful to say Aunty or Uncle rather than use just the first name of an adult. Parties at the Joyces' house were legendary for the sheer amount of food and drink that was put out for guests. Andrew (my cousin who lived next door) and I would gorge ourselves until we physically couldn't stuff in any more. Then we'd sneak a few alcoholic drinks until Andrew had to go home to be sick, happy, happy days!

I remember the Millennium vaguely well, although I probably shouldn't. I was 28 years old and a student. I ended up going to London and boozing with Col (the same Col who went to Australia and lived with us), while just about every other person in London made their way to the River Thames to see the then Prime Minister Tony Blair set off fireworks on the Millennium Wheel (now the London Eye) with the point of a laser. Col and I spent the late afternoon drinking cans of lager and cider, after which we headed southwest to Wimbledon for the main event rather than north into Central London. I think I must have been stopping at Col's flat in Streatham, although I'm actually a little hazy on that particular detail. At some point we realised that our limited money wouldn't last the evening in expensive Wimbledon so we left the pub to buy vodka from a shop to then sneak back into the pub. The only problem was that once we had acquired the vodka, none of the door staff on any of the pub doors would let us back in. This was possibly due to the fact that by this point, I was wearing a road cone on my head, which I tried to pass off as fancy dress. "I am dressed as roadworks," I remonstrated with the surly bouncers in my thick northern twang. None of them were having it, so Col and I ended up swigging neat vodka out of the bottle, whilst we walked all the way back to Streatham, which took hours. The journey was punctuated with me shouting, "happy New Year to one and all," through the road cone, which I had turned into an impromptu megaphone. As we worked our way through South West London's suburbia, I also shouted through the road cone, "if you're having a New Year party, please can we come in? Happy New Year." It didn't work, we were not invited into anyone's homes, and I honestly can't imagine why. It was about 8 minutes after midnight that we realised that we were now in the 21st Century and the next Millennium, so smashed were we that we hadn't even realised that fireworks had been going off for nearly 10 minutes. Happy New Year indeed!

These days New Years are much more civilised affairs, and the PW and I would much rather go somewhere abroad and turn the New Year into a holiday. In recent years we have spent the New Year in Amsterdam, Copenhagen, Geneva, Gdansk, Katowice, Kraków, Prague and Wrocław. This year we are having a twin-centred New Year holiday to Poznań and Eindhoven. I take advantage of the fact that flights and hotels are cheaper than one might expect at this time of year, particularly to cities in countries with colder climates. A visit to Poland at New Year never disappoints, the Christmas decorations are still up, the Christmas markets are in full swing and the atmosphere is still very festive. As well as this, Poland compared to the UK is inexpensive, so the British pound converted to the Polish złoty goes a long way. Eindhoven will be a different matter, the Christmas markets will have gone and the value of sterling against the euro has plummeted since the Brexit referendum, but don't get me started on that. However, it is fair to say that Eindhoven is a decent city and it's somewhere new for the PW to see. I have been to both cities before, but the PW has been to neither, and I like to use my local cultural and geographical knowledge to show her around such places. My name Stuart literally means 'steward' and in life I get a kick out of fulfilling this role.

We fly from Doncaster to Poznań with Wizz Air. Due to my struggles with movement I booked us a taxi from our home in North Leeds to Doncaster Airport, which only takes an hour from our house. This is instead of taking a taxi from our house to Horsforth Station; a train from Horsforth Station to Leeds Station; a train from Leeds Station to Doncaster Station and a bus from Doncaster Station to Doncaster Airport. The £80 taxi is only £30 more expensive than it would have cost us both to travel by public transport, but it is 90 minutes quicker and physically less demanding on my very sore knee joint. The official name of Doncaster Airport is actually Doncaster Sheffield Airport, but I personally find that name irritating and annoying as the airport is nowhere near Sheffield, in fact it is much closer to Rotherham, Retford and Scunthorpe than it is to Sheffield. A sensible name for the airport would have been 'South Yorkshire Airport', but of course in an era of overpaid marketing stupidity, sensible names are rarely used. The airport (as a civilian airport) began life as 'Robin Hood Airport', which is an even more stupid name, seeing as though Robin Hood's fictional associations were with the city of Nottingham, which is 50 miles (80 kilometres) away. If any airport were to be called Robin Hood Airport, it should have been East Midlands Airport, which is only 13 miles (21 kilometres) from Nottingham. Doncaster Airport prior to being a civilian airport was called RAF Finningley and has a very long runway that is capable of handling the largest aircraft in the world. I have fond childhood memories of going to Finningley Air Show to see huge United States Air Force 'Galaxy' aircraft, as well as the Royal Air Force's Red Arrows, skydivers, helicopters and even electro synth-pop star Gary Numan flying a Harvard trainer aircraft low over the runway, I remember him waving from the open side cockpit window!

Marketing stupidity isn't the only annoyance that I have about Doncaster Airport, it has a railway line that goes right past its perimeter, so why on earth doesn't it have its own railway station? I'll tell you why, because it is in the under-invested North of

England. In any other European country, this airport would have had a railway station and probably a tram link. My own local airport, Leeds Bradford Airport suffers the same problem, as it has a nearby railway line but no railway station, despite talk of one for years. Leeds Bradford Airport like Doncaster Sheffield Airport also suffers from having a stupid name, when the airport is entirely situated in Leeds and not one square metre of it is in Bradford; again a more sensible name would have been West Yorkshire Airport, but like I said previously, when you let idiot overpaid marketers make decisions, this is what you end up with. When it comes to rail links to make airports sustainable viable via public transport connections, I can only think of Manchester and Newcastle Airports in the north of England that have this luxury. In the south of England, Heathrow, Gatwick, Stansted, Luton, Southend and Southampton Airports all have rail links, while Bristol Airport is currently planning one. The underinvestment in public transport in the north of England is yet another consequence of years of Tory neglect of the north.

Anyway I'll stop digressing and get back to the story. We arrive at Doncaster Airport in plenty of time, the journey taking exactly an hour. The airport is very quiet, as there is only one departure every 2 hours. It is difficult to see how this airport is financially viable, I'm certain that a proper rail link would make it more attractive to passengers and therefore airlines would expand the airport's portfolio of destinations; as the saying goes, you need to speculate to accumulate. I know that the airport also supports itself by handling a lot of freight from around the world. My dad once told me that there is a weekly Boeing 747 cargo plane from Nigeria to Doncaster, I wonder what we import from there? The super-sized Airbus A300-600ST (nicknamed the Beluga) has also landed at Doncaster. This is truly one of the world's largest and most unlikely looking flying machines, do a Google image search for it and see for yourself.

We go to check our bags in at the Wizz Air check-in desk. We have one full-sized 20kg suitcase each and then a small hand luggage bag each. I am using my crutch and hobbling quite badly. I ask at the check-in desk if there is any way that I could board the aircraft first as I will struggle in the melee of passengers (it's always a melee on the budget airlines). The check-in assistant is very amenable and makes me a 'special assistance' passenger. I've never been designated this before, but it means that we won't have to go down the steps from the terminal to the runway and will instead go in a lift.

After going through the usual security and ticket checks we are in departures. It is quiet, a flight to Budapest has just closed and our aircraft is due to board in 90 minutes. That means plenty of time for a cheap Wetherspoon's gin, yes Doncaster Airport has a Wetherspoon pub in the departures area, and the irony of this isn't lost on me. The Brexit backing pub is solely in an area where people are travelling into Europe, not trying to get out of it.

We enjoy a gin and tonic each, which I have to drink slowly, stirring out the bubbles with a straw. A lady who works for the airport approaches us after seeing my crutch, and asks if I'm one of the special assistance passengers for Poznań? I confirm that I am. She checks our tickets and passports while we are sitting in the pub and then let's me know that a gentleman will be along shortly to take us to the lift. What a way to travel, this is better than first class, no standing for ages waiting for the plane to land and disembark, no queueing, no pushing, we've been checked for departure with drinks in hand, this is certainly a relaxing way to travel.

10 minutes later a gentleman does indeed approach us and take us downstairs in a lift. But once downstairs the special VIP assistance gets even better. There are no stairs for us to climb to board the aircraft, we don't even have to walk to the aircraft, we are being taken to the aircraft in an 'ambulift'. An ambulift is a bit like a delivery lorry on a scissor lift, but instead of space for freight, the lorry has seats inside it. We are escorted from the terminal to a platform on the back of the lorry that raises us up into the ambulift. From there we take our seats inside the ambulift and are driven to the back door of the aircraft, where the magic happens. At the push of a button the whole back of the lorry raises on a scissor lift. A door then opens and we step directly into the aircraft, it's great, and that's another new experience to tick off my life experience

list. There is a certain irony in losing weight to become less disabled, but in doing so becoming more disabled due to my knee.

We are seated peacefully before the melee of passengers scrum down into the aircraft. This is my first flight since I had the operation, and I am more than pleased to report that losing 30 centimetres from my waist means that I no longer need to use an extension belt with my aircraft seatbelt, which now fits me comfortably with room to spare. The arm between the PW's seat and my seat easily folds down into place, where as I usually have to stuff it down against my fat muffin top, and the fold-down table in front of me folds down all the way instead of resting on my rotund Buddha like belly, which is now much less prominent. The PW remarks that she has much more room than she usually has when sitting next to me on an aeroplane, as my frame usually invades her space and is squashed against her. Flying in general, but especially on budget airlines, is going to be a much more pleasant experience for me from this point onwards, and the person sitting next to me! The whole seat feels roomier, when in fact it is no bigger than it was the last time I took a flight with Wizz Air, and the extra space I can feel is because there is physically less of me taking up space.

The flight is comfortable and fast, from take-off to landing is around 1 hour and 45 minutes. I like these short-haul flights, the beauty of Europe is that culturally you can be somewhere completely different to where you are from in little more than an hour's flying time. I have often thought about living in Australia, Canada or the USA, but honestly I would miss the rich cultural heritage and diversity that Europe has to offer. There isn't anywhere else on the planet that can offer such a rich variety of cultures in such a geographically concentrated area like Europe does. I have visited most countries in Europe, and I haven't been to a country that I disliked. There are certainly some cities that I'm not so keen on, Paris and Amsterdam for example are just too big and busy, I can't relax and enjoy myself in them, and they are also extremely overpriced. I would much rather visit a city like Limoges in France than the nation's capital Paris, and likewise, I'd much rather visit a city like Breda in the Netherlands, than its capital city Amsterdam.

Poznań is not on the tourist trail of as many visitors to Poland as are some higher profile cities such as Kraków, Warsaw, Wrocław or Gdansk. Indeed, when I mentioned to one of my Polish students that I was visiting Poznań for New Year, he pulled a face as if I had farted in front of him and asked me, "what on earth are you going there for?" Let me tell you why: there are plenty of things to see and do in a geographically small area, so it is easy to explore on foot; there are many stunning buildings, including churches, the cathedral, and the buildings around the market square; the craft beer scene is growing rapidly and is superb; the food is fantastic, particularly my favourite Polish food pierogi (dumplings); the city is inexpensive compared to some of the higher profile Polish cities; and whilst Poznań is a busy city, it is not too congested and overly busy as to be off-putting to a slow moving fat man who hobbles with a crutch.

The PW and I are staying in the Novotel Poznań Centrum, which is a new and very contemporary high-rise development. We have a lovely new room on the top (16th) floor, which has a nice big walk-in shower in the bathroom. The room has a panoramic view over the city and a super king-sized and very comfortable bed. We've paid the bargain price of around £40 per night to stay here; try and beat that sort of price in a Novotel in most cities, believe me you will struggle. Novotel hotels usually look very stylish, and many of them feel better than I might expect for the price that I have paid. We are staying on a room-only basis, as the price of breakfast would be wasted on me, as I can only eat very small amounts.

It is dark by the time we have arrived and I am exhausted. My body clock seems to synch with the colour of the sky. The PW sensing my weariness unpacks my case for me, while I sit like a pudding on the bed. She knows that by doing this, I'll have a bit of recovery time energy wise. I am still tired though and make the suggestion that maybe we stop in tonight and hit the sights of Poznań early tomorrow morning. The PW rebuffs this notion immediately, it is Saturday night, the PW is in a new city, the PW wants to explore, the PW has Poznań Wanderlust. I know that there is no point in pressing the matter any further, so I mentally and physically prepare myself for a night out. In days of old I would have been chomping at the bit to get out and get into the pub.

Uber is available in Poznań, so in order to avoid putting stress on my aching knee, we order an Uber to a craft beer bar on the far side of the main old market square. The car arrives and is tiny, even with my reduced frame size, I struggle to get into the vehicle, particularly with one knee that is reluctant to bend. The journey is uncomfortable but remarkably cheap; a 10-minute ride costs 10 złoty, which is around £2. In cities that don't have Uber, I would normally study how to use the public transport system before visiting, but when rides are as cheap as this, I just don't bother. Poznań has an excellent tram, rail and bus system, but it is easier for me to take advantage of cheap Uber rides that go door to door albeit in tiny cars, than it is to use public transport.

The craft beer bar, which is called 'Chmielnik' isn't overly busy. Craft beer has really taken off in Poland, the younger 'hipster' generation really go for it, as do the tourists, but for the older generation, who are used to plain fizzy and cheap lager, paying double the price for something that is much stronger in terms of ABV and also with new and experimental flavours is a bit of a non-starter. The average older and middle-aged Polish Tyskie drinker would probably rather drink his own pee than a 7% marshmallow porter. The selection of beers in this bar like many craft beer pubs in Poland is very extensive. We take a seat towards the back of the bar where I can stretch out my sore right leg. Even with my reduced body size, I only just fit into the very tight seat. Prior to me losing weight, I would never have fitted into such a seat before and would have ended up slightly embarrassed and standing. I order a 6.5% porter, which is served in a 250ml or a 500ml glass, however the price of the 250ml glass is only 2 złoty (40p) less than the 500 ml serving (rather than being half the price), so naturally the value for money Yorkshireman in me orders the 500ml serving, which is just under an imperial pint in size (a pint is 568 ml). The PW settles on having a fruit beer, after first trying to order a cider, then a white wine, then a gin and tonic. This craft beer pub, really is a beer pub.

The drinks go down slowly, after which we head to the old market square, or Stary Rynek as it is called in Polish. The square is an impressive sight, as it and much of the old town date back to the 13th Century, when it was settled and constructed by Germanic settlers. Many of the surviving buildings that stand in the market square today were constructed in the 17th century, during the Catholic inspired Baroque architectural trend, which swept much of Europe around this era. These ornate buildings with their curves and intricate design, were deliberately artistic and served as public art pieces as well as functional building spaces, inspiring wonder and awe amongst those who saw them, as well as a greater appreciation of the Catholic Church, which was intrinsically linked to their construction. The most dominant building in the square is the old town hall, which is now a museum. The square has a cobbled surface, which isn't particularly crutch- and hobble-friendly, and I spend more time looking downwards at where I am placing my crutch and my feet than I do looking at the illuminated buildings, statues and Christmas lights. I have been here before though, so I'm not too disappointed. The PW is in a state of open-mouthed wonderment at the fairy-tale buildings and lights, snapping away at them all with her camera. If she is happy then I am happy.

After a circuit of the square we visit a bar within the square. This time it is a traditional bar, and the décor is nice but the bar has limited beer choices. I order a bland Czech black beer, while the PW has a glass of white wine. We then make our way out of the square and down a very busy street called Wrocławska, which is certainly orientated towards nightlife, and has a great many themed bars and restaurants. The demographic on this street is certainly much younger than in the market square, which is only a few metres away. We find a bar on this street called Jabeerwocky, which is another craft beer pub with 15 different craft beers on tap to choose from. My beer of choice in this venue is a 7.3% stout, which is absolutely delicious. I savour every mouthful of this rich, thick, sweet and highly calorific liquid. I think back to my self-disappointment after my last meeting with dietician Mary, but only briefly, I want to enjoy this evening.

The night rolls on, the PW is hungry, and the bar serves small hot snacks, so we order a portion of onion rings, a portion of chips and a cheese, onion and tomato burrito. The food is beige coloured, which usually means fatty and calorific, and of course it is both, but it is also delicious. I manage three onion rings, one chip and a few bites of the burrito before the feeling of fullness registers. That is dinner for me for tonight, and it tasted incredible, everything tastes great! The PW finishes off the chips and onion rings as well as one of the burritos, but in true Yorkshire lass style wraps up two burrito pieces in a tissue to take home for breakfast. She would make any Yorkshireman proud, would that lass. From Jabeerwocky we set off back towards our hotel on foot, and even though walking is painful, I need to move to help the food go down and for my stomach to settle. It is around a 1 mile (1.6 kilometres) walk, which takes me nearly 30 minutes, with the PW patiently walking by my side. The beer, food and exercise are a perfect recipe for a very deep and satisfying sleep.

"Hello, sleepy-head," says the PW's voice; my eyes are closed, CPAP mask affixed and the air is gently blowing into my dry mouth. The PW says this at some point every day, but usually to our cat Indy, though today she is saying it to me. I open my eyes slowly. The room is in semi-darkness, but I can see that the PW is standing at the foot of my bed wearing her gym attire. "I've just done an hour in the gym," she tells me, "I ran for 15 minutes too." The PW is a physical woman, she has far too much energy, I hadn't stirred once all night, I never even stirred when she got up to go to the gym. My smart watch tells me that I slept for a total of 8 hours and 12 minutes, and of this 6 hours 25 minutes was a deep sleep.

The small breakfast burrito is like a party in my mouth, the red onion tastes like something from the vegetable Garden of Eden. That small amount of food is enough to fill me up and fuel the fire for a walk into Poznań's Old Town. Breakfast is followed by a cocktail of drugs and vitamins, I have had to be extremely organised and dispense everything into a dosset box; at home the PW is happy to be nurse and dispense my morning and evening daily meds, but it seemed silly bringing all the boxes and tubs of pills here when I could just count out the ones that I need. I have a morning dosset box packed with 8 mornings' worth of pills and a night dosset box packed with 8 nights' worth of pills. My morning's pills are as follows: two turmeric tablets; one multivitamin; one vitamin D; one iron tablet, and one glucosamine with chondroitin tablet. My night pills are as follows: one turmeric tablet; one magnesium tablet; one simvastatin tablet; one lansoprazole tablet, and; one glucosamine with chondroitin tablet. Besides these, I am taking two codeine tablets and two paracetamol tablets every waking 4 hours for the pain in my knee and wrist. I also have my Oramorph with me in case of emergency, I'm not even sure if I'm allowed to bring morphine into Poland without special permission, perhaps I'm now a drug smuggler? I'm sure with the amount of pills inside me that I must rattle when I walk. My toilet bag looks as though I am a travelling pill salesman, so thankfully I haven't had to open it at customs.

The walk is slow and quite painful on my right knee which grates with movement and occasionally gives me a jolt that feels like I've been stabbed in it. My feet also hurt. I have the new insoles from Wharfedale Hospital in my trainers and they don't feel particularly comfortable. On the face of it they don't seem to be correcting my odd penguin-like walk in any way, and the raised ridges in them seem to be on the wrong side, but I will persevere with them for now. We walk past an open window and the delicious smell of food wafts out. I breathe it in like a Bisto kid (remember them?) and get a hunger pang. I haven't really had any hunger pangs since my operation but this one is memorable because I can identify it being triggered by the smell of food. I wasn't hungry in any way at all, but for a few seconds after the pang, I feel hunger, which is a feeling I haven't had for 3 months now. Moments later the feeling of hunger subsides but it leaves me wondering when I will start to feel hungry again. Janine did tell me that feelings of hunger would return at some point, I just didn't expect it to be so soon.

My walking is painfully slow, I really am using the crutch for support and not just balance; upon reflection my right knee doesn't seem to be any better now than it was in Edinburgh, and that was 5 weeks ago. I mention this to the PW, and she agrees but also points out that my fatigue is now much less than it was then and that I am getting tired much less, so my body overall is recovering well from the operation. I also must consider how bad my knee was when I went to Stoke. It is certainly better now than it was then, so I definitely am making some sort of recovery, albeit slowly.

We spend the day going from church to church to building of interest, to statue, to notable street. The PW is in her element, camera in hand snapping away; the PW is a happy photo walker. I spend every opportunity I can sitting down on benches either on the street or in churches. Whilst my weight is less, my sore knee is giving me no respite and coupled with this, the soles of my feet are hurting from my new insoles, which might as well be made from Lego. It's a disappointment that I'm not really feeling the benefit of being 4 stones lighter on my first post-op foreign jaunt due to my other physical problems. Respite comes in a pub and I manage three beers, but then feel full and need to walk it off again. It doesn't take long for the fullness to subside, I seem to be handling liquids quite well. As we walk the streets in the early evening darkness, a lovely food smell again awakens my appetite. There is no mistaking this smell, it is my favourite food smell of all, curry. Fate has brought us to Poznań's only Indian restaurant. The PW loves her curries too, and we haven't eaten anything today since breakfast, so we go inside.

Ordinarily my Indian restaurant routine would be as follows: a pint of Indian lager; two poppadoms and the pickle tray; onion bhaji starter; chicken or mixed meat balti or jalfrezi main; boiled rice, and a Peshwari naan bread. Now that level of delicious and greedy Indian food consumption is all but a distant memory. The PW orders a glass of wine to drink, and I have nothing to drink due to the 30-minute food and drink rule (which I'm trying to stick to). We then order one mixed vegetable bhaji starter, one chicken balti curry and one portion of boiled rice and this is to share between us. I ask the waiter if we can have the starters and main together at the same time and explain that we are sharing. I feel the need to have to explain and add that, "I only have a small stomach and cannot eat much." The waiter didn't need to know that, but it's almost as if I felt guilty or duty bound into giving an explanation. The food comes after a short wait, and it looks incredible, smells incredible and tastes like the best thing that I've ever eaten. I absolutely love going out to eat Indian food; try as I might (and believe me I have), the flavours are something that I simply cannot replicate at home, and I've missed eating out in Indian restaurants more than I have realised. I manage to eat a couple of the bhaji starters and around three spoonfuls of chicken balti, but then the feeling of fullness hits and I must stop, otherwise I will make myself ill. I am completely satisfied by what I have eaten and not in the least bit disappointed in only eating a small amount, I've had my fix of spicy deliciousness and I'm happy. The PW is also happy as she now gets to finish off the meal without my interference. Again after the food I feel like I need to walk to aid my digestion, and we walk for 30 minutes back to the hotel. When I'm at home I wouldn't consider going for a walk after a meal to aid digestion, but when I'm away, it's the first thing that I think of doing. Maybe I should incorporate this good habit into my home routine too?

The following day we take an Uber to Poznań Cathedral, a magnificent gothic building, which dates back to the 14th Century. It is located northeast of the city centre on the island of Ostrów Tumski, and the island is surrounded by waterways (the Warka and Cybnia rivers) making it only accessible by bridge (of which there are several). The cathedral is a must-see building in Poznań and has extensive decoration within its sculpted walls, stained glass and numerous art pieces. I have been before in the summertime, and it was even more spectacular then as the bright sunshine outside better illuminated the building's innards. Today it is a dull and gloomy day and the lighting within the cathedral is quite dim, which is a shame as the full glory of the art work within the cathedral is slightly subdued. Neither the PW nor I are religious, but we do both appreciate the art and architecture that churches and cathedrals provide. I find them to be akin to religious and historically themed museums and art galleries. Every such building that I have encountered is an experience that usually has an educational component to it that you need to be there to appreciate.

After leaving the cathedral we negotiate the quiet cobbled streets of Ostrów Tumski, and again with my crutch and dodgy knee this is more of a challenge for me than it needs to be. The buildings of Ostrów Tumski are ornate, some baroque and others more neo-classical, some walls are painted with historically themed intricate murals and there are numerous photo opportunities, which again slows down my journey. We haven't eaten yet today and the PW is hungry, and we spot a very small and traditional looking Polish restaurant called 'Hyćka Restauracja' so head inside. The restaurant is very small and quaint but of a good standard. The raw brickwork of the walls is exposed but cleaned, and there is an atmosphere of high quality as well as tradition about the place. The PW orders pork, potato dumplings and pickled cabbage, and I order pierogi. When in Poland I have to eat pierogi, the traditional Polish dumplings, it would be rude not to. My favourite are with a meat filling, usually pork and/or beef, but also the Russian dumplings with cheese and potato are good, as are the vegetable-filled ones. Basically all pierogi are delicious. When I was in Warsaw some years ago with my mates, we went to a pierogi restaurant and I ate three plates of dumplings, 24 in total. We all ate a ridiculous amount. Today my plate arrives with seven pierogi on it. Each mouthful is wonderful, the soft pasta like case bursts to give the flavours from the meat and herbs within. I savour them by eating slowly and chewing meticulously; my days of throwing food down my throat and mass pierogi eating are behind me, and out of the seven pierogi on the plate, I only manage to eat two and a half before feeling full. The PW eats one and a half for me, and the remaining three pierogi are taken away in a pierogi doggy bag, they are simply too good to leave!

From the restaurant I need a walk to help me digest the food, so we walk along the shores of Lake Malta to Posnania, which is a huge out-of-town shopping centre in Poznań. The distance is around 1.3 miles (2km), but with my crutch and hobble on the rough path it takes me 40 minutes. The wind blowing from the lake penetrates my clothing and bites into me. I feel cold now like I haven't felt in years, that is what happens when you lose a good sized layer of insulating blubber. At least the cold takes my mind off my aching knee and feet. When we arrive at Posnania I am ready to drop, I just want to sit down somewhere warm, and wonder if there is a sofa/sauna shop.

Upon entering the shopping mall the blow of hot air above the entry doors is most welcoming. The mall is ultra-modern and very new, it would compete with any shopping mall anywhere in the world. I am not a shopper, but the PW is, and now like a shark that can smell blood in the water she is in a hyper hunting mode, set to strike at any January sale bargains that catch her eye. It so happens that just inside the entrance to Posnania is a micro-brewery pub called 'Bierhalle' with free Wi-Fi and comfortable padded seats that will do nicely. The PW deposits me in Bierhalle while she goes to shop. I happily sit there with a 6.5% stout as do numerous other men that have also evidently been deposited here by their better halves, who are also taking advantage of the January sales. Sheffield United v Manchester City is on the TV, it's the third time that I've seen this match on TV in 2 days. The Poles certainly love the English Premier League, and I'd rather watch this game again though than shop.

Shopping for me these days is almost entirely online. Amazon and eBay are two of my main shopping hubs. I buy virtually everything except clothes and groceries from Amazon, and I buy most of my clothes from eBay. Once I grew beyond a 3XL I found that the only shop in Leeds that sold my sizes was Great Clothes, which wasn't that convenient for me to get to. There is also High and Mighty in Leeds city centre, but it is expensive and doesn't usually sell what I'm after. I'm not much of a fan of Jacamo either, I find their sizing to be out of kilter with my sizing. That means I play the eBay clothes size lottery, I've bought 4XL and 5XL T-shirts that have drowned me and looked like dresses, I've also bought 7XL T-shirts that realistically are the equivalent of a UK medium size. I tend to find that the American and German sellers are usually good in terms of sizing, the UK sellers in my experience have been very hit and miss (I've bought 4XL that realistically is a 2XL), and the sellers in the Far East are usually rubbish, I'm sure some of them just sew a range of size labels into clothing that is all the same size. If something arrives and it is too small, I rarely send it back, I just can't be bothered, and there is always that old chestnut that, "I'll lose weight so it will fit me," which never happens. Now, though, it might. I wonder if when I have lost the weight that I want to lose and can fit into 'normal' sized clothing that is available on the high street, I will get a renewed appreciation of shopping? Will I become a happy shopper like the PW?

After 90 minutes of retail action, the PW returns to me in Bierhalle laden with bags of January sale bargains. Jumpers, necklaces, hair clips, brooches, Christmas decorations, ornaments and pet treats are all displayed before me along with a short story for each item that includes their before sale and sale pricing. The PW as a true Yorkshire lass is certainly price wise. She thinks that she has done well, and I'm sure that she has, so she celebrates with a pilsner, while I try a honey beer. All that shopping has worked up an appetite with the PW, so she orders a burger and fries, which is something that the old me would have ordered in a place like this, all that grease definitely complements the beer. Not wanting to be left out, I order a herring starter, which consists of 9 pieces of pickled herring and some onion and caper mayonnaise dip. This is something that old me would never have ordered in a million years in a place like this, but I'm fairly sure that I will be able to manage to eat it, particularly with it being a small portion, plus the fish is a good source of protein. As it happens I manage to eat four pieces of herring before feeling overly full and I give the rest to the PW to have with her burger, turning it into an impromptu surf and turf.

After the meal I feel like I need another walk to get the food moving along my oesophageal conveyor, again it is 1.3 miles (2 km), back to the hotel, so off we trot (although my trot is a hobble). The walk takes around 40 minutes, and en route we call at Zabka, (convenience store) to buy in some snack items for breakfast. When we eventually get back to the hotel the feeling of fullness has gone as the walk has helped my digestion, but I am in agony, my right knee and both feet are killing me. I look forward to a day when I don't have to suffer this. I wonder if I will ever be pain free? That night I have my codeine, paracetamol and morphine just to get myself comfortable so that I can sleep.

New Year's Eve 2019 is upon us, the 365th day of this tumultuous year, the year that my life changed for the better forever. I scroll through Twitter, but nearly everyone who is writing about 2019 is slagging it off. Yes, politically it has been very shit, but personally I have had another great year that I am very thankful for. I quickly have enough of the moaning, it's bringing me down. After our breakfast of crackers, pepperoni, cup-a-soup and a ginger biscuit (a very flavoursome random breakfast), we get an Uber to Park Cytadela, which is Poznań's largest city based park. The park also plays host to the Cmentarz Bohaterów (a military cemetery) as well as a military museum.

I struggle out of yet another tiny Uber car into cold and windy air that chills my fingertips and body within seconds, and realise this is going to be an uncomfortable day, made even more uncomfortable by the 50 steep steps in front of me to get into the park. That really isn't what I need right now. Fortunately, the PW spies a sloping path, which will be much more manageable for me. The walk uphill is tough and I have to stop numerous times to get my breath, I'm really not used to this level of exercise anymore. The path takes us through the military cemetery, which is both spectacular in its commemorative artworks but very sad in that these are nearly all for young men who died in battle because of aggressive dictators and the failures of governments. There is a large Commonwealth War Graves area with headstones for British and British Empire Service personnel, who were mostly killed in the Second World War. The majority of Commonwealth War Graves here are for men aged 19-25. It is truly saddening that so many young lives were lost so far from their homes. I wonder how many family members of these men have ever had the opportunity to visit these graves, that is assuming that the families are aware that their relatives are buried here in the first place. The cemetery is well maintained and there is an atmosphere of respect here as well as remembrance. RIP brave warriors.

At the top of the hill I spot a bench, and that becomes my first pit stop of the day. My knees and feet are hurting a lot and the 5 minutes of respite that I get sitting down is very welcome. The PW strolls up and produces a chocolate bar for me, saying, "energy boost." She'd kept that well-hidden, but it hardly touches the sides on the way down. It's ironic how my banana stomach can seemingly process: crisps, chocolate;

and cakes without a problem, yet I can't even manage to eat more than four small pieces of herring. It goes to show how empty a lot of 'naughty' snack items are in terms of substance and sustenance, and it also makes me realise how the operation that I've had might not be any good for somebody who is addicted to such junk items, which thankfully I'm not. Yes, I like them, of course I do, they give a hit of flavour, salt, sugar and fat, they release dopamine in my brain that makes me happy, but I don't go out of my way to eat these foods anymore, they are to be only occasional treats and thankfully we rarely have them in the house at home. I know that I need to remain mindful when it comes to food like this though, and that will be for the rest of my life.

After the rest we push on, and there are numerous interesting sights within the park including a monument to all war dead; some decommissioned tanks; a memorial bell to those who died in the Hiroshima bombing; landscaped gardens, and public artworks including sculptures and statues, which are mostly themed around life and death. This park certainly is a place to make you think about the fragility of life and your own mortality as well as the consequences of war and conflict. After an hour or so of hobbling around the park, the cumulative effect of the pains in my knee and feet combined with the cold penetrating my body to the bone lowers my mood and I'm ready to head home. The PW can read me well, and we head back to the hotel for some rest and relaxation before going out for the evening's New Year celebrations.

Outside of London and Edinburgh, the UK doesn't seem to celebrate New Year very well. Certainly in my home city of Leeds, there is nothing official happening from the city council for the general public in terms of a city centre event counting down to midnight with fireworks afterwards, it just doesn't happen. In Poland, the New Year is celebrated widely. Cities up and down the country have special events, with elaborate stages, entertainment and of course fireworks, lots of fireworks. The main event in Poznań is being held in plac Wolności, one of the city's main squares. Fireworks have been going off all day long, and from our room on the 16th floor of the Novotel tower we have seen them going up and heard them banging continuously for the past few hours, to the uninitiated it must sound like a war zone. Having looked online, we see that the Poznań event seems to begin at 22:00, and there are several Polish musicians and local dignitaries on the bill. We head out at 23:00 hoping to get into the main square before midnight. We were not alone in adopting this strategy, as seemingly half of Poznań has had the same idea, and many of the revellers are very drunk and worryingly many of them are carrying huge fireworks of their own, I begin to sense the ingredients of a disaster. The approach to letting off New Year fireworks by revellers in Poznań is quite basic; simply find a spare patch of road or footpath, put the fireworks there and let them off, I'm not exaggerating. If there are people too close to the firework, it is their responsibility to get out of the way. If you are driving, tough luck, hopefully your car will protect you. The roads are littered with smouldering firework launchers, boxes and shells, as well as broken glass, and as midnight draws closer these only increase in number. We reach the main square to see huge queues to enter it, and an arena has been created with security fencing and an entry wristband is required, which has created a bottleneck. I'm wary of being in crowds after my experience last year in Wrocław, particularly with my bad knee and crutch. I suggest to the PW that we go around the arena to see if we can find a good spot that is away from it. A narrow path has been created between the arena fencing and the buildings down one side of plac Wolności, so we venture down it. As we are almost halfway down, a male artist takes the stage inside the arena at 23:30 and there is a surge on the path towards the security fencing, where people are looking for gaps to see the artist. These people stop and cause a blockage, but all the while, more people are entering the path, and suddenly it begins to feel tight as gaps between people disappear.

I have studied event disasters before, where mismanagement of crowds has caused crushing that has led to the deaths of event attendees. I have taught lessons about the Hillsborough disaster of 1989, where 96 people lost their lives and the Love Parade disaster of 2010 where 21 people suffocated in an underground tunnel after being crushed. I haven't had a drink and am stone cold sober unlike the mass of bodies around me, so I can see that this crowd crush situation is not far from becoming a potential tragedy, and I grab hold of the PW's arm and tell her to follow me. Against the flow of bodies, we hug the security fencing and push our way out of the footpath and away from the arena. This takes us a couple of minutes to do, during which time my adrenaline kicks in, giving me strength and hyper alertness, the pain in my knees and feet disappears as I guide the PW to the relative safety of another part of plac Wolności, where we only needed to worry about being hit by fireworks and not being crushed to death. I took charge, my 'steward' instinct kicked in, I wasn't useless for a change. I have been in some scary crowd situations before now, and that experience was right up there amongst; getting pepper sprayed by German police while being held in an underground tunnel after I got caught up amongst a load of Schalke 04 fans in Cologne; being stuck in Malta's national football stadium after a riot between Malta fans and fans of The Lebanon's national football club, and last New Year's traumatic experience in Wrocław's main square. All those experiences were memorable, but none of them would I want to repeat.

At the stroke of midnight there is a firework frenzy, which is both spectacular and terrifying. The official fireworks look amazing, but I'm more concerned about the rockets, bangers and flares that are going off in the street right next to where I am standing to fully appreciate the beauty of what is in the sky above me. Eventually the official fireworks end, and we begin to make our way back to the hotel, past exploding fireworks on roads and paths littered with broken glass. People are staggering all around, and almost every spare metre of wall is taken up by men relieving themselves of what they have been drinking for the past couple of hours. We see one brave and foolish girl walking barefoot, her boyfriend carrying her stiletto heels, and think she must have been in some severe pain to be doing that, because all I can hear underfoot is the crunch, crunch, crunch of glass. The clean-up operation for this event must cost a fortune. As we get further from the main square, the streets become emptier of people and the broken glass underfoot becomes less audible. The roads are still all littered with discarded firework launchers, many of which are still smoking. I don't think health and safety matters as much in Poland. The sight of our hotel is very welcome as it represents sanctuary and safety, and it is my first New Year since adulthood that I've been stone cold sober, not having had a single drink. As we enter the Novotel, I vow to the PW that we won't come to Poland again for New Year, as whilst it is a great country and the fireworks are a spectacle, it's all just a bit too traumatic. Still digesting what we have experienced this evening, we haven't really discussed our New Year's resolutions. When we get back to our room and in bed, the PW tells me that her resolutions are to: maintain her current weight; swim at least once per week; use her craft room at home more often in order to start making art and craft things, and make me go the cinema at least once per month. I only have one resolution, to finish 2020 weighing less than what I begin it.

For the second part of our New Year holiday, we fly from Poznań to the Dutch city of Eindhoven. At online check-in I book Wizz Air special assistance for this flight, which means for the PW and me that we get a security fast-track and escorted to the aircraft, being first to board at Poznań. At Eindhoven we are last to depart the aircraft, but have an ambulift to get us down from the aircraft, before a short walk to baggage collection. Once again on this flight, I fit nicely into my seat and have no problem securing my seatbelt, which fits nicely.

We stay at the Pullman Eindhoven Cognac Hotel, which is located centrally in the city centre. We have a very modern room, that is quite boutique in style, with a wet-room walk in shower, perfect for me in terms of accessibility. This hotel like the Novotel in Poznań is a part of the Accor group, and is a more high-end luxury brand than Novotel, but is still very business orientated.

Eindhoven is quite a modern city; the buildings are mostly low-rise and much of the architecture seems to be post Second World War, and it has a smaller and more compact city centre than Poznań. There is no real 'old town' area in Eindhoven, and the streets are mostly very crutch- and hobble-friendly, with extensive pedestrian areas that are block paved rather than cobbled. Eindhoven has a thriving shopping area, with several malls all within the city's central business district (CBD). The city's nightlife is also extremely vibrant with several nightlife zones within the CBD that have numerous bars, pubs, cafes, restaurants and clubs. Besides these, there are several local breweries with their own craft beer bars. Eindhoven is a destination that is geared towards shopping and alcohol tourism. As we venture out from the hotel, it is getting dark and the weather is very wet, windy and cold, which is a perfect recipe for sending us into one of the numerous bars, many of which sell delicious Belgian beers.

Now I'm not supposed to drink fizzy drinks, and to be fair the beers that I try aren't that fizzy, but in Eindhoven just like in Poznań there is certainly some degree of fizz to the beers that I drink, either through forced carbonation or the brewing fermentation process. I attempt to remove the fizz before swallowing the tasty froth liquid through swilling the beers around in my mouth. This is probably a futile and pointless thing to do, but it makes me feel a little less guilty about drinking them. I feel no ill effects from the beers whilst I am drinking them and afterwards, and have no problems at all. I like Belgian beers, because they are typically a high ABV. Many of the beers that I drink are between 6% and 11%, but they are served in bottles in reasonably sized 250ml and 330ml measures, rather than in pints. Because I am taking less liquid in, I can manage to drink up to five beers before I have had enough. This is definitely more than I could manage in Leeds when we went out for Christmas drinks with Rob, Julia and Linda. I hope that my stomach doesn't stretch, and that I'm not doing too much too soon. I am on holiday, and I do drink more regularly on holiday, but I am aware that I need to remain mindful of my drinking as that is a major source of calorie intake.

Over the next couple of days I incorporate the odd coffee, water, glass of wine, apple juice and Aperol Spritz amongst my drinks, reducing the number of beers that I drink. These drinks aren't all necessarily 'better' for me than beer (wine and Aperol Spritz are quite calorific), but certainly a coffee or a soft drink is a good thing to have. I'm not concerned about my alcohol intake, because I know that my normal home routine will no longer involve regular drinking. I also know that I don't feel a compulsion to drink alcohol, I've just done it this week because I'm on holiday and it seems like an appropriate thing to do. I know that there is an issue with increased alcohol intake amongst some post bariatric surgery patients but I'm not worried about becoming an alcoholic, my binge drinking prior to surgery was on a whole other level to what I am consuming now, which I feel is a bit more geared towards quality and enjoyment rather than quantity and getting drunk.

My eating in Eindhoven is quite meagre, but I do try and ensure that I have sufficient protein in my daily intake. Again the naughty junk items like crisps, nuts and waffles go down far too easily, so I limit my intake of them. When we eat out I either order a starter, or I order a main that will be OK to eat later if we get a doggie bag. Tapas works well, the small dishes are a good size for me, and I can manage around one and a half tapas, providing it is soft and digestible. Fish and vegetable tapas are easily digestible as are meats that have been slow cooked or stewed. Sharing boards and platters also work well, but are often not particularly healthy, in that much of the food on them is either fried or processed (or both). I eat a small amount of crusty bread from one of the sharing boards, and to my surprise it goes down easily after being well chewed and seems to digest much easier than I had been led to believe that it would do.

The PW tends to either share my plates or order a main and pick at what I leave, or take it away for us to have later. My initial anxieties about the awkwardness of eating out in restaurants seems to subside the more that I do it, but still sometimes I feel that I need to offer the waiting staff some kind of explanation if I don't finish my food, the most common one being that, "I'm completely full, I only have a small appetite." I'm still a big guy and I see some surprised looks when I say this, but after a while it just becomes routine and I get used to it. If I do overeat, I quickly get a full and very sick feeling, which is unpleasant. It is difficult to describe, but try and imagine feeling that the stomach is full, and food is sitting in the oesophagus awaiting entry to the stomach. The feeling is sickly, I want to burp but I can't, and I feel like I could throw the food back up, but I don't want to be sick in public. Sometimes exercise helps to move things along, sometimes I feel the need to lie down, sometimes I have to close my eyes and concentrate on not being sick. The PW quickly learns the signs when I do overdo it and makes the suggestion that I stop eating before feeling full, which of course helps a lot. This is all part of the learning process. I must add, that everything that I eat and drink still tastes great, and my taste buds are extremely appreciative of just about every flavour that they encounter.

While we are in Eindhoven I actually manage to put on my own walking boots. The PW has been putting my socks and footwear on me for 2 months now due to my inability to bend my right knee. I think back to only a few weeks ago in Stoke, when I had to wear flip-flops to a university meeting because I couldn't get my trainers on. Whilst my knee is still sore it must be improving, otherwise I wouldn't be able to put on my boots. I still can't put my socks on myself, but hopefully that is just now a matter of time. It's easy to take for granted being able to do something so mundane and routine like putting on socks, but when you can't do it anymore it makes you realise how essential this task is and how extremely frustrating it is to be unable to do it. I like to think that I'll never take the routine and mundane aspects of life for granted again.

A bit of respite in the weather sends us on an exploration of the streets of Eindhoven. The PW has a spot of retail therapy and so do I. We encounter a shop called Smart Planet, which as well as selling psychedelic paraphernalia (much of which relates to cannabis), also sells CBD oil. CBD in this case is an abbreviation of cannabidiol, which is an extract from the cannabis plant that doesn't contain Tetrahydrocannabinol (THC), so has no psychoactive effect and doesn't make you feel 'high'. I've read quite a bit about CBD oil's effectiveness as a medication for treating both pain and epilepsy. In the US, the CBD oil based drug Epidiolex was approved by the Food and Drug Administration (FDA) in 2018 for the treatment of epilepsy. In the Netherlands CBD oil is perfectly legal and well recognised for its pain fighting benefits. In the UK it isn't possible yet to buy CBD oil of any decent strength, but I'm not in the UK, I'm in the Netherlands, and the shop in front of me might have the solution to the seemingly perpetual aches and pains that I suffer, so I step inside. The shop has a mixture of customers, from young and obvious stoners who are looking at bongs, to people my age and older who are looking at alternative medicines. I know nothing much about CBD oil, so I approach the counter and ask the assistant for some advice. He asks me what my pain is related to, so I point at my crutch and wrist support and tell him "arthritis." The assistant shows me a range of CBD oils, which he says get good reviews from customers for fighting pain. The oils range from 5% to 20% cannaboid content, the higher strength ones being more associated with helping pain relief. I have lived with pain on a daily basis for over 20 years. I cannot remember my last pain-free day, and I would love to find something other than tablets that can help relieve this. Pain is depressing, it lowers my mood, makes me snappy and is something that I would much rather live without. I ask how much a 10ml bottle of 20% CBD oil is, and I'm slightly taken aback at the €150 price, but if it works it might be worth it, I'll never know unless I give it a go.

Back at the hotel I study the CBD oil bottle and literature; the bottle comes with a tiny dropper. I am supposed to take two drops using the dropper under my tongue, two or three times per day. I then have to leave the drops there for 2-3 minutes before swallowing. It seems simple enough so I administer my first dosage of CBD. Despite the fact that I am dropping this under my tongue, the taste is still easy to detect, and it is the first thing that my taste buds have detected since the operation that they didn't like. I can't describe the taste, it is disgusting, burnt rubber, graveyards, coal sheds, mouldy leaves, a garage floor all come to mind. I have to tell myself that something that tastes this bad can only be good for me. So now as well as the occasional dose of morphine, and codeine, I'm on the cannaboids. It's a good job that I'm not an athlete because I don't think that I would pass a drug test. I do not notice any immediate effect from the CBD oil, and it is likely to need to build up within my system for it to have any effect at all. I'll persevere with it until the bottle is empty before deciding if it's any good for me or not.

We take the train from Eindhoven to Amsterdam Schiphol Airport from where we are flying back to Leeds after a nice 8-day twin-centred New Year break. At Amsterdam Airport I have pre-booked special assistance, as I am aware that there are a number of steps and no passenger lift at pier H, which is mostly reserved for budget airlines. We are flying back to Leeds with Jet2 and as with Wizz Air, booking the special assistance was a very simple process. At Amsterdam Airport we head to the special assistance lounge, where I give in my boarding pass and passport for identification. I am found on their database straight away and allocated a helper. The whole airport is extremely busy with mostly full flights as this is the final day of the Christmas and New Year holiday period, and the special assistance lounge is no different, the staff are extremely stretched but cope well. After a short wait, my helper arrives and because my difficulty is with stairs it is recommended that I be transported in a wheelchair. At first I object as I can manage a hobble and I would feel a fraud if in a wheelchair, but the PW insists that I should do what is recommended.

This is my first wheelchair ride since being in hospital. Almost everyone who enters the special assistance lounge at Amsterdam Airport on their feet, leaves in a wheelchair, and that could sound sinister, but it isn't. The airport is huge, in fact Amsterdam Airport is the busiest in Europe in terms of aircraft movements and covers an area of 27.87 square kilometres. On this extremely busy day with numerous queues throughout the airport, special assistance gets me priority and queue jump at check-in and security, which is very welcome as without special assistance, the standing queue times would have been significant and painful on my feet and knee. After security we are taken to a waiting area, and then transferred onto an electric golf buggy type vehicle to be driven through the airport to pier H. It is a long drive and ashamedly it was fun. I'd always wanted to be driven through a bustling airport, and yes of course I filmed some of it and then unashamedly took a selfie.

Another ambulift awaits us at pier H to get us on board the aircraft, which on this occasion has already been boarded before our arrival, which in my limited ambulift experience is unusual. We are last to board the aircraft, shortly after which the doors are closed and the aircraft taxis for an unusually long time, before take-off and then the short 1 hour flight to Leeds. Once again I fit more than comfortably into my seat and once again the seat belt leaves me with ample room.

At Leeds, the PW and I are first to leave the aircraft, which is again unusual in my limited ambulift experience, but this is because the ambulift arrives before the buses to ferry the rest of the passengers to the terminal. We are fast-tracked through security and have collected our baggage while the rest of the flight's passengers are probably still on board the aircraft, special assistance rocks!

A welcome cup of tea is traditionally brewed and served by the PW when we arrive home from any holiday, and today is no different. As I unpack my bags and separate clean clothes from dirty clothes, UK electric adapters from European electric adapters and numerous wires from around each other (why do they always do that), I consider the past 8 days and can officially say that my first post bariatric surgery foreign jaunt went much better than expected. I had been worried about how I would cope with eating, drinking and mobility, but ultimately everything worked out just fine. The PW was incredible as always, I would not have coped as well without her (I'd definitely have kept the same socks on). The special assistance was hugely helpful, and I will not be ashamed to use it again in future if I feel that I need to. My next foreign holiday is actually in 11 days with 'The Big Lads'. Our 'Big Lads on Tour (BLT)' jaunt (an annual fixture) for 2020 is to Porto in Portugal, a city with numerous steep hills and cobbled streets, a perfect nightmare for my feet and knee. I won't have the PW with me, and how I will cope is a bit of a worry if I'm completely honest, but I'll just have to do what I can, even if I can't change my footwear! This year's BLT certainly won't be the huge drinking and eating tour for me that it usually is and I'm likely to become a spectator to some of the overindulgence more than a participant.

I switch on the TV to the 24 hour BBC news channel to see that Australia is on fire, Donald Trump is trying to start Gulf War 3 with Iran and Boris Johnson is hiding away in the Caribbean. I switch the TV off, some things I can still do without. I can say with some confidence that my own New Year 2020 has been a very good one and I have my fingers crossed that the rest of this year will be. It is both ironic and unfortunate that I seem to have become more physically disabled since having the operation and losing weight, but hopefully my knee will recover and as I become lighter, hopefully the pain in my legs and feet will lessen, and I will feel more the benefits of weighing less.

In terms of health, I'll end this chapter with a summary of my first few days back at home of 2020. On the Monday I have my annual diabetes health-check at my local GPs; my blood pressure is the best I've ever known it at 110 over 70, my pulse was a quite reasonable 70, I gave blood and urine samples, but I won't know the results of these for a few weeks, but the headline is that my weight on my first official weigh in of 2020 is 21 stones 3.25 pounds (297.25 pounds/134.83 kilos). Following my Christmas weight loss plateau, I have still managed to lose 3.25 pounds (1.47 kilos) over my New Year holiday, which is despite eating mostly unhealthy restaurant food and drinking alcohol each day. It is possible that my increased movement hobbling around Poznań and Eindhoven may have played a part in this by boosting my metabolism. In any case, it is a great result for me, I don't think that I've ever lost weight on a foreign holiday before. Since beginning the LRD in October, my total weight loss to date is 4 stone, 2 pounds (58 pounds/26.31 kilos).

On the Tuesday I am back in Wharfedale Hospital to see a physiotherapist about my right knee. It is a short 30-minute appointment, which goes very well. After I give the physio the full background story behind the history of my knee troubles, and after she sees how limited the movement in my knee is, she decides that I'm beyond physiotherapy help and puts me straight onto the surgery list. This is a great result. I had envisioned months of useless exercise being prescribed to me using a big red elastic band, so being recommended to go straight for surgery will hopefully mean that getting to the root of my knee problems will now happen much more quickly.

I began my banana journey in the hope that I would live a longer and better quality of life and hopefully I will go on to achieve that goal. It is fair to say that there are no certainties in life, apart from the fact that death is an inevitability that we will all face. As we grow older, the clock is counting down to the time that we depart this mortal coil. So I'm ending this chapter and pretty much this book on a very sad note that highlights our fragility and mortality in the face of the inevitable and how we never know what is around the corner. Going back to work on the Wednesday I found out that one of my colleagues, a member of my teaching team and a friend, Dave Morby died suddenly and unexpectedly at home in the New Year. Dave was in his early 60s with a background in leadership and management. He was a former soldier who had lived in Germany, a country that we both have a fondness for and talked about over many coffees on campus. He was a physically fit man who led an active life, he was a regular traveller and he loved his sport. Dave's presence in the classroom was greatly appreciated by the students, who would praise him in student focus groups and course review meetings. It is true to say that Dave has positively helped a number of students in life, both at university and in their careers beyond. He was a proper Yorkshire gentleman, and he will sadly be missed by many, including his wife Ali and his daughter Louise, both of whom are colleagues of mine also, rest in peace, Dave.

We never know what is around the corner, so live your life to the full, spend less time looking at your phone and on social media, have experiences, tell stories as every one of them is a learning experience shared, touch the lives of others in a good way and have a legacy. If you need help, don't be afraid to ask for it, speak to experts and not just Facebook 'friends', accept that if you can't do something for yourself, you should let others that are better placed to assist and guide you. If I hadn't gone on this banana journey my life would have still been good, but now it will be better, much better. I will eventually be able to do many things that others take for granted including movement, climbing stairs, exercising, maybe one day I'll even go for a jog. As I look forward to what will hopefully be a longer and brighter future for myself, I do wonder where my final weight will settle, I'd love to get to 17 stone (238 pounds/108 kilos), which I know is a weight that suits my body frame well. I know that I will have to remain mindful with regards to eating and drinking for the rest of my life. My self-belief sometimes wavers, but at present I am determined to face with positivity the challenges ahead of me, I do know for a fact though, that the future will never be certain in my banana life.

Afterword

It is January 2021, just over 14 months after I began writing this book. I had initially set myself a deadline of February 2020 to complete it and in all honesty, I had written 80% of this book by that point, but then something happened which threw me off-track and in the end, it has taken me 11 months to write the last three chapters.

You see around about the time that I was going into hospital for my surgery, a chain of events began, which would have a profound effect on me and also the entire planet. About 5,500 miles (8,850 kilometres) away from Leeds in a forest in China's Hubei province, a bat in a tree did a shit that landed on the forest floor. A pangolin came along and ate the shit, the shit made the pangolin sick. The sick pangolin was caught by a trapper and taken live to a wet market in Wuhan to be sold for either food or medicine. I don't know the exact fate of the sick pangolin, but I do know that its illness was passed on to at least one human, who then passed it on to another human and another and another and another.

It's so funny to look back on the Twitter of New Year's Eve 2019 and see the number of tweets from people moaning about what a terrible year 2019 had been. For me it was a brilliant year, a life-changing and life-saving year. The 2019 haters would soon be getting quite a shock as in a chain reaction that is a kind of 'butterfly effect' (Google it), a coronavirus pandemic, which was named Covid-19, swept Planet Earth, making 2020 probably the most difficult year for a great many people globally. At the time of my writing, so far almost 2 million people have died globally of Covid-19 and today, the 4th of January, 2021, England has just announced its third lockdown after a total of 2.65 million Covid-19 cases and over 75,000 Covid-19 related deaths.

Industries such as tourism and events have collapsed, while others such as music (streaming) and the media have profited. People even started to wear masks in order to gain entry into banks. One year ago, disposable plastic was the enemy, today its indestructability and ability to repel liquids makes it a saviour. People are avoiding touching one another, with a mantra of 'hands, face, space', and the pubs have been closed for weeks. Birthday parties are happening on Zoom and it just isn't right to blow out the candles on the cake anymore. Staying at home in bed instead of going to work suddenly became the right thing to do. I never thought the comment, "I wouldn't touch them with a six-foot barge pole," would become a national policy, and I never expected a Tory Chancellor of the Exchequer to create a socialist furlough scheme, but here we are! 2020 has been a very strange year indeed and in all likelihood, 2021 will undoubtedly be similar. In fact, I don't predict normality returning in the UK until 2022, and in some parts of the world, it will likely be much later.

I really feel sorry for those people who were nearing their operation date (for any operation) and have had it thrown out because the hospitals became full of Covid-19 victims. I particularly feel an empathy for those who were due to undergo weight-loss surgery and have now found this de-prioritised as the NHS is brought to its knees in the face of this terrible disease after years of Tory cuts and underfunding.

The nation clapped every Thursday throughout the first lockdown in a co-ordinated show of support for our NHS and key-workers who on a daily basis put themselves at risk. I do wonder out of those Thursday night clappers how many of them voted for the Tories and how many of them will continue to do so in future. Sadly, there are probably still a significant number of Tory voters out there, voting for the party that has singlehandedly done the most damage to this country both financially and socially of any political party ever. And why? Because most of the newspapers tell them to, and because our main news outlets have been taken over by Tory spin-doctors and apologists. It stinks.

Why hasn't Dido Harding been mauled in the media for the abject failure that is track and trace? Why have Tory mates of Tory MPs been allowed to profiteer billions to deliver second-rate personal protective equipment (PPE) that didn't work? Why is Gavin Williamson the 'Frank Spencer' of MPs in charge of education, literally how did that happen? "Ooh, Betty, the Covid did a whoopsie in the schools." The schools are safe, no they're not, yes they are, no they're not. U-turn has followed U-turn from the top downwards, as an incompetent Prime Minister surrounded by unskilled (but easy to manipulate) MPs in his cabinet are given senior posts that affect millions of people's lives. Advice from scientists is ignored and then reacted to far too late in an abject failure of leadership from the Prime Minister, whom I now refer to as Bovid and his idiot Cabinet. Harry G. Frankfurt's definition of bullshit has never been truer and the history books will not be kind to these charlatans. I'm just glad that *Spitting Image* has returned to portray these puppets and monsters as they actually are.

My final political rant of this book is now over, and focusing back upon my banana journey, what happened after the New Year of 2020? As rumours of a new disease in China began to appear in the media, I continued to lose weight but at a slower pace. Sadly my weight-loss plateaued only 4 months after the surgery, the lowest my weight has been so far is 20 stone and 5 pounds (129 kilos), which represents a weight-loss since I began the LRD of exactly 5 stones (32 kilos). Since February 2020 my weight has yo-yoed in a range between 20 stone 5 pounds and 20 stone 10 pounds. I haven't let myself become obsessed with the weighing scales and I only weigh myself monthly. Everybody's weight-loss journey is different. Some people whom I have read about on social media that had the operation the same time as I did have lost twice as much weight as me, whilst others have lost half as much as me.

I am a little disappointed not to have lost more weight, but I have to look at the bigger picture. This is a marathon and not a sprint, and my 5-stone weight loss so far has come with some major benefits. Physically I feel much more energised and capable, I'm wearing clothes that haven't fit me for 20 years, I get complimented on how well I'm looking and I can walk long distances without the constant need to sit down. My sleep apnoea is at an all-time low of 1 apnoea event per hour, and I'm hoping that within the next two years and with a little more weight loss I'll be able to return my CPAP machine. My blood sugar has dropped from a diabetic 52 to a healthy 36 and my cholesterol has dropped from 5, which is borderline high cholesterol, to 4.2 which is within a normal range. I would still like to lose another 3 stones (19 kilos), and I have certainly not given up hope of doing so. Psychologically however, I still suffer from body dysmorphia. I still see a huge fat person when I look in the mirror, even though I'm only looking at a moderately fat person now. The PW constantly reminds me that I should love myself more, but I haven't quite got there yet.

Bariatric surgery is not a quick fix or a magic bullet for weight loss, it is a tool that will help you to lose weight sustainably if you follow the guidance and don't fall back into previous bad habits. I've tried to do the right thing, my portions have got larger over the past year, but are still only 'child-sized' from a small breakfast bowl. I can eat anything I like, there are no foods that won't stay down and I've never experienced dumping syndrome, although filter coffee does usually lead to a good clear out around an hour after drinking it. I have noticed that I must eat much more regularly than I did before the operation and when I don't eat for long periods, I feel pain in my stomach and I get extremely cold. On the hunger scale I can go from not being hungry whatsoever one second, to feeling absolutely starving and shaky the next as my sugars can drop very quickly. I had hoped that hunger would be gone forever but that hasn't been the case. I have to eat at short notice quite often, and if I go for a walk, I know to take a cereal bar or a sandwich with me, as I know that I will probably need to eat something whilst I am out of the house. When I eat, I get a runny nose and I often hiccup, and this is now normal to me, but is something that didn't happen to me before the operation. My stomach also growls much more now and is definitely more audible than it was prior to surgery.

I probably eat takeaway food only once per month. The PW and I have been really enjoying cooking, particularly in light of lockdown after lockdown, which turned mealtimes into an event to look forward to. I don't think I do too bad diet-wise, I'm certainly not eating anywhere near the quantity of naughty foods that I was before, but with that said, if I fancy a packet of crisps or a piece of cake, then I'll have one. I must stress that I do not do this regularly though.

I can and do walk long distances, and I've enjoyed many a film-walk with my Go-Pro throughout 2020. The inability to travel internationally has led to the PW and me exploring our locality in great detail, something which I have been documenting on Instagram as well as building *Leeds The Movie*, which I plan to release in 2023 (see www.leedsthemovie.co.uk for further information about this project).

The first lockdown of March 2020, along with unseasonably sunny and warm weather provided me with an impetus to work on my garden, and completely reignited my passion for gardening. Our garden looked better in 2020 than it has in any other year. I would be out planting and pottering from 07:00 and sometimes earlier fitting my garden in-between working from home and numerous Zoom meetings. I could easily achieve 10,000 steps per day without leaving my front gate. I actually enjoyed lockdown, I have enjoyed the freedom and flexibility of working from home and I have never appreciated my beautiful home and garden so much. Working from home has still been stressful, I signed up to become a teacher and educator and ended up being a television presenter, with pre-recorded lectures now the norm. But you know what? I've enjoyed the experience and I've developed as a person with it. I have had to spend extended hours sitting at a computer, and I have gone days at a time without enough exercise, but overall I definitely moved around more in 2020 than I did in 2019, and I'll move around more in 2021 than I did in 2020.

The one thing that I haven't given up following surgery is beer. I'm going to be completely honest and put this out there. I am definitely drinking less beer than I did before surgery, but I am still drinking beer each week (mostly at the weekend), and beer is calorific. I know that this will not be helping me and whilst beer alone isn't the reason for my weight-loss plateauing, I am trying to remain mindful of how much goes down my throat. Sunny lockdown evenings in the garden throughout 2020 wouldn't have been nearly as nice without a good ale to savour.

So what of the other 'rules'? Well I'm still taking my tablets every day, twice per day morning and night, I'm leaving 30 minutes between eating and drinking, I'm trying not to overeat as that is what stretches the stomach and I am trying to exercise more, particularly with walks and gardening. I barely drink fruit juice, squash or other cold (non-alcoholic) drinks these days and have become much more of a tea and coffee drinker throughout the daytime than I have ever been before. I don't know if that is related in any way to my surgery or journey, but it just seems to have happened to me in 2020.

There is one thing that I really do need to report though and I have the PW to once again thank for saving me. The pain in my knees has gone; after seeing a specialist it turns out that I have rheumatoid arthritis rather than osteoarthritis, which is why the pain was mostly on the outside of my knees. Rheumatoid arthritis can normally be treated easily with NSAIDs, such as aspirin or ibuprofen, except I can't take these anymore. At least not in tablet form as it will damage my delicate banana stomach. The PW suggested if liquid ibuprofen that you give to babies might be safe for me to take. I emailed Mr Mehta to ask his opinion of this and he told me that it would be completely fine. I contacted Dr Williams, and liquid ibuprofen is now on my repeat prescription. Within one week of me taking the first dose of liquid ibuprofen in February 2020, my knees were almost completely cured of pain and inflammation. I couldn't believe that something so simple was the solution to fixing the agony that I went through. The PW is truly a pharmaceutical wizard.

I'd like to end by saying that if you are unhappy with your weight and it is impacting upon the quality of your life, do consider seeking help outside of Facebook and social media. There are many dedicated and wonderful professionals out there (particularly in the NHS) and speaking with real people definitely helped me. I have found everyone on the Leeds weight-loss service to be extremely supportive, they have literally added years to my life, and for this I cannot thank them enough. In a similar vein I'd just like to reiterate what an absolutely fantastic asset and resource the NHS is. Please remember this when you next vote, because the more that the NHS is chipped away and privatised and the more that friends of politicians get their hands on it, the less it will be around in future. If 2020 has taught us anything, it is that we NEED the NHS.

I'd like to thank again Mr Mehta and his team, all of the staff at Jimmy's, the Leeds weight-loss service particularly Janine, Mary and Dr Barth, as well as my own GP Dr Williams and every other NHS superhero that I have encountered directly or indirectly along my journey.

I'd ultimately like to thank the PW who has made me a better person both physically and mentally.

It's been emotional, onwards and upwards (although not the weight hopefully).

About the author

Stuart Moss has been working in higher education for 20 years, prior to this his work background included marketing and human resource positions in visitor attractions, hotels and telecommunications.

Stuart has a range of publications, including two co-authored text-books on the subject of employability, as well as two edited text-books about the entertainment industries, and strategic management within the entertainment industries. Besides these, Stuart has numerous book chapters, journal articles and over 30 international conference key-notes to his credit. Stuart is a seasoned public speaker and is often described as having a presentation style that is energetic, passionate and motivational.

Stuart has recently become a volunteer litter picker, which means his activity levels have greatly increased, but it's true to say that he still spends far too much time on social media, he can be contacted through the following methods.

Email: stuartmoss@gmail.com
Web: http://www.stuartmoss.co.uk
LinkedIn: stumoss
Twitter: @stuartmoss
Instagram: stumoss